Complementary Medicine FOR DUMMIES®

by Jacqueline Young

BICENTENNIAL 1807 WILEY 2007 BICENTENNIAL

John Wiley & Sons, Ltd

Complementary Medicine For Dummies®

Published by
John Wiley & Sons, Ltd
The Atrium
Southern Gate
Chichester
West Sussex
PO19 8SQ
England

E-mail (for orders and customer service enquire: cs-books@wiley.co.uk

Visit our Home Page on www.wileyeurope.com

Milton Keynes Council	
1962576	
Askews	Sep-2007
615.5	£15.99

WILEY

About the Author

Jacqueline Young is uniquely qualified to write this book. She has worked in both the fields of orthodox and complementary medicine internationally for over 20 years, practising, studying, teaching, writing, researching, and serving on committees.

Jacqueline is a qualified clinical psychologist, oriental medical practitioner, naturopath, and nutritionist. She is also trained in a whole host of complementary therapies including herbal medicine, homeopathy, flower remedies, Tibetan medicine, Ayurveda, applied kinesiology, massage, shiatsu, iridology, nature cure, sound therapy, and various types of bodywork and healing. In between she qualified as a Sivananda yoga instructor and found time to squeeze in a brown belt in karate!

On the academic front Jacqueline holds a Bachelor's degree in Psychology and a Master's degree in Clinical Psychology and has completed postgraduate education in nutrition, epidemiology, and clinical education. She's done her bit serving on professional committees involved in setting national standards for clinical psychology, acupuncture, and nutrition. She's taught complementary medicine to doctors, nurses, postgraduates, the general public, and school children – and anyone else who's interested.

Jacqueline has practised her skills in hospitals, clinics, and health centres in several countries. She is an enthusiastic medical volunteer for Care & Share International with whom she has had the privilege of running complementary medicine clinics in a tent high in the Himalayas and in Bhopal, India.

She's written several books on complementary medicine and often contributes to national magazines, newspapers, radio, television, and Web sites including BBC Health.

Jacqueline practises in central London, and is the Education Director for the Revital Health Education Centre (www.revital.com). Outside work she is still trying to master the art of growing really tasty vegetables that even her son will eat!

She's exercised her brain, and stretched the patience of friends and family and her publishers, in writing this compendium and hopes you'll find it handy to have around and a useful guide on your healing path.

To contact the author (feedback, comments, and constructive suggestions always welcome) write to: PO Box 2211, Barnet, Herts, EN5 4DZ, United Kingdom, or e-mail youngfeatures@aol.com.

Dedication

This book is for all those people who are willing to have an open yet discerning mind about complementary medicine. It is also dedicated, with thanks, to all my complementary medicine teachers, patients, students, and colleagues.

Yes, we need to explore and research complementary therapies so that we can be confident about their safety and effectiveness. Yet at the same time we should not allow barriers to be erected that may obstruct new learning and deny access to therapies that could provide a powerful healing force in our world.

Author's Acknowledgements

I am very grateful to my family and friends who have supported me in the long time it took to write this book. Mum, Don, Mark and Ken, Issy and Jamie, Tanya, Olesya and Tommy, Irina and Alina, Titi, John and Marjie, Fred and Chris, Annie and Jake, Michael and Jasmine, Jarek and Suzie, Selina and Theo, Nic, Kirsten and Emilie, Ikuyo, Connie, Drid and Jane Garton – you've all played your part, even when you didn't know it. My son, Michael, deserves a special mention because he has endlessly had to spare me to the computer, but we've had fun making up for it in other ways on other days too! So does Alfonse – because he always makes me laugh!

I also acknowledge my precious 'departed family' – you live on in my heart and are one of my motivations to work in the field of health and healing: My irreplaceable best friend Mary, my dear friend Maria, and my inspirational friend and godmother to my son, Penny Brohn. All were overcome, but not beaten, by the cruel ravages of cancer, and Penny's outstanding and pioneering work on the role of complementary medicine in cancer care lives on (www.pennybrohncancercare.org). I also credit my much-loved father, Alan Young, who introduced me to yoga and home grown veg, and my dear grandparents, who loved a good cup of comfrey tea.

I'm also grateful to my 'professional family' – all the brilliant conventional, unconventional, and/or integrated medical colleagues who have kindly contributed to this book: Prof. David Peters, for kindly reviewing the entire text, and the following people for making some time to read through individual chapters, or to talk over points with me: Professor George Lewith MA, DM, FRCP, MRCGP; Dr Julian Kenyon MD, MB, ChB; Dr Neil Slade PhD, LCH, RSHom; Professor Laurie Hartmann PhD, DO; Deirdre Stubbs DO; Ulrik Sandstrøm BSc, DC, ICSSD, FCC; Richard Blackwell BMedSci, LicAc, MSc

(Acupuncture); Etsuko Kobira MIFA; and Anne McIntyre FNIMH. Also Dr Jovan Djurovic DO for his chiropractic exercise, Mike Burrows for his eloquent quote in the dedication, and Dr Rory Hafford MSc, PhD, Dip. Psych. for his willingness to contribute. I was always pleasantly surprised when chapters came back with virtually no red ink but take full responsibility that any remaining errors or omissions are my own.

I owe a great debt to my 'publishing family' too: Alison Yates, Commissioning Editor; Rachael Chilvers, Project Editor; and Mike Kelly, Developer at Wiley have been patient and helpful throughout and contributed a great deal. Thanks to Julia Lampam and Jamie McOuat (Publicity and Rights) for working their magic too.

And the last word goes to my good friend, Ted Katchuk OMD, Assistant Professor of Medicine at Harvard Medical School, USA, and also godfather to my son, for one of my favourite quotes. When asked in a magazine interview, 'What is the greatest danger to complementary and alternative medicine?' he swiftly replied, 'Lack of humour'. I think he may be right. Hopefully some of the anecdotes and cartoons in this book, in between the more serious stuff, may put a bit of humour back in!

Publisher's Acknowledgements

We're proud of this book; please send us your comments through our Dummies online registration form located at www.dummies.com/register/.

Some of the people who helped bring this book to market include the following:

Acquisitions, Editorial, and Media Development

Project Editor: Rachael Chilvers

Development Editor: Mike Kelly

Content Editor: Steve Edwards

Commissioning Editor: Alison Yates

Executive Editor: Jason Dunne

Executive Project Editor: Martin Tribe

Brand Reviewer: Jennifer Bingham

Copy Editor: Kate O'Leary

Proofreader: Lesley Green

Cover Photo: © GettyImages/ Digital Vision

Cartoons: Rich Tennant, www.the5thwave.com

Production

Project Coordinator: Jennifer Theriot

Layout and Graphics: Carl Byers, Brooke Graczyk, Stephanie D. Jumper, Melanee Prendergast, Christine Williams

Proofreaders: Todd Lothery, Susan Moritz

Indexer: Aptara

Publishing and Editorial for Consumer Dummies

> **Diane Graves Steele,** Vice President and Publisher, Consumer Dummies
>
> **Joyce Pepple,** Acquisitions Director, Consumer Dummies
>
> **Kristin A. Cocks,** Product Development Director, Consumer Dummies
>
> **Michael Spring,** Vice President and Publisher, Travel
>
> **Brice Gosnell,** Associate Publisher, Travel
>
> **Kelly Regan,** Editorial Director, Travel

Publishing for Technology Dummies

> **Andy Cummings,** Vice President and Publisher, Dummies Technology/General User

Composition Services

> **Gerry Fahey,** Vice President of Production Services
>
> **Debbie Stailey,** Director of Composition Services

Contents at a Glance

Table of Contents

Foreword

I have known and worked with Jacqueline Young for over 10 years and have great respect for her ability to condense often very complicated issues into simple and understandable text. *Complementary Medicine For Dummies* does just that. All sorts of claims and counter-claims are made about whether therapies work, are safe, or are just simply a 'confidence trick'. Jackie guides us through this morass of information in a thoughtful, sensible, and humorous manner so that you really will understand what's going on and what you might be able to safely use to help yourself.

One of the great strengths of complementary medicine is its ability to empower. Understanding why you might be using a particular approach to improve your health and maintain wellbeing allows you to take back sensible control of your health and use the best of both conventional and complementary medicine. That's what most people want for themselves and indeed what most medical practitioners want for both themselves and their patients.

I hope you enjoy *Complementary Medicine For Dummies* but above all else I hope you find it valuable, empowering, and humorous.

George Lewith

Dr George Lewith, MA DM FRCP MRCGP
Reader in Complementary Medicine, University of Southampton
Visiting Professor, University of Westminster
Complementary Medicine Research Unit
Primary Medical Care
Aldermoor Health Centre
Aldermoor Close
Southampton
SO16 5ST

Introduction

● ●

Complementary medicine is growing in popularity all the time, and is becoming a significant part of modern-day healthcare, with millions of treatments taking place each year. It reaches back into the distant past, drawing on health wisdom from ancient cultures such as the Greeks, Egyptians, and Chinese, and yet is also bang up-to-date with new health innovations and the latest technological advances.

Complementary medicine also excites lots of controversy, with animated debates between those who are convinced it works and those who believe that it's all hocus-pocus and quackery.

I take a middle path, giving you the low-down on each of the therapies, presenting you with evidence on their effectiveness (or the lack of it), and leaving you to make your own informed opinions and choices.

My aim is to give you easy access to all the information you need to know to use complementary medicine safely and effectively, with a few entertaining stories, quizzes, and useful health tips thrown in along the way.

If you care about your health you're bound to find something to interest you in this book that you may be inspired to try out. I'm passionate about complementary medicine and have devoted most of my working life to practising, teaching, writing about, discussing, researching, and studying it! I'm excited to have this opportunity to share my enthusiasm with you and to guide you through the complementary medicine maze.

About This Book

The field of complementary medicine is vast, ranging from well-established therapies regulated by law through to the more unconventional ones.

I make things easy for you by covering a massive range of therapies one by one and dividing each up into bite-sized chunks that provide you with information such as what the therapy is all about, how it works, what it may be good for, what evidence supports its use, what to expect in a typical consultation, and much more. You can find out whatever you need to know with the minimum of effort and yet be fully informed with the most up-to-date and comprehensive information available.

I also include a couple of chapters on complementary diagnosis so that you can discover how to read your body's health signs, such as what it means if your tongue develops a thick, white coating, and the different types of diagnosis used by practitioners.

This book covers the most popular therapies, from ancient to modern, and as many as possible of the lesser known ones too. For easy reference, you'll find a handy A–Z of therapies towards the back of the book, plus lots of Web and phone links throughout the book to help you find out more.

Your health matters, and having comprehensive, reliable, and up-to-date complementary medicine reference resources all in one book, is invaluable. Why suffer unnecessarily if a therapy can help ease your discomfort, promote your health, or even help prevent future health problems? Yet where do you start if you haven't a clue about what therapy to go for? And what if you wisely don't want to waste your money or risk putting yourself in the hands of someone incompetent who could cause you harm?

This book can help you by doing the following:

- ✒ Introducing you to the range of complementary therapies practised today.
- ✒ Helping you discover which type of therapy may best suit you or ease your current health problem.
- ✒ Telling you about the latest information and research evidence to help you decide whether the therapy is safe or effective.
- ✒ Showing you how to know whether a person is qualified and providing you with the most up-to-date resources for trained practitioners.
- ✒ Suggesting questions you need to ask to be sure that you're in good hands.
- ✒ Letting you know what to do if things go wrong.

Conventions Used in This Book

This book is a jargon-free zone; I set out the information in a practical way so that you can quickly and easily get the information you want on the therapy you're interested in. When I introduce a new term, I *italicise* and define it.

The only other conventions in this book are that Web addresses are in monofont, and the action part of numbered steps and the key concept in a list are in **bold**.

Foolish Assumptions

I'm assuming the following about you:

✔ You want to know more about complementary medicine and what may be good for you.

✔ If you're a sceptic, you're willing to have an open mind and consider the facts.

✔ If you're a convert, you're prepared to read the information carefully and make intelligent choices.

✔ You're willing to spend time delving into this book for the sake of your health but you want the information to be handy, relevant, and accurate.

How This Book Is Organised

As with all *For Dummies* books, you don't have to read this book from cover to cover. You can simply dip in wherever and whenever you like and find the information that you need. You can search for a particular therapy, look up an ailment, investigate a type of diagnosis, find a self-help tip to try out in an idle moment, or just enjoy looking at the cartoons.

The Table of Contents and the Index can help you find where you want to go and I've added lots of links throughout the book to take you from one relevant section to another.

Here's an overview to help point you to where you want to go.

Part 1: Finding Out about Complementary Medicine

This part is a good place to start if you're new to complementary medicine. It gives you an overview of what complementary medicine is all about, who uses it, what it may be good for, how to choose an effective therapy, and so on. It also introduces you to the diagnostic techniques used in complementary medicine and tells you about some you can use for yourself, such as reading your tongue.

Part II: Exploring Traditional Healing Systems

In this part, I explore the ancient healing wisdom and health practices of some of the great traditions that have survived and flourished to this day. You can find essential information on Chinese, Tibetan, and Japanese traditional medicine; the Ayurvedic tradition from India; and the European Nature Cure tradition. But this part isn't a dry, historical read. It's a vibrant account of how these traditions are being practised today and what you can expect if you consult one of their practitioners.

Part III: Using Popular Complementary Therapies

This part gives you the information you need to know about five of the most popular complementary therapies practised in the West today: Acupuncture, herbal medicine, homeopathy, nutritional medicine, and naturopathy.

Part IV: Treating Your Body

In Part IV, I home in on the myriad of therapies that have been developed to work directly on your body. Starting with the most popular and regulated, osteopathy and chiropractic, I move on to the joys of massage and all the other therapies in between. Delve into this part if you want to know your Alexander technique from your Bowen therapy or to explore therapies from applied kinesiology to zero balancing.

Part V: Healing Your Mind and Spirit

Many therapies focus on treating or rebalancing your mind and emotions. In this part, you can explore relaxation therapies, aromatherapy, healing, psychological therapies, energy medicine, and the creative therapies. You'll find here everything from the Buteyko breathing technique to Reiki, from colour and sound therapy to spiritual healing.

Part VI: The Part of Tens

This nifty part – an element of every *For Dummies* book – gives you a bird's eye view of elements of complementary medicine, including tips for healthy living, superfoods to incorporate into your diet, and herbal remedies to boost your health.

You'll also find a handy A–Z of therapies that you can use as a reference guide or to direct you to the appropriate place in the book.

Icons Used in This Book

These icons help you find your way through the maze of complementary medicine, highlighting important bits and showing you where you can find some entertaining tales.

The fun part! These icons spotlight some of the juicy tales in the history of complementary medicine, from the fighting over cornflakes by the Kellogg brothers (Chapter 8 if you can't wait to find out) to Daniel David Palmer (the founder of chiropractic) being run over by his son. They also include a few real-life accounts about people who've tried out different therapies and some of my own experiences, too.

Can't tell your acupressure from your chiropractic? Never heard of a meridian or a hydropathist? Don't worry – wherever you see this icon you find each term explained in straightforward English.

This icon draws your attention to important points to keep in mind.

This icon highlights lots of useful complementary medicine tips, from what to do with homeopathic remedies when you're flying, to how to make an aromatherapy gargle for a sore throat.

This icon highlights all the need-to-know stuff to keep your experience of complementary medicine safe, such as which herb may make your contraceptive pill ineffective or when not to use certain essential oils. Watch out for these safety tips.

Where to Go from Here

Where to go from here? Wherever you like. You can dive into Part I and explore tongue and face diagnosis, or leap to Part II to find out about ancient health secrets. Or you can select a therapy of your choice and go to the relevant chapter, or simply flick through the pages reading whatever takes your fancy.

If you're not sure where to start, take a look at Chapter 1 for an overview of complementary medicine and suggestions on where to go next. Just turn the page and join me on an exploration of all you've ever wanted (or needed) to know about the wonderful world of complementary medicine.

Part I
Finding Out about Complementary Medicine

The 5th Wave   By Rich Tennant

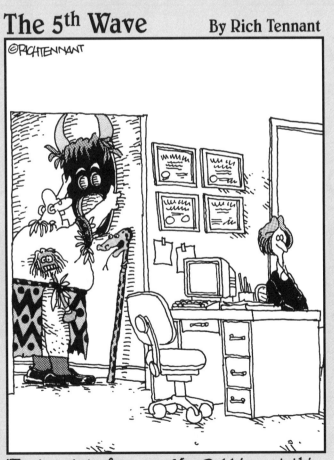

"Fortunately for you, Ms. Dobbins, at this clinic we firmly believe in alternative medicine."

In this part . . .

Welcome to the wonderful world of complementary medicine. The chapters in this part introduce you to diagnosis in complementary medicine (both professional and self-diagnosis), its long history, and the safety and effectiveness of complementary medicine. I also point you in the right direction for choosing an effective therapy for you.

Chapter 1

Understanding Complementary Medicine

Complementary medicine is an increasingly popular form of healthcare in the Western world. Millions of consultations take place every year, and according to some surveys, almost one in three people have tried it. People with chronic conditions, such as long-term pain, make use of complementary medicine particularly frequently.

Gradually, acceptance of complementary medicine is increasing in orthodox medical circles with more and more doctors training in, or referring patients for, complementary therapies or incorporating complementary practitioners into their practices. You can find complementary medicine in hospitals, specialist clinics, hospices, schools, beauty clinics, and gyms.

At the same time, people are becoming more discerning about the complementary therapies that they use and asking for proof of effectiveness and safety. Practitioners are increasingly well trained and many of their professional associations have been working hard to raise standards.

In this chapter, you can find out exactly what complementary medicine is, who uses it, and what the most popular forms of complementary therapy are. You'll also find out how to decide which therapy may be appropriate for you and how you can assess its safety and effectiveness.

Finding Out about Complementary Medicine

This section starts right at the beginning by sorting out the confusion over names used to describe this form of therapy.

What do all the names mean?

At one time, people often used the term *alternative medicine* because people tended to select this therapy as an alternative to mainstream medicine – that is, the medicine practised by doctors and nurses and offered in GP surgeries, hospitals, and so on. Mainstream medicine is generally referred to as *orthodox*, *allopathic*, or *conventional* medicine. So, alternative medicine has also sometimes been called *unconventional* or *unorthodox* medicine.

Some practitioners liked the term alternative medicine, because they believed their approach did provide a real alternative to orthodox healthcare. However, others felt the term was too confrontational, creating a 'them' and 'us' situation between medics and alternative medicine practitioners. These people preferred the term *complementary medicine*, because they saw their work as complementary to orthodox medicine and believed the two were perfectly capable of working alongside one another.

Gradually, the term *CAM – complementary and alternative medicine –* evolved to reconcile these two perspectives and has been quite widely used. However, as CAM therapies become more incorporated into the mainstream, people are dropping the word 'alternative'. Also, the term CAM is itself now making way for the buzz phrase *integrated medicine*, referring to what Prince Charles calls 'the best of both worlds'. This incorporates the best of both orthodox and complementary approaches to provide the most appropriate form of healthcare for different health problems and individuals.

For this book, I use the terms complementary medicine and complementary therapies because these are currently two of the most widely used and recognised. However, I myself see complementary medicine as part of the wider whole of healthcare – drawing on the best of tried and tested ancient medical traditions, pioneering new and modern forms of healthcare, and integrating with existing medical practices. I also believe that rigorous training standards, research, and evaluation of the different therapies are essential to ensure that they're safe and effective for public use.

From ancient to modern – Ayurveda today

Ayurveda – the ancient medical system of India – is a good example of how a traditional medical system now takes a place in both the complementary and orthodox worlds. It dates back well over 2,000 years but is still the most widely practised form of medicine in India and is now also popular in several Western countries. Ayurveda's herbal remedies, massage, and healing practices are hugely popular – with celebrities, sports personalities, and even royalty giving them glowing endorsements. Yet, doctors are starting to take it seriously as well. As one example, the plant *Gymnema sylvestre* has been found to help balance blood sugar levels and some now believe that it may have a useful role to play in the treatment of diabetes. Other researchers have investigated the role of single or combination Ayurvedic remedies for health conditions such as liver and heart problems.

What is complementary medicine?

What actually comes under the complementary medicine umbrella? Ancient traditions provide the roots of complementary medicine: the medical systems of China, India, Tibet, and so on that also incorporate influences from the traditions of ancient Greece, Persia, and elsewhere. Some people believe that these traditions shouldn't even really be classed as alternative or complementary because they've been practised for thousands of years. However, their revitalisation and popularity today puts them firmly in the frame of modern health approaches. Good examples of these are Ayurveda, Traditional Chinese Medicine (TCM), Tibetan medicine, and Kanpo (Japanese herbal medicine).

Some of the most popular complementary therapies today developed directly from these ancient roots – for example, acupuncture is a part of Traditional Chinese Medicine and has developed over thousands of years. Others have been developed more recently, such as osteopathy, which developed from the work of US Army doctor Andrew Taylor Still in the 19th century.

Five types of therapies are particularly well-established in the UK: Osteopathy, chiropractic, acupuncture, herbalism (Western and other forms such as Chinese, Tibetan, and Japanese herbal medicine), and homeopathy. In the US, Australia, and Germany naturopathy is also a predominant and well-regulated form of treatment. Other therapies, such as nutritional therapy, are growing in popularity too.

Some of these complementary therapies have become increasingly mainstream. Osteopathy and chiropractic, for example, are now regulated by law in the UK, included under many health insurance schemes, practised on the National Health Service (NHS), and used for referral by GPs for health problems such as back and neck pain. In fact, for some people these therapies are no longer regarded as complementary at all but are considered as professions allied to medicine.

However, this situation doesn't mean that all therapies are immune to controversy. A subtle form of osteopathy, known as *cranial osteopathy*, has been particularly under attack (read more about this in Chapter 14), and homeopathy, developed in the 18th century in Germany by Dr Samuel Hahnemann, excites major disagreement as to whether it is effective or 'all in the mind' (jump to Chapter 10 to work out your views on that one).

Other less well-established therapies are regarded by many as truly weird and wacky. These include crystal, colour, and light therapy, chakra healing, and so on. Yet each of these therapies also has many serious and committed practitioners and research may yet confirm their effectiveness.

In this book, I aim to cover as many as I can of the therapies that you are likely to come across, or want to consider using, and to present a balanced view for each. Go to Part II to find out more about the traditional medical systems, to Part III for more on some of the most popular therapies, to Part IV for more on manipulation and massage therapies, or to Part V for healing and other mind/body therapies. I tell you exactly what each therapy involves and what it may be good for, but I also point out potential dangers and how you may distinguish the charlatans from the professionals.

What's the evidence?

Complementary medicine can generate huge amounts of controversy, with the argument ranging between those who are convinced that it works to those who are dead set against it and determined that it's all 'quackery'. Probably a middle path is a more reasonable approach, where each therapy is considered in the clear light of evidence examining its effectiveness.

Critics often argue that little or no good research supports the use of complementary medicine, but this simply isn't true. Many of the well-established therapies, such as acupuncture, herbal medicine, naturopathy, osteopathy and chiropractic, have quite a number of good quality scientific studies on their use. Research has been carried out around the world, including in Europe, the US, China, Japan, and India. However, researchers often find it difficult to get funding for this kind of research (only a tiny portion of public or private money is spent on complementary medicine research compared to medical research in most countries) and many early studies have design flaws. More good quality research is underway and much needed.

Other therapies, however, have little or no scientific research to back them up, although they may have lots of anecdotal evidence – that is, accounts of people who claim to have benefited from the therapy. However, this type of evidence is not enough to 'prove' that the therapy is effective and is rarely enough to convince sceptics. Lack of evidence may be a reason to approach the therapy with caution but it doesn't necessarily mean that it is ineffective.

All in the mind?

Some critics argue that complementary medicine is all *placebo*, that is, that the treatments work simply because the patients want them to work rather than through any value of their own and that benefits are 'all in the mind' or are due to the increased personal attention and time spent with patients in complementary consultations. The growing body of scientific evidence doesn't really justify such a claim and yet all treatments involve placebo to some extent. For example, studies have shown that, even in orthodox medicine, patients do better if they have strong confidence in their doctor or the treatment/medicine that they're receiving. So some researchers argue that placebo is a power to be harnessed rather than dismissed.

Prince Charles famously said, 'The unorthodoxy of today may well become the orthodoxy of tomorrow', and so it may prove that some of the therapies that are so maligned and ridiculed now prove to be accepted and commonplace in years to come.

Going carefully but breaking down barriers

Carefully investigating what sort of evidence is available before deciding to undergo a particular therapy is certainly worthwhile. However, also remember that orthodox, or conventional, medicine is itself relatively new, and many of its treatments have also developed through trial and error and even accident (such as the discovery of penicillin!). Many of its medicines, such as aspirin, are based on old herbal remedies and even extensive medical research cannot always guarantee safety. In fact, certain orthodox treatments have triggered terrible side effects (consider thalidomide) and the British Medical Journal has concluded that many have only limited or unknown proven effectiveness. So complementary medicine deserves the chance to be carefully considered and investigated, along with other forms of medicine, rather than being rejected simply because it is unconventional. Building barriers may in fact obstruct new learning that could be beneficial to health!

Using Complementary Medicine

Complementary medicine is now a massive growth industry, with its usage and range of therapies and products increasing all the time. Complementary medicine is used by people of all ages and for a wide range of complaints. Traditionally, women have been the most common users of complementary medicine, but men are catching up and children are often seen by complementary medicine practitioners too.

Complementary medicine: A holistic approach

A special feature of many complementary therapies is their *holistic approach*. Rather than focusing solely on your ailment, the practitioner is likely to be interested in your overall health and will spend time with you, asking about your diet and lifestyle, attempting to build up a picture of how one aspect of your health impacts on another.

This approach is in line with the World Health Organisation's definition of health as a 'complete state of physical, mental, and social well-being' and not simply the absence of disease.

Because of this holistic focus, people with the same ailment may be treated quite differently according to their individual make-up or needs. For example, two asthma sufferers may have similar symptoms and yet be given different types of herbs, homeopathic remedies, or acupuncture treatments by the same practitioner according to the diagnosis of their overall state of health and the perceived underlying cause of their condition.

The aim of this holistic approach is often the restoration of *homeostasis* or body balance, which is believed to facilitate the body's own self-healing mechanisms.

Typical users are people who are generally interested in health and diet and who are strongly motivated to look after their own health. They may also be disenchanted with, or have been failed by, conventional medicine, such as those with chronic illnesses for which Western medicine has little to offer. Other users include people with serious illnesses who want to use complementary medicine alongside orthodox medicine – such as people with cancer who may undergo chemotherapy and also choose to utilise nutritional therapy or healing therapies alongside this treatment.

In the UK, patients have access to complementary therapies via the National Health Service (NHS) in GP surgeries, hospitals, and clinics. As one recent example, in Northern Ireland in October 2006 a new scheme was announced by the Health Minister offering £200,000 worth of complementary services as part of health service treatment.

Things you need to check out: Safety and effectiveness

If you decide to try out any form of complementary medicine for yourself, first consider the following:

✔ Find out as much as you can about the therapy. Check the appropriate section in this book to find out what it involves, what it may be good for, what evidence supports its use, and what the safety warnings or possible side effects are.

✔ Check out the qualifications and experience of any practitioner you're thinking of consulting. Don't be afraid to ask questions and to ask for an explanation of letters after the practitioner's name, their membership of a professional and/or regulatory body, and their years of experience – particularly with your specific type of health problem. Check out individual chapters in this book for more details on all these issues for each therapy and its practitioners. Don't use unqualified, unregistered practitioners that aren't members of a reputable professional body.

✔ Check that the practitioner is fully insured and follows standards for safe practice, such as using disposable needles for acupuncture and disposing of them properly (again, more details on safety appear in each chapter of this book).

✔ Ask about and consider the number of treatments that you're likely to need, what sort of improvements you may expect, and what the likely costs are. Investigate whether the therapy is available on the NHS or covered by health insurance if you have any.

✔ Consider consulting or informing your doctor about having complementary medicine. Very few people do inform their doctor about this, fearing that such information won't be well received, but many doctors are now better informed and open to complementary medicine, and most complementary practitioners are happy to communicate with GPs too.

✔ If in doubt, seek advice from one of the professional organisations mentioned in the various chapters of this book.

What's complementary medicine good for?

Complementary therapies can have a real role to play alongside orthodox medicine, especially for the treatment of long-standing conditions that don't readily respond to conventional treatments, such as back and neck pain, osteoarthritis of the knee, nausea, stress, anxiety, and depression.

In fact, lots of people would like to see complementary therapies made more readily available. A recent National Health Service poll asked if the NHS should fund certain complementary therapies and 7,030 people responded. The affirmative results included 84 per cent for acupuncture, 74 per cent for reflexology, 71 per cent for homeopathy, 52 per cent for shiatsu, and 19 per cent for crystal therapy. Just 4 per cent of poll participants wanted none of the therapies made available. (Chiropractic and osteopathy were excluded from the poll because they are now regulated.)

Many therapies make claims to treat a wide range of illnesses, and gradually research trials are taking place to check these out. Some trials have not given any substantial proof that the therapy works, but others have indicated that real benefits may exist. Examples are trials that suggest that acupuncture can help neck pain, osteopathy can ease back pain, and homeopathy can relieve hay fever, although even these studies aren't immune to criticism.

In each chapter in this book, I list the type of ailments for which some research evidence exists that the therapy may be beneficial.

'Natural' does not necessarily mean 'better', 'safe', or even 'effective'. Complementary therapies should not be regarded as a substitute for orthodox medical care in case of serious health concerns. Well-trained complementary practitioners are taught how to spot serious medical conditions that require medical referral but not all therapists have had this training. If you're in any doubt about your condition, consult your GP.

Choosing the Right Complementary Therapy

Choosing the right complementary therapy is always tricky. You need to consider the nature of your ailment, the track record for resolving it with different therapies, any evidence of effectiveness, and any possible side effects or negative outcomes. In practice, the most common ways that people choose a therapy is by word of mouth from friends or colleagues, by recommendation from a GP or other practitioner, or by reading or learning about the therapy from a book, TV, radio programme, or the Internet.

To start you off, Table 1-1 may help point you in the right direction, but delve into the chapters in the rest of this book to find out more.

Table 1-1	Finding the Right Complementary Therapy
Problem	*Therapy**
Painful or aching joints, stiffness, sports injuries	Consider one of the manipulation or massage therapies in Part IV or acupuncture (Chapter 9).
Tired all the time, menstrual or menopausal problems, problems with memory or concentration	Consider nutritional therapy (Chapter 12).
Feeling sluggish, bowel or urinary problems, skin problems	Consider naturopathy (Chapters 8 and 13) or herbal medicine (Chapter 11).
Respiratory problems such as hay fever or asthma, migraines, headaches, or childhood ailments	Homeopathy (Chapter 10) or herbal remedies (Chapter 11) may bring relief, or try Traditional Chinese Medicine (Chapter 4).

Problem	Therapy*
Stressed out, anxious, irritable, and not sleeping well	Explore relaxation, breathing, and healing therapies. Aromatherapy can help, too. (All are covered in Part V.)
Digestive problems, blood sugar imbalance, Type II diabetes, gall bladder problems	Ayurveda, Japanese, or Tibetan medicine (Chapters 5, 6, and 7) or nutritional therapy (Chapter 12) may bring relief.
You're really motivated and in search of some self-help tips that you can try out at home	Check out the health tips in Part VI.

* Please note that this table represents a very simplified set of recommendations to get you started. Many therapies treat the same types of health problems and a lot depends on your personal preferences. Remember that many of the above problems may also require medical investigation to rule out serious health concerns.

Counting the Cost of Complementary Therapies

Because the majority of complementary therapy treatments aren't covered by the NHS or health insurance, the costs can soon mount up. Typical costs per session are around £25 to £35 but can be as little as £15 (such as in teaching clinics) or as much as £100 or more for top private specialists in expensive locations.

So instead of throwing your hard-earned money away, give yourself a budget to work with and ask your practitioner a few questions such as the following:

- ✔ How many treatments am I likely to need before I start to see results?
- ✔ What kind of improvements can I reasonably expect?
- ✔ How much experience have you had in treating my particular condition?
- ✔ What sort of success has your treatment led to?
- ✔ What is the total cost of my treatment likely to be?
- ✔ Are any other additional costs expected, such as supplements, herbs, or other remedies or goods?
- ✔ Do you do any discounts for block booking a series of treatments?

Staying healthy

Even if you get the best therapist and therapy in the world, your health and healing still rest to some extent in your own hands. Help yourself by practising the following:

✔ Start each day in a positive frame of mind.

✔ Eat healthily and sensibly, with lots of fresh vegetables, fruits, whole grains, nuts, seeds, and other healthy proteins, and avoid junk foods, saturated fats, and excess sugars and salt.

✔ Drink plenty of fresh water; eight glasses sipped during the course of the day is a good amount to aim for.

✔ Get regular exercise of both the vigorous (aerobic) and gentle, stretching (such as yoga, pilates, and t'ai chi) varieties. Two to three sessions a week of at least 20 minutes – enough to build up a bit of a sweat – is a good goal.

✔ B-r-e-a-t-h-e well! Lots of people simply stop breathing when they are concentrating, or they breathe very shallowly. Focus on your breath at regular intervals during the day and ensure even, free breaths. (Check out the section on Buteyko breathing in Chapter 18 if you want a way to really improve your breathing habits.)

✔ Limit your vices! Moderate alcohol intake and stop or at least cut down on the cigarettes.

✔ De-stress. Practise stress management and aim for a good work-rest-play life balance with time for socialising, creativity, and enjoyment.

✔ Get plenty of good quality sleep.

✔ End each day with gratitude for everything in your life.

Of course, getting exact answers to each of these queries may not be possible, because a lot depends on how your body responds to the treatment, but at least you gain a reasonable idea of what to expect.

Full benefits may take time, so don't give up after only one treatment if you haven't experienced earth-shattering results. But equally, don't go on and on with treatment hoping it will make a difference if nothing is happening.

Chapter 2

Diagnosing in Complementary Medicine

. . . .

In This Chapter

▶ Understanding complementary medicine diagnosis

▶ Asking questions about your health

▶ Examining the tongue and pulse for clues to your health

▶ Exploring complementary medicine testing and diagnostic devices

▶ Looking at the evidence for diagnoses

. . . .

Complementary medicine practitioners use a range of techniques to assess your health and diagnose the root cause of your illness or imbalance. They use this diagnostic information to determine the best course of treatment for you.

Some diagnostic approaches are more art than science, with their roots going back hundreds or even thousands of years. These approaches include tongue and pulse diagnoses, as used by practitioners of traditional Chinese, Japanese, Tibetan, and Ayurvedic (Indian) medicine. These diagnostic methods involve great sensitivity and skill on behalf of the practitioners who claim they're really useful tools in 'reading' the body. However, many modern medics reject these techniques because they haven't been scientifically proven.

Other diagnostic methods are more firmly rooted in science and some 21st century complementary medicine practitioners use many diagnostic techniques that are also used by orthodox medical doctors, such as laboratory tests, blood analyses, and x-rays.

In this chapter, I give you a guided tour of the different types of complementary medicine diagnosis and point out how reliable they may (or may not) be.

Finding Out about Diagnosis in Complementary Medicine

In this section, I discuss the following main forms of diagnosis used by complementary practitioners:

- ✔ **Questioning:** Includes questions about your physical and emotional health, symptoms, lifestyle, diet, and sleep patterns

- ✔ **Observation:** Includes examination of your tongue, your general appearance, and gait, as well as iris diagnosis and micro-diagnosis

- ✔ **Palpation:** Includes checking pulse and pressure points, *hara* (abdominal) diagnosis, and foot reflexology

- ✔ **Physical diagnosis:** Includes muscle testing and mobility testing

- ✔ **Clinical signs:** Includes examining changes in the appearance of your skin, hair, nails, and eyes

- ✔ **Charting and calculations:** Includes food diaries, sleep diaries, and Tibetan medical astrology

- ✔ **Testing:** Includes laboratory tests and electro-diagnostic measurement devices

- ✔ **'Energetic' diagnosis:** Includes methods for sensing the electro-magnetic field around your body

Questioning

Many practitioners start by asking you to describe any current symptoms that you're concerned about. They're interested in when the symptoms started, their nature and severity, and what alleviates or aggravates them. Your practitioner will also want to know of any treatment you may have had so far and its effect. The practitioner will also ask about your medical history, including any previous ailments, accidents, or surgery, and details of any present or past medication.

Always remember to inform your practitioner of any pharmaceutical drugs, nutritional supplements, and herbal, homeopathic, or other medicine you're currently taking, or any other therapies you're undergoing, in case of any possible interactions.

A tale of holistic diagnosis

Jane came to see me suffering from persistent, unexplained tiredness (a common medical syndrome called TATT, or 'tired all the time'). Her doctor had carried out various medical investigations but nothing abnormal had revealed. Jane had been advised to take some time off and get some rest. She'd followed this advice but felt no better. A dietary analysis showed that she was eating and drinking a huge amount of energy-sapping foods, that is, foods that are low in nutrients and high in stimulants. She lived on coffee, fizzy drinks, sugary sweets, pizzas, and ready meals. She was also unhappy in her job and felt stressed because she had the workload of two people after a colleague had left and not been replaced. Her sleep habits were also erratic because she often worked late into the night.

Tongue diagnosis revealed nodules at the rear and a red tip, which are signs in Traditional Chinese Medicine (TCM) that the person is under stress and has kidney/adrenal weakness. The adrenals are small glands that sit on top of your kidneys and control the release of the hormone adrenalin, which speeds up your heart rate and increases the oxygen supply to the muscles in times of need such as fight, flight, or fright.

Palpation of the pulse revealed a weak pulse overall and a deep, faint pulse in both the 'kidney positions' on her wrists (TCM practitioners take pulses for each of the internal organs at different points on the wrist). A laboratory saliva test confirmed that she had adrenal insufficiency – that is, her adrenals were worn out due to continued over-stimulation from dietary stimulants and stress.

Thus, from a holistic point of view her tiredness could be seen as due to a combination of (i) dietary insufficiency (a lack of essential nutrients), (ii) adrenal insufficiency (over-stimulation of the adrenal glands due to stress and dietary stimulants), (iii) inadequate rest and poor sleep, and (iv) work stress and job dissatisfaction.

Jane's immediate symptoms were remedied by means of dietary change, nutritional supplementation, adrenal support, and natural sleep aids. Jane also made the decision to change her job and to join a gym. Within a month she was bursting with energy, her tongue and pulse were normal, her sleep was good, and she was happily in training for a charity trek on Mount Kilimanjaro!

The practitioner may also be interested to know about the health history of your immediate family (in particular your parents, grandparents, and siblings), and may use this to determine your health risk factors and predisposition to disease. For example, women who have more than one female relative diagnosed with breast cancer have an increased risk of developing it themselves. In these situations, the practitioner can then advise you on steps to take to decrease whatever your risk may be. In some traditional medical systems, such as Traditional Chinese Medicine (TCM), knowledge of your parents' and grandparents' health history, and the order of your birth in relation to your siblings, is used to determine how much 'source *qi*' (pronounced *chee*) – that is, core vitality – you have.

Other questions are likely to cover your diet, lifestyle, stress levels, mental and emotional health, and your daily habits such as sleep, exercise, and recreation. Homeopaths, for example, use answers to lifestyle questions to build a picture of your ideal constitutional remedy (for more about this, see Chapter 10 on homeopathy).

Most complementary practitioners consider you from a holistic viewpoint. They use these different bits of information to build a picture of your current symptoms in the context of your overall health and well-being.

You don't have to have a health complaint to go to a complementary medicine practitioner. Some people are symptom-free but choose complementary medicine because they believe that it can help them optimise their health and prevent disease. In such cases, the questioning may be more focused on your existing lifestyle and health and desired optimal health goals.

Observation

In observational diagnosis, the practitioner may examine a particular part of the body to identify signs that reflect something going on in another part of the body, or may observe the movement and appearance of the whole body to determine more general underlying factors. This section includes descriptions of some of the more common types of observational diagnosis.

Tongue diagnosis

Tongue diagnosis is used by most traditional Chinese, Japanese, Tibetan, and Ayurvedic (Indian) medicine practitioners. You're asked to stick out your tongue so that the practitioner can observe its shape, colour, coating, and any movement. According to these traditional medicine systems, different tongue shapes and appearances can give valuable information about specific internal organ function as well as general health. For example, a thick, yellow coating in the middle of the tongue is considered indicative of sluggish bowels and constipation.

Chinese and Japanese tongue diagnoses are the most detailed, with more than 100 different types of tongues identified, all relating to different patterns of individual organ balance. Tibetan and Ayurvedic medicine use a more simplified form of tongue diagnosis that concentrates on establishing the general balance within the body's constitution, rather than focusing on individual internal organs. Western medicine also uses a simple form of tongue diagnosis.

Little scientific evidence supports the more detailed form of tongue diagnosis used in the traditional medical systems and by many complementary medicine practitioners today. Chapter 3 has more details on tongue diagnosis.

Iris diagnosis

Also known as *iridology*, in this form of diagnosis the practitioner examines your iris (the coloured part of your eye) by means of either a special measurement device or a hand-held magnifying glass designed for eye inspection.

The practitioner looks for specific marks and signs in particular parts of the iris that are believed to correspond with specific parts of the body. This form of diagnosis is often used by naturopaths or nature cure practitioners and sometimes by people solely trained in this technique. Some slight evidence supports the use of this technique but more research is needed.

For more about this intriguing form of diagnosis, read Chapters 8 and 13 on nature cure and naturopathy.

Micro-diagnosis

The face, ears, abdomen, back, feet, fingers, and toes can be used diagnostically to reflect the body as a whole. This is called *micro-diagnosis*. For example, in TCM face diagnosis, the areas under the eyes are linked to the kidneys, so grey bags under the eyes are believed to be indicative of adrenal exhaustion. In Japanese finger diagnosis the thumbs are linked to the lungs, so deformed or weak thumb nails may be indicative of past or underlying lung conditions such as asthma. However, the evidence for this is only anecdotal so this form of diagnosis is not accepted by many doctors.

More on this type of diagnosis appears in Chapter 7 on Japanese medicine.

Appearance and gait

Before diagnosis, the practitioner observes you from the moment you enter the room, noticing your gait and general appearance in case either has a bearing on your symptoms. For example, you may visit an osteopath because of back pain and as you walk in, the practitioner may observe that you have a very lopsided gait. Further physical investigation may reveal that one leg is longer than the other and that this leg discrepancy causes pelvic and lower-back imbalance, which causes the back pain. By re-adjusting pelvic alignment and recommending the use of special inner soles for your shoes, called *orthotics*, your back pain may be dramatically relieved.

Alternatively, a practitioner may observe that a person's gait is very stooped and their appearance dishevelled, prompting the practitioner to ask questions about mood and self-care. This combination of observational diagnoses and questioning may reveal that the person is actually suffering from depression even though this had not been mentioned as a symptom. Depression can then be addressed by the practitioner.

This type of observational diagnosis can have preliminary importance but then needs to be backed up with other diagnosis to confirm the significance of the observation.

Palpation

Palpation involves applying light pressure to different parts of the body to determine the body's response, or to feel for areas of tenderness, pain, heat, and so on. The most commonly used forms of palpation are pulse diagnosis, pressure point diagnosis, and abdominal diagnosis.

Pulse diagnosis

Traditional Chinese, Japanese, Ayurvedic, and Tibetan medicine practitioners rely strongly on pulse diagnosis. In Western medicine, only a single pulse is taken at the wrist to determine the rate of blood flow with each heartbeat. However, in the traditional medical systems, pulses are taken at three points on each wrist and at different depths. Each position is said to correspond to a different internal organ and to give information about its functioning.

The well-known Tibetan physician, Dr Yeshe Donden, was invited to carry out a ward round at an American hospital. He was presented with patients without being given any information about their medical condition or medical history and invited to diagnose them simply with his pulse-taking skills. The American doctors were amazed when, without any questions to the patients, Dr Donden was able to accurately diagnose health problems, including a faulty heart valve.

Western medicine finds it hard to comprehend this concept of tuning into the body using just the artery on the wrist and because this technique is difficult to measure and verify scientifically, many medics dismiss it.

More information on different types of pulse-taking appears in the chapters of Part II.

Pressure points

Many complementary medicine practitioners palpate the skin in order to determine points of sensitivity or pain known as *pressure points*. Pressure points can give information about the condition of underlying tissues and organs but may also be used to give information about related internal organs according to *meridian* or other body maps. For example:

> ✔ Osteopaths, chiropractors, and massage therapists palpate to locate areas of inflammation and to get information about structural alignment and the health of the joints and surrounding tissues.

✔ Reflexologists use painful points on the feet to diagnose internal organ health according to a zone system that links specific points on the feet with specific internal organs and body parts.

✔ Acupuncturists palpate to locate points where the flow of vital energy, or *qi*, may be blocked in the acupuncture meridians (energy channels).

Painful pressure at certain points is believed to indicate malfunction in related internal organs. For example, a point on the upper side of the foot, above the groove between the big and the fourth toes (known as the Liver 3 point) is said to become very sensitive if a person has a hangover and a weakened liver due to excess alcohol!

Little evidence supports these forms of diagnosis, other than the fact that they've been used for thousands of years. Many medics reject these forms of diagnosis, and more research is needed.

For more on these approaches see the relevant chapters that cover osteopathy, acupuncture, and reflexology.

Abdominal palpation

Another form of palpation is *abdominal diagnosis*, also known as *hara* diagnosis or *ampuku*. This involves firm pressure to different parts of the abdomen, which is used both diagnostically and to give treatment. No real scientific evidence supports the use of this technique, although it's been used clinically for hundreds of years, which many feel is a testimony to its effectiveness.

For more on abdominal diagnosis check out Chapter 7 on Japanese medicine.

Physical diagnosis

Physical examination is an important part of diagnosis for several types of practitioners, especially osteopaths and chiropractors. These practitioners usually ask you to bend your spine and move your joints in different ways to determine your level of mobility and your range of movement.

Kinesiologists and Touch for Health practitioners use muscle testing as part of their examination. This testing involves 'challenging' a muscle by applying gentle pressure that you have to resist. Kinesiologists believe that the muscles are linked to specific internal organs and body systems and that muscle weakness reflects internal organ or body system weakness.

Chapters 14 and 15 cover osteopathy and chiropractic, and Chapter 16 explains kinesiology.

Clinical signs

Clinical signs are like signposts on the road to a destination (the diagnosis). These signs may be changes in the appearance of your skin, hair, nails, eyes, and so on, or perhaps a bloated abdomen or swollen glands. All these signs may be linked to specific diseases or imbalances according to the various complementary medicine approaches. So, for a practitioner of Traditional Chinese Medicine, spots around the mouth would be linked to problems with the large intestine and digestion, according to the meridian pathways. Ridged nails may indicate a zinc deficiency to a nutritionist.

Complementary medical practitioners who've completed a full, professional training course of several years (usually a degree course that also includes practical training in clinical skills) are also carefully trained to recognise specific physical, emotional, or mental signs that may indicate serious diseases requiring medical attention – for example, excessive thirst and weight loss are potentially linked to diabetes, while chest pain and breathlessness may be linked to heart disease.

Sometimes, clinical signs may all be linked together to confirm a diagnosis. To an acupuncturist, for example, headaches, irritability, abdominal fullness and bloating, a love of sour foods, and an aggravation of symptoms in the spring are all linked to a liver imbalance. This diagnosis is according to the system of correspondences of Five Element Theory (to find out more about this, see Chapter 4) and makes perfect sense to a TCM practitioner, but wouldn't make a lot of sense to an orthodox medic with no background in TCM.

Charting and calculations

Several complementary medicine disciplines use charting or paper calculations as part of their diagnosis. A nutritionist is likely to ask you to complete a food diary and uses it to analyse your nutritional status and the suitability of your diet. Tibetan and Ayurvedic physicians sometimes calculate your birth chart and use astrology to determine what sort of diseases you may be predisposed to. Naturopaths may ask you to keep sleep, food, and lifestyle records that may be analysed for patterns as part of the diagnostic process.

Testing

Laboratory or home-kit testing used by complementary practitioners can include blood, saliva, hair, urine, and stool tests. These tests may be used to determine many things including vitamin and mineral status, allergies, food intolerance, hormone balance, the presence of parasites, and more.

Manipulative therapists, such as osteopaths and chiropractors, may use x-rays and scans to check on structural balance; they may also use equipment to check blood pressure or small hammers to test muscle reflexes.

Many of these forms of testing are also used by medical doctors and are well-accepted in orthodox medicine although some of the newer tests, such as tests for food intolerances remain controversial despite growing scientific evidence to support their use.

Other methods of testing may involve specially designed devices such as the equipment used to examine the eyes in iridology or the electro-acupuncture devices used to measure the flow of vital energy (*qi*) in the acupuncture meridians (see Chapter 22 for details on these energy medicine devices). These are less well-accepted in orthodox medicine and have little scientific evidence to support their use.

Energetic diagnosis

Energetic diagnosis involves assessing the *aura* or electro-magnetic field believed to surround each person and may be determined using the hands or a measurement device.

In manual diagnosis the practitioner runs their hands above the surface of your body to detect subtle changes in the electro-magnetic field according to changes in sensations felt in the hands that may indicate health problems.

In other cases a diagnostic measurement device may be used. An example of this is Kirlian photography, whereby images of the energetic field around the body are alleged to be captured photographically, (see Chapter 22 for more about such energy medicine techniques).

These methods of 'energetic' diagnosis are controversial and aren't accepted within conventional medicine because no real scientific evidence supports them.

Complementary versus Orthodox Medical Diagnosis

Many different forms of diagnosis are used in complementary medicine. Different therapies employ different techniques and the diagnoses may not always agree. The diagnoses can also be quite different from orthodox medical ones.

Practitioners must take great care to ensure that they don't miss spotting any serious medical conditions.

Taking the necessary precautions

Certain symptoms are regarded as red flags that require proper medical investigation. A well-trained complementary medicine professional should spot these and refer you on to your GP or other medical specialist. However some complementary therapists who have only undergone a very short training, such as a short course in a particular type of massage, may not know how to spot these warning signs.

If you have any of the symptoms listed below, or are in any doubt about a diagnosis you've been given, seek a second opinion from a medical practitioner or another well-qualified complementary medicine practitioner:

- ✔ Chest pain or discomfort, especially if accompanied by sudden shortness of breath.
- ✔ Persistent cough or coughing up of blood.
- ✔ Prolonged difficulty breathing or swallowing.
- ✔ Unexplained bleeding, such as from the vagina or anus.
- ✔ Persistent headaches or head pain.
- ✔ Blurred vision or other persistent visual disturbance.
- ✔ Unexplained lumps, swellings, or persistent pain.
- ✔ Changes in size or appearance, or presence of lumps, in breasts or testicles, plus any discharge.
- ✔ Unexplained dizziness, mental changes, or memory loss.
- ✔ Persistent stomach or abdominal pain.
- ✔ Changes in size, shape, or colour of any mole on the skin or any sudden itching or bleeding from a mole.
- ✔ Sudden skin changes, such as a rash, especially if accompanied by high fever.
- ✔ Unexplained swelling of the legs or abdomen.
- ✔ Severe allergic reactions.
- ✔ Prolonged, unexplained weight loss and/or loss of appetite and/or excessive thirst.
- ✔ Difficulty urinating, such as experiencing blockage and being unable to maintain flow (men) or increased frequency and painful, burning urination (women).
- ✔ High fever or loss of consciousness.
- ✔ Prolonged, unexplained fatigue.
- ✔ Compulsive repetition of simple daily tasks, excessive mood swings, paranoia, or delusions.

All these symptoms may be indicative of serious health conditions and need to be investigated fully.

Weighing up the evidence

Although many of the complementary medicine diagnostic techniques have little, or no, scientific evidence to support their use, don't forget that many of them have been used for hundreds or even thousands of years.

Many practitioners who've practised for years to refine these diagnostic skills are convinced of their effectiveness and feel it may be only a matter of time before scientific research is able to confirm their accuracy.

Chapter 3

Reading Your Body

. . . .

In This Chapter

▶ Understanding self-diagnosis

▶ Examining your tongue

▶ Reading your face

▶ Looking at other types of self-diagnosis

▶ Finding out more about self-diagnosis

. . . .

Self-diagnosis is all about discovering how to read the body's everyday signs and signals that reflect your state of health. Analysing your own body isn't a substitute for orthodox or complementary medical diagnosis in the case of illness. Rather, self-diagnosis is a way of monitoring your health and possibly preventing disease by detecting early signs of imbalance.

In this chapter, I describe some common forms of self-diagnosis that have their roots in complementary therapies and traditional medicine. You'll find out how to read your tongue, face, and various other body parts. Their signs can give you important health clues.

You can use some of these diagnostic techniques to have a bit of fun and develop quite a handy party trick or even a new chat-up line – 'Would you like to stick out your tongue at me and let me read it for you?' (Well, maybe not!) Seriously, though, you can use these self-diagnostic techniques to increase your awareness and get to know your body much better.

Finding Out about Self-Diagnosis

Self-diagnosis has its roots in traditional medicine, going back to a time when physicians and healers weren't readily available and people had to take greater care of their own health. Reading your own body also goes back to a time when people lived lives that were more in tune with the natural cycles, rather than dominated by the artificial, urban environments in which many of us now live, more cut off from nature, fresh air, natural daylight, and the changing seasons.

In those ancient times, people were able to read their environment by knowing what weather to expect from observing the behaviour of birds and insects or observing the form and movements of clouds. They also seem to have been able to read the body any try to remedy any upsets.

This chapter offers some examples of these ancient techniques that you can use to understand your own body better.

Exploring Tongue Diagnosis

Stick out your tongue in front of a mirror and look at its shape, colour, coating, and any movement.

According to Traditional Chinese Medicine (TCM), the *tongue proper* (that is, the shape and colour of the tongue itself) links to the various organs and also reflects general circulation and overall hydration of the body. The tongue coating, which lies on the surface, can indicate your health condition or the nature and stage of a particular disease.

A normal tongue is light red in colour, has free motion, and has a thin layer of clear, or slightly white, coating that is neither too dry nor too moist.

Reading signs of the tongue proper

Take a look at your own tongue and use the guide below to detect signs that, according to TCM, may indicate some imbalance:

- A pale tongue indicates problems such as frequent colds, kidney or adrenal weakness, or joint problems.
- A red tongue indicates conditions such as pain, inflamed joints, irritable bowel, and allergies.
- A deep red tongue can indicate the late stage of fever.
- A purple tongue can indicate blood stagnation and poor circulation of vital energy as seen in premenstrual syndrome (PMS) and fatigue syndromes.
- A full, flabby, soft tongue with teeth marks shows weak digestion, catarrh, and heavy, aching limbs.
- A tongue with a red tip indicates stress and circulation problems and sometimes heart problems.
- A tongue with a lot of cracks can indicate dehydration and/or exhaustion of body fluids due to fever (although a few people are simply born with a cracked tongue).

✔ A 'thorny' tongue with lots of little raised red bumps on the surface can indicate 'internal heat', often inflammation of the liver or intestines, and may also be due to vitamin B deficiency.

✔ A tongue that can't stop quivering, or that is deviated to one side, can indicate liver imbalance, for example, due to too much stress, alcohol or sweet foods, or an excess of catarrh and phlegm.

Observing tongue coatings

The *tongue coating* lies on the surface of the tongue (it isn't the colour of the body of the tongue itself). Here's what the tongue coating can tell you:

✔ A thin white coating can indicate a fairly recent 'cold' or 'deficiency' condition such as a common cold.

✔ A thick white coating suggests food retention and sluggish digestion.

✔ A sticky white coating indicates excess phlegm.

✔ A thick yellow coating can be a sign of digestive problems such as constipation. If the coating is dry, the problem is usually with the stomach and intestines; if it is wet you may have excess phlegm.

✔ A thin yellow coating can signify a lung infection.

✔ A greyish or black tongue coating (yes, the coating can actually be black!) usually indicates a significant health problem. If your tongue is either of these colours, consult a health professional as soon as possible.

✔ A peeled tongue, sometimes called a 'geographic tongue' because it looks like a map, can indicate a crisis point in a long illness.

Always observe the tongue in good daylight and exclude obvious false phenomena such as a purple tongue after sucking a blackcurrant lolly or a red tip after burning it on a hot drink.

Organ correspondences

In Chinese and Japanese medicine, the tip of the tongue is said to correspond with the heart, and the area just behind it, at the front of the tongue, corresponds with the lungs. The middle of the tongue corresponds with the stomach and spleen while the sides reflect the liver and gall bladder. Finally, the back or 'root' of the tongue corresponds to the kidneys and urinary bladder (see Figure 3-1).

A tongue story

A couple of years ago one of my students, Moira, took my course on self-diagnosis in the Oriental medical traditions and was surprised to be diagnosed with a 'cold condition' during pair work on tongue diagnosis. Her partner had observed a pale tongue and a thick white coating, especially in the area at the front of the tongue corresponding to the lungs, and had concluded that this indicated a lung cold. Moira was rather sceptical about the merits of this diagnosis because she felt perfectly healthy at the time. However, a few days later she phoned saying: 'Do you know, that tongue diagnosis was accurate after all! That evening I felt shivery and by the following morning I had a runny nose and phlegmy cough and ended up with a terrible cold for three days!' Apparently, the imbalance had been reflected in her tongue *before* the actual symptoms manifested fully – a situation often observed by practitioners in clinical practice. She now checks her tongue every morning when she brushes her teeth and at the first sign of any white coating she takes some vitamin C and the herb Echinacea (designed to boost the immune system) and takes care to get plenty of rest and fluids. She's found that this early warning system and preventive action works for her and she hasn't had a cold since.

For example, nodules at the back of the tongue can indicate kidney weakness and fatigue or bladder problems, a red tip can indicate stress and maybe raised blood pressure or other circulatory problem, a yellow coating in the centre can indicate stomach upset or other digestive problem, and so on.

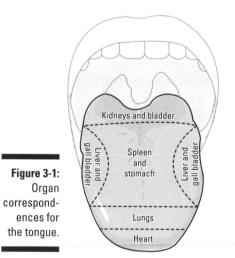

Figure 3-1:
Organ correspondences for the tongue.

Tongues in Ayurvedic and Tibetan medicine

In Ayurveda, abnormalities in the tongue reflect abnormalities in the three *doshas*, or 'vital energies'. A dry, rough, cracked tongue with a dark coating indicates *vata* (wind) disturbance; a red, hot tongue with a burning sensation indicates *pitta* (choler or bile) disturbance; and a pale tongue that's wet, slimy, and white-coated indicates *kapha* (phlegm) disturbance. (For more about what these disturbances reflect, take a look at Chapter 5.)

In Tibetan medicine, a red tongue indicates 'hot' diseases and a white tongue 'cold' diseases. *Loong* ('wind') disturbances are reflected in pale tongues with white coatings; *Tripa* ('bile') conditions have red tongues with yellow coatings, and *Peken* ('phlegm') diseases have flabby, tongues with greasy, wet coatings. (For more about these signs, check out Chapter 6.)

Exploring Face Diagnosis

Face diagnosis features in Chinese, Japanese, Ayurvedic, and Tibetan medicine. This form of diagnosis involves looking at the shape of the face and the arrangement and appearance of individual facial features, such as the eyes, mouth, nose, and ears, to determine the health of the internal organs and predisposition to disease.

In Traditional Chinese Medicine (TCM), facial signs are interpreted in terms of the person's *yin* and *yang* balance – that is, the balance of 'male' and 'female' energies in the body (to find out much more about *yin* and *yang*, have a look at Chapter 4).

Checking out face shape

A face shaped in a downward pointing triangle with a large forehead, pointed chin, and features spaced apart is said to indicate a *yin* constitution and a person with a tendency toward 'deficiency' conditions such as fatigue and muscle weakness. Conversely, a face with a square jaw, small forehead, and features set close together is thought to indicate a *yang* constitution and a predisposition toward inflammatory or painful conditions such as joint pain and irritable bowel disorder.

Investigating the eyes

The eyes are believed to give away vital information about diet, digestion, and general health. Large eyes are said to reflect high intake of *yin* foods, such as sugar, while small eyes indicate a diet dominated by *yang* foods, such as meat and animal products.

Sparse eyebrows are said to indicate an excess of sugar in the diet, while short eyelashes suggest a predominance of meat and animal products.

Puffiness or dark rings under the eyes can indicate problems with kidney or adrenal function and/or fluid retention.

Eye whites showing under and around the iris reflect a condition known as *sanpaku* ('three whites') in Japanese medicine. *Sanpaku* is said to indicate an excess of sugar in the diet and an unhealthy lifestyle.

Examining the nose

Narrow noses with small nostrils are believed to indicate weak lungs while bulbous, red noses can be linked to over-indulgence in food and drink and heart problems. Long noses are thought to be a sign of a *yin* constitution while short noses can indicate a *yang* constitution.

Observing the mouth

A small mouth with thin lips is said to indicate a *yin* constitution while a large mouth with thick lips is thought to be more *yang.* Dark, purple lips indicate poor blood circulation, and are often seen in people suffering from premenstrual pain, while pale, dry lips can indicate poor stomach function.

Considering Other Forms of Self-Diagnosis

Other forms of self-diagnosis used by complementary medicine practitioners that can also be used by you to monitor your own health include urine and stool diagnosis. Many people don't like to pay any attention to urine and faeces, yet they can be really useful in monitoring your health.

Ayurvedic urinalysis

In Ayurvedic medicine, urine analysis can help determine your constitutional 'type'. Chapter 5 explains the lifestyle advice that you can adopt to help your health and has more about Ayurveda. Here's a sample of urine analysis (no, not a physical one!):

✔ If your urine is frequent, clear, and odourless, then you may have a predominance of *vata* – follow the lifestyle advice for *vata* types.

✔ If your urine is scanty, deep yellow or brown in colour, and has a burnt odour, then you may have a predominance of *pitta* and should follow the lifestyle advice for *pitta* types.

✔ If your urine is copious, whitish in colour, and has a stale smell, then you may have a predominance of *kapha*. Follow the lifestyle advice for *kapha* types.

Stool analysis

Stool diagnosis, as used in various therapies, can help you monitor your health and remedy imbalance:

✔ If your stool is pale and contains undigested pieces of food, then Traditional Chinese Medicine (TCM) suggests that this is due to poor digestion and a weak spleen and stomach. To remedy this situation, you need to use acupuncture, acupressure, and/or Chinese herbs, and eat predominantly warm and easily digestible foods.

✔ If your stool is hard and dry, then according to nutritionists, this can indicate dehydration and a lack of essential fatty acids (EFAs). Drinking more water and increasing EFAs in your diet, such as from oily fish, seeds, nuts, and plant oils, can help to remedy the situation.

✔ If your stool contains parasites, such as small threadworms, then herbalists recommend using sweet wormwood (*Artemisia annua*), a powerful, bitter herb, plus other digestive and bitter herbs to eradicate the parasites and support gut ecology.

Taking the Necessary Precautions

None of the forms of self-diagnosis described above can be taken as definite indications about your state of health. They're based on the ancient medical traditions and have been used for centuries. However, little scientific evidence backs them up at this time. I suggest that you use them as a way of increasing your self-awareness and of getting to know your body better.

Please remember that self-diagnosis is never a substitute for professional diagnosis by a doctor or other experienced health professional. If in any doubt about a sign or symptom that your body has revealed, always seek advice from a medical or qualified complementary medicine practitioner.

Part II
Exploring Traditional Healing Systems

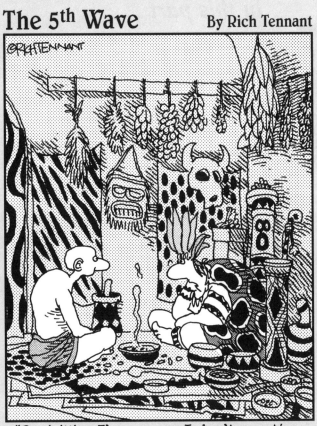

The 5th Wave   By Rich Tennant

"Penicillin? I'm sorry – I don't practice alternative medicine."

In this part . . .

The ancients weren't all long beards and weird tattoos. Ancient healing wisdom and health practices of some of the great traditions survive and flourish to this day.

In this part I take you on a world tour to China, Tibet, Japan, India, and Europe. Sit back, and enjoy some armchair travels to discover the therapies that originated in these places, what they're good for, and how to find reliable practitioners.

Chapter 4

Uncovering Traditional Chinese Medicine (TCM)

· ·

In This Chapter

▶ Discovering the origins of TCM

▶ Understanding TCM concepts of health and disease

▶ Diagnosing in TCM

▶ Exploring TCM therapies and how they work

· ·

*T*raditional Chinese Medicine (TCM) is one of the oldest forms of medicine in the world. From its beginnings thousands of years ago in ancient China, TCM has spread around the globe and is now one of the most widespread forms of complementary medicine in the West.

In this chapter I tell you a bit about where TCM came from and translate for you some of the strange terminology used by TCM practitioners. You can try a quiz to help you to work out what type of TCM element imbalance you may suffer from, and read TCM self-care tips for how you may remedy any imbalance. I also give you a guided tour of TCM therapies and let you know what they can be useful for. Finally, I offer tips for finding yourself a TCM practitioner.

A (Very) Brief History of TCM

Traditional Chinese Medicine is thought to have started over 2,500 years ago. Its history is blended with myth and legend. TCM is said to have originated from two legendary emperors who were medical pioneers and keen to live long and healthy lives (see the sidebar 'The founders of TCM').

The founders of TCM

Legend has it that over 2,500 years ago a Chinese emperor called Shennong tasted every herb and plant he could lay his hands on and noted its effects. His insights are said to have led to the first ever text on Chinese herbal medicine, *The Shennong Bencaojing* (*Classic of Herbal Medicine*), although in reality this actual text was written some time later. Shennong became known as the father of herbal medicine in China and is often portrayed clothed in leaves and holding or chewing medicinal plants.

Around the same time another Chinese leader known as the Yellow Emperor, or Huang di, is supposed to have had long conversations with his physicians about medicine. Their question-and-answer sessions are supposedly recorded in another ancient text known as the *Huang Di Nei Jing* (*The Yellow Emperor's Classic of Internal Medicine*) and Huang di is known as the father of traditional Chinese medicine.

Nowadays some scholars believe these figures were mythical, rather than real, but in any case the knowledge said to come from them still forms the basis of TCM practice today. You often see their pictures in TCM practitioners' waiting rooms!

Early Chinese people are believed to have used herbs as medicines and to have warmed stones as a form of heat treatment. Inscriptions on tortoise shells over a thousand years old give evidence of the use of water and simple herbal remedies for healing. Over time (in the Zhou dynasties from 1100–256 BC), medicine developed into an organised system and absorbed influences from the philosophical and religious traditions of Confucianism and Daoism. This led to the development of the concepts of *yin* and *yang* and the *five elements* or *phases* (described in the next section). The system of diagnosing by means of the tongue and pulse and observing other body signs was also created.

Over many centuries great Chinese medical texts were compiled and *acupuncture* (needle treatment), *moxibustion* (heat treatment with a warming herb), and herbal medicine became widespread.

The arrival of Christian missionaries in China in the 19th and early 20th centuries led to the introduction of Western medical ideas and a downsurge of interest in TCM. However TCM was revived by Chairman Mao as part of his Revolution and it now flourishes alongside Western medicine in modern day China.

Understanding TCM Concepts of Health and Disease

TCM has its roots in the Daoist concept of living in harmony with nature and of all living things stemming from one primordial force. This force is represented by the *Tai Ji*, a symbol representing oneness made up of two interconnected, dynamically changing and also opposing forces known as *yin* and *yang*.

Exploring yin and yang

In the *Tai Ji* symbol (see Figure 4-1), the white area represents *yang*, which is said to have the qualities of masculinity, expansiveness, activity, heat, brightness, and hardness, while the black area represents *yin*, which is said to be feminine, contracting, passive, cold, dark, and soft.

Figure 4-1:
The
yin/yang
symbol.

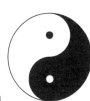

Yin and *yang* were seen as two great interdependent and creative forces that manifest in all living things, including the body and the environment. These forces are in a constant state of change. For example, night (*yin*) turns into day (*yang*), which later again becomes night (*yin*), and so on.

For this reason the white (*yang*) portion of the circle also contains a black dot to represent some *yin* within the *yang*, while the black (*yin*) portion of the circle also contains a white dot representing some *yang*. So if you look again at the symbol in Figure 4-1 you may see that it is not really a fixed design but rather can be seen as constantly moving and dancing, as black (*yin*) turns into white (*yang*) and back into black (*yin*) again.

In terms of your body *yin* and *yang* represent the following:

- ✔ The outside of the body is seen as *yang* while the inside is *yin*.
- ✔ The upper portion of the body is *yang* while the lower portion is *yin*.
- ✔ The internal organs are also divided into *yin* and *yang*.
- ✔ The great 'storing' organs of the body – liver, heart, and lungs – are *yin* organs.
- ✔ The active organs involved with movement and transportation of substances, such as the stomach, intestines, and urinary bladder, are seen as *yang*.

Table 4-1 offers a breakdown of how all the internal organs shape up in terms of their *yin* and *yang*.

Table 4-1	The Yin and Yang of Body Parts
The Yin Organs	**The Yang Organs**
Lungs	Large intestine
Spleen	Stomach
Heart	Small intestine
Pericardium (the membrane around the heart, but in TCM this 'organ' is related to circulation and responds to stress)	'Triple warmer', or *san jiao* (related to the upper, middle, and lower parts of the body, known as the 'three burners' and responsible for circulation and temperature balance; also helps regulate sexual function)
Kidneys	Urinary bladder
Liver	Gall bladder
	Brain
	Uterus (along with the brain, the uterus is regarded as an extraordinary yang organ)

In TCM, good health relies on a balance of *yin* and *yang* so all your *yin* and *yang* organs need to be functioning well and working in harmony together.

Understanding the power of qi

In TCM, *qi* (pronounced 'chee') is the name for the vital energy believed to power everything in the universe, including our bodies. The Chinese character for *qi* represents a union of earthly and heavenly energy. (Chapter 9 has more about *qi*.)

According to TCM if you have good *qi*, you'll be healthy and energetic and live long, but if your *qi* is abnormal, wayward, or blocked, disease may develop.

Qi courses through the body via a network of channels known as *meridians*. The twelve main meridians are divided into *yin* and *yang* pairs:

✔ Lungs and large intestine

✔ Spleen and stomach

✔ Heart and small intestine

✔ Pericardium and triple warmer

✔ Kidneys and urinary bladder

✔ Liver and gall bladder

Traversing the meridians

JARGON ALERT

The meridians course all over the body like a great rail network and are punctuated by hundreds of major and minor *acupoints*, rather like main line stations and lesser-used country ones.

The underlying theme for TCM is the restoration and preservation of free-flowing and abundant *qi*.

Much research has been carried out in different countries to verify the meridians and the links between *qi* flow and disease but these have not yet been firmly proven to the satisfaction of scientists (I discuss this research in Chapter 9 in a bit more detail).

Exploring the Five Elements

In addition to *yin* and *yang* and *qi*, TCM has a clever system of correspondences worked out called the *Five Elements* or *Five Phases*. This system is used to understand the relationships between the internal organs of the body, mental and emotional states, the environment, and so on. These relationships may be generating and supportive (the black arrows in Figure 4-2) or they may be destructive, whereby one element predominates and can overcome another (the grey arrows in Figure 4-2). This system is illustrated in Figure 4-2.

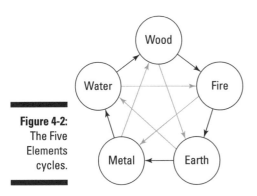

Figure 4-2:
The Five
Elements
cycles.

Compare Figure 4-2 with Table 4-2. According to the Five Elements:

- ✔ The heart is associated with fire because it pumps blood around the body to warm and nourish it.
- ✔ The nutrients carried in the blood pumped by the heart support the function of the stomach and spleen (that is, fire nourishes earth).

✔ The kidneys are associated with water because they control fluid metabolism.

✔ If the kidneys malfunction, blood pressure may rise, which in turn affects heart function. In other words, if the body is dehydrated (lacking in the element water) the heart can't function efficiently. In TCM terms the fire of the heart is raised, leading to elevated blood pressure and even heart attack. In this scenario, the fire element becomes too strong because the water element is insufficient to keep it in check.

You can also apply the five element principle in TCM to tastes, colours, and seasons. These correspondences, shown in Table 4-1, are used as a valuable diagnostic tool for TCM practitioners. For example, you may complain to your TCM practitioner of the following symptoms:

✔ Suffer from earache and aching bones

✔ Feel worse in the winter

✔ Crave salty food

✔ Often feel anxious

Your practitioner would think to the correspondences in the five element table and – hey presto! – it would become obvious you may have an imbalance in your kidney/urinary bladder meridians or some weakness in the organs themselves (take a look at the bottom line of Table 4-2 to see for yourself how this links to the symptoms described above).

Table 4-2:		Five Elements Table of Correspondences			
Element	*Taste*	*Colour*	*Organs*	*Sense organs*	*Weather*
Wood	Sour	Dark blue	Liver and gall bladder	Eyes	Wind
Fire	Bitter	Red	Heart and small intestine	Tongue	Heat
Earth	Sweet	Yellow	Spleen and stomach	Mouth	Dampness
Metal	Pungent	White	Lung and large intestine	Nose	Dryness
Water	Salty	Black	Kidney and bladder	Ear	Cold

Western medical doctors find this system of correspondences a bit mystifying, but TCM practitioners swear by its accuracy and clinical efficacy. Therefore, even if you go to a TCM practitioner complaining of backache you may still be asked about your food preferences, emotional state, and even colour preferences. Now you know why.

Taking the Five Elements quiz

You can use the Five Elements quiz in Table 4-3 to identify your possible element imbalance and then discover simple TCM ways of restoring balance.

Work through the questions in Table 4-3 and tick a 'yes' for each question that applies to you.

Table 4-3	The Five Elements Quiz		
The Element of Water		*Yes*	*No*
Do you often suffer from puffy bags under the eyes, a puffy face, or swollen ankles?			
Do you often get low backache?			
Do you often suffer from cystitis or other urinary infections?			
Do you often have problems with your ears and/or sore throats?			
Do you have problems with your bones or aching joints?			
Do you crave salty foods?			
Are your symptoms often worse in winter?			
Are your symptoms often aggravated by cold and wet conditions?			
Do you often feel anxious or fearful?			
Do you feel drawn to the colours midnight blue or black?			
Total Water Score (this represents the health of your kidneys and urinary bladder)			**/10**
The Element of Wood		*Yes*	*No*
Do you often suffer from nausea and lack of appetite?			
Do you often get headaches and/or migraines?			
Do you often suffer from PMS and/or cramps?			
Do you often have problems with your eyes?			

(continued)

Table 4-3 *(continued)*

The Element of Wood	Yes	No
Do you have problems with tendon injuries and aching?		
Do you crave sour foods?		
Are your symptoms often worse in spring?		
Are your symptoms often aggravated by wind?		
Do you often feel irritable and angry?		
Do you feel drawn to the colour green?		
Total Wood Score (this represents the health of your liver and gall bladder)		/10
The Element of Fire	**Yes**	**No**
Do you often suffer from palpitations?		
Do you often suffer from insomnia?		
Do you have any history of blood pressure or heart problems?		
Do you often have problems with your tongue, such as soreness?		
Do you have problems with your circulation?		
Do you crave burnt, smoked, or bitter foods?		
Are your symptoms often worse in summer?		
Are your symptoms often aggravated by heat?		
Do you often get overexcited or feel panicky?		
Do you feel drawn to the colour red?		
Total Fire Score (this represents the health of your heart and small intestine)		/10
The Element of Earth	**Yes**	**No**
Do you often suffer from digestive problems such as indigestion?		
Do you often have abdominal bloating?		
Do you sometimes have undigested food in your stools?		
Do you sometimes have problems with your mouth or lips?		

The Element of Earth	*Yes*	*No*
Do you have problems with aching muscles?		
Do you crave sweet foods?		
Are your symptoms often worse in late summer?		
Are your symptoms often aggravated by moist, damp conditions?		
Do you often worry?		
Do you feel drawn to the colours yellow and orange?		
Total Earth Score (this represents the health of your stomach and spleen)		**/10**
The Element of Metal	*Yes*	*No*
Do you often suffer from colds, coughs, or chest complaints?		
Do you sometimes have breathing difficulties or shortness of breath?		
Do you suffer from constipation?		
Do you have a poor sense of smell?		
Do you have problems with your skin, hair, and nails?		
Do you crave spicy, strong tasting foods?		
Are your symptoms often worse in autumn?		
Are your symptoms often aggravated by dry conditions?		
Do you often feel depressed or grieving?		
Do you feel drawn to the colour white?		
Total Metal Score (this represents the health of your lungs and large intestine)		**/10**

Helping yourself: Five Elements self-care

Count up your ticks for each section of the quiz in Table 4-2. The one with the most 'yes' ticks indicates the element where you seem to have the most imbalance and which most needs your care, attention, and support.

Here are some TCM-based self-care approaches, which can help you rebalance the five elements:

If you scored highest for the Water element, the following may help:

- ✔ Avoid cold and wet conditions.
- ✔ Keep your body warm and well wrapped, especially your feet, abdomen, and lower back.
- ✔ Avoid crop-tops (T-shirts and tops that leave the midriff and lower back exposed) and going barefoot.
- ✔ Limit salt intake.
- ✔ Drink plenty of water and eat lots of root vegetables, pulses, and warming foods.
- ✔ Wear yellow and orange.

If you scored highest for the Wood element, the following may help:

- ✔ Avoid windy conditions and draughts.
- ✔ Exercise regularly to reduce stress and irritation.
- ✔ Stay calm and practise patience.
- ✔ Limit intake of sour foods and drinks.
- ✔ Drink plenty of water and eat lots of green, leafy vegetables, salads, and raw foods.
- ✔ Wear white.

If you scored highest for the Fire element, the following may help:

- ✔ Avoid heat and stay cool.
- ✔ Wear light clothing and layers you can remove easily to adjust body temperature.
- ✔ Reduce stress and practise meditation.
- ✔ Avoid burnt or smoked foods.
- ✔ Drink plenty of water and increase intake of fresh fruit and vegetables, oily fish (up to three portions a week), and seeds and seed oils (such as flaxseed oil).
- ✔ Wear midnight blue and black.

If you scored highest for the Earth element, the following may help:

✔ Avoid damp conditions.

✔ Chew food slowly and eat in a relaxed environment without doing other things.

✔ Avoid excess worrying.

✔ Limit intake of sweet and sugary foods.

✔ Drink plenty of water and eat warming, easily digestible foods such as soups or casseroles.

✔ Wear green.

If you scored highest for the Metal element, the following may help:

✔ Avoid dry conditions.

✔ Practise breathing exercises and stretches.

✔ Think positive and seek help for your depression or grief if this is a problem.

✔ Limit intake of spicy, strong-tasting foods.

✔ Drink plenty of fluids and increase your intake of seeds (such as sunflower, sesame, or pumpkin seeds) and oily fish (up to three portions a week).

✔ Wear red.

Diagnosing in TCM

The four main types of diagnosis used by TCM practitioners are:

✔ **Observation** of tongue, face, skin, nails, and hair

✔ **Palpation** of pulse and acupoints

✔ **Listening** to sounds of the body such as the voice, a cough, and digestive gurgles

✔ **Questioning** about general health and lifestyle, your and your family's medical history, current symptoms, bowel health, and sleep habits

Taking your pulse

When training, TCM practitioners take many thousands of pulses in order to be able to feel the differences between them. Six pulses are on each wrist, with one representing each major organ and meridian. Practitioners palpate the pulses with the three middle fingers of their hand on the insides of each of the patient's wrists, just above the wrist crease. TCM practitioners use both light and firm pressure to detect surface and deeper pulses and different speeds and qualities are noted for each.

Each pulse has its own descriptive quality such as 'tight like a bow string' (a type of pulse indicating a liver problem) and my own personal favourite, 'like pearls rolling on a plate' (a type of pregnancy pulse).

TCM therapies are designed to balance *yin* and *yang* and the *five elements* and to ensure the free flow of *qi*.

You can think of the different aspects of TCM therapy as a tree with several branches, leaves and fruits:

✔ The soil in which a tree stands carries the nutrients that determine its health and growth. So in TCM the primary therapies forming the basis of health are *dietary therapy* and *lifestyle advice*. TCM recommends you eat seasonal, fresh, and lightly cooked food. Eat moderately, chew your food well, and select foods according to their *yin* and *yang* properties. Some examples of these are given in Chapter 12.

✔ The trunk of the tree represents the body and both exercise therapies and breathing. These are seen as important for maintaining vitality, memory and a good flow of *qi*. These movement and breathing therapies include tai chi and qi gong and are also mentioned in Chapters 16 and 18.

✔ The branches of the tree represent the limbs and body parts and the different therapies that can be used to correct their imbalances and stimulate healing. These include the hands-on therapies such as acupressure and tui na massage (see Chapter 17) and remedial therapies, such as acupuncture, cupping, moxibustion, and herbal medicine (see Chapters 9 and 11).

✔ The leaves and fruits of the tree represent emotional and spiritual health, and the therapies that support these such as meditation practises (also mentioned in Chapter 18).

You can consult a TCM practitioner for many different kinds of ailments but common ones are: pain relief; joint and arthritic problems; respiratory conditions such as asthma; skin problems such as eczema; headaches and migraines; PMS; and insomnia.

A lot of research has been carried out on Chinese acupuncture and Chinese herbal medicine. Much of this has been done in China and is not readily available in translation but a growing amount of this type of research is now being conducted in the West too. The positive research studies support the use of TCM as a valuable form of modern healthcare that has stood the test of time but more research is needed.

Research provides encouraging evidence for some, but not all, of the conditions listed and is summarised in Chapter 9 on acupuncture and Chapter 11 on herbs. I also give Web resources for accessing research evidence.

For details on how to find TCM practitioners of acupuncture see Chapter 9; for a Chinese herbal medicine practitioner see Chapter 11. For more on finding a massage practitioner who may practise *tui na* see Chapter 17.

Chapter 5

Revealing Ayurveda's Science of Life

A yurveda, the ancient medical tradition of India, has become increasingly popular in the West in recent years. It is regularly featured in the media and even seems to be the therapy of choice for some celebrities.

Some find Ayurveda's language a bit confusing, so in this chapter I show you how to tell your *vata* (wind) from your *kapha* (phlegm) and how to identify your predominant constitutional 'type'. This information gives you a chance to explore Ayurvedic recommendations for appropriate lifestyle and diet for each constitutional type. These recommendations are designed to balance your body and promote your health.

In this chapter, I also take you on a tour of the way in which an Ayurvedic practitioner diagnoses health problems and introduce you to the wonderful world of Ayurvedic therapy and its treatments for cleansing the body and purifying the mind.

Along the way I share with you a few stories of my experiences at Ayurvedic clinics in India illustrating how this amazing system of medicine works in practice.

A (Very) Brief History of Ayurvedic Medicine

The word 'Ayurveda' is derived from *āyus* meaning 'life' and *veda* meaning 'knowledge' and is often translated as the Science of Life. Ayurvedic medicine's roots go back thousands of years. Legend has it that this medical art and science originally came as a divine gift from the Hindu god Brahma and that its wisdom is contained in the *Vedas*, the ancient Hindu sacred texts. However, little real evidence exists for this idea as these texts actually include only a few mentions of medicine or health practices. Instead, nowadays Ayurveda is believed to have developed over time, through trial and error, absorbing information from various sources along the way.

Even so, the earliest medical texts for Ayurveda are around 2,000 years old. Two great compendiums written by the early physicians, Charaka and Sushruta, known as the *Charaka Samhita* and the *Sushruta Samhita*, and a later one by the physician Bhela, contain a vast array of information ranging from diagnosis, therapy, and surgery to health tips for daily life. These books are so detailed and useful that they're still used today in the training of Ayurvedic physicians.

The great Ayurvedic medical texts

According to legend, the king of the Hindu gods, Indra, received medical teachings direct from Lord Brahma and then passed them down to the sage Atreya, who in turn passed them on to his student, Agnivesa. Charaka, a famous physician who lived around the first or second century AD, rewrote Agnivesa's work and, over time, others also contributed to his new medical compendium, the *Charaka Samhita*.

The compendium has 120 chapters divided into eight sections: *Sutra* (pharmacology, diet, and philosophy), *Nidana* (eight main causes of disease), *Vimana* (nutrition and pathology), *Sarira* (anatomy and embryology), *Indriya* (diagnosis and prognosis), *Cikitsa* (therapy), *Kalpa* (pharmacology), and *Siddhi* (general therapy). *Charaka Samhita* also discusses the idea of rebirth.

Sushruta is said to have received the knowledge for his compendium, the *Sushruta Samhita*, direct from the god Dhanvantari, who also received them from Indra. However, historical analysis suggests that the text was in fact a compilation from various authors, including the sage, Nagarjuna. His compendium eventually had six sections: *Sutra* (the origins of medicine and medical training), *Nidana* (pathology, prognosis, and surgery), *Sarira* (embryology and anatomy), *Cikitsa* (therapy), *Kalpa* (dealing with poisons), and *Uttara* (children's diseases, eye disease, dentistry, and demonic attack!).

Two later texts, *The Heart of Medicine, or Astangahrdaya,* and the *Tome on Medicine,* or *Astangasamgraha,* probably compiled by Vagbhata around AD 600, brought all the strands together and first described Ayurveda as a complete system of medicine. These texts were translated into many languages, influencing Tibetan, Chinese, and Arabic medicine, and are still important today.

Dhanvantari, the god of Ayurveda

In Hinduism, the three gods that make up the holy trinity (*trimurti*) are known as *Brahma*, the Creator; *Vishnu*, the Preserver; and *Shiva*, the Destroyer. These gods take on different incarnations for different purposes and one of Vishnu's incarnations is said to be Dhanvantari, the god of Ayurveda. Legend has it that when the oceans of the world were being churned by the gods, he rose out of the depths carrying a vase filled with the nectar of immortality that could cure all diseases and began to teach the art and science of Ayurveda for health and healing. Statues of him can be found in many Ayurvedic hospitals and clinics and he is worshipped by Hindus for his healing powers.

Early Ayurvedic medicine concentrated on herbal remedies and dietary and lifestyle recommendations but also developed pioneering forms of surgery.

Ayurveda was not encouraged during British rule in India in the 19th century but was revived with that nation's independence movement. Nowadays it enjoys the support of the Indian government and is a dominant form of medicine in India, with Ayurvedic colleges, clinics, and pharmacies across the country. Its popularity has also spread to the West where you can find many Ayurvedic practitioners and various Ayurvedic training courses. Ayurvedic beauty and rejuvenation treatments have also become popular in beauty salons.

Deciphering Disease in Ayurvedic Medicine

In Ayurveda, the body is seen as a mini-universe where the five great elements of the cosmos – ether (*akasha*), air (*vayu*), fire (*agni*), water (*jala*), and earth (*prithvi*) – known as the *panchamahabhutas* combine to form three humours.

The humours, known as *doshas*, each have their own special qualities and manifest in the body in different ways to determine your individual constitution (*prakrti*) or type.

Your type is also affected by the strength of your 'digestive fire', known as *agni*, which is the ability of your body to digest food and absorb nutrients efficiently, and *kostha*, which is the regularity and efficiency of your bowel function and indicates how well your body can expel waste materials.

The law of karma

Hindu beliefs include the concepts of *reincarnation*, of being reborn in a new form after death, and the law of *karma*, the law of cause and effect. These beliefs have also crept into Ayurvedic medicine and so karma, resulting from inappropriate actions in a past life, is also considered as a possible cause of disease and is taken into account in therapy. When I worked in Ayurvedic clinics in India, I encountered many patients who cheerfully accepted this to be the case because they also believe that good deeds and prayers in this life can help to dissolve the karma and ease their condition.

Ayurveda also pays a lot of attention to your mental and emotional state and the strength of your spirit. Three tendencies, or *gunas*, are said to interplay to determine mental state:

- ✔ **Sattva** represents purity and balance and predominates when you feel calm and peaceful and have a clear and ordered mind.

- ✔ **Rajas** is behind activity and dynamism and triggers desires for material things or for meeting physical needs and the fear of losing them. For example, *rajas* is the force behind the mechanism of feeling hungry, thinking about food, and then obtaining it and eating it or fearing you won't have enough or someone will take it away.

- ✔ **Tamas** relates to solidity but is also associated with slowness and mental ignorance. This can relate to mental dullness or confusion, lethargy, or self-destructive tendencies such as depression.

Imbalances in the humours and the *gunas* caused by faulty lifestyle, poor dietary habits, lack of exercise, and negative thoughts are believed to be the root cause of disease.

The three *gunas* can also be applied to foods and their effects on the mind and body. For example, *sattvic* foods such as fresh, organic fruit and vegetables are light and easily digestible and said to have a calming effect on the mind; *rajasic* foods are spicy and hot and heat the body and can disturb the mind, triggering anger and irritation; and *tamasic* foods are cold and heavy (such as ice cream) and can slow the mind and trigger lethargy and dullness.

Understanding Your Health the Ayurvedic Way

In Ayurveda establishing whether your basic type is *vata* (wind), *pitta* (choler or bile), or *kapha* (phlegm) is important. You can then make simple changes to your diet, lifestyle, and daily habits to help restore balance in your body and improve your health. This section describes how to figure out your personal type.

Go through the checklists in Table 5-1, answering the questions. Then tally your totals for each checklist. The one that has the most 'yes' answers is your current type according to Ayurvedic medicine.

Table 5-1	Figuring Out Your Type		
CHECKLIST A		*Yes*	*No*
Are you slim and do you find it hard to gain weight?			
Does your skin tend to be dry and rough?			
Are your nails dry, brittle, and easily breakable?			
Is your hair dry, thin, and brittle?			
Are your eyes small and deep-set?			
Is your appetite irregular and do you suffer from digestive problems?			
Are you talkative, active, prone to anxiety, imaginative, and creative?			
Are you often forgetful?			
Do you often feel tired when you wake up?			
Do you lack regular routines and often feel stressed?			
TOTAL 'YES'		___/10	

(continued)

Table 5-1 *(continued)*

CHECKLIST B	Yes	No
Are you of medium build and height and quite muscular?		
Is your skin oily, smooth, and warm?		
Are your nails lustrous, strong, and flexible?		
Is your hair straight, fine, and neither dry nor greasy?		
Are your eyes medium-size and bright?		
Do you have a good appetite, often feel hungry, and have a fast metabolism with some loose stools?		
Are you quick-tempered and impatient, but also determined and industrious?		
Do you often feel hot, flushed, or red-faced?		
Are you always on the go and do you often feel 'hyped up'?		
Do you find it hard to get to sleep and sometimes wake during the night?		
TOTAL 'YES'	___/10	

CHECKLIST C	Yes	No
Are you of large build, with a tendency to put on weight, and not very tall?		
Is your skin pale, moist, and generally cool?		
Are your nails smooth, wide, thick, and shiny?		
Is your hair curly, thick, and easily greasy?		
Are your eyes quite large and long-lashed?		
Are you a slow eater with a steady appetite and slow digestion?		
Are you generally quiet, thoughtful, and slow to react?		
Do you find it easy to sleep and lie-in or take naps?		
Are you generally laid-back and unstressed?		
Do you often feel lethargic and dislike exercise?		
TOTAL 'YES'	___/10	

Here's a guide to your Ayurvedic type:

✔ Most ticks for Checklist A in Table 5-1 means that you're predominantly a *vata* type. This means that you are always doing something and tend to suffer from stress, anxiety, and digestive problems like IBS (irritable bowel syndrome).

✔ Most ticks for Checklist B means that you're predominantly a *pitta* type. This means you're quite a dynamic and fiery person with a quick intelligence but you don't suffer fools gladly and may be domineering. You may suffer from digestive problems and headaches.

✔ If you have most ticks for Checklist C, then you're predominantly a *kapha* type. This means that you're practical, down-to-earth, and resilient but also tend to be a bit lethargic and may suffer from fatigue, bloating, sugar-cravings, and water retention.

For details on how to balance your type, look for the tips in the later section 'Restoring Balance with Ayurvedic Therapies'.

Making Diagnoses in Ayurvedic Medicine

Ayurvedic practitioners use an eight-fold examination (*astavidha pariksha*) to investigate your health:

✔ **The pulse (*nadi*):** Your wrist pulse is used to determine pulse qualities. A *vata* pulse is fast and slippery, a *pitta* pulse is jumpy and irregular, and a *kapha* pulse is slow and steady.

✔ **The tongue (*jihva*):** This looks at the colour and coating of your tongue. A *vata* tongue is dry, rough, and cracked with no coating; a *pitta* tongue is red with an oily, yellow coating; and a *kapha* tongue is swollen and moist with a greasy, white coating.

✔ **The voice (*sabda*):** *Vata* types have rough, throaty voices; *pitta* voices are erratic and may break during speech; and *kapha* types have deep voices and often have to clear their throat when speaking.

✔ **The skin (*sparsa*):** The physician looks at the colour and texture of your skin and may palpate certain points to check for tenderness or redness. *Vata* types have dry, rough, sensitive skin that is cool to touch; *pitta* types have reddened areas of skin that feel hot to the touch; and *kapha* types have clammy, moist, cold skin.

✔ **Vision (*drka*):** The Ayurvedic practitioner checks the whites of your eyes and registers any other visual abnormalities. *Vata* types have dry, sensitive eyes with dull eye whites; *pitta* types have a burning sensation in their eyes and yellowed eye whites; and *kapha* types have heavy, drooping eyelids and frequent watery eyes.

- **General appearance (*akrti*):** This covers your posture and gait. *Vata* types are often thin and wiry and move rapidly; *pitta* types are often strongly built and restless; and *kapha* types are often heavily built and rather slow moving.

- **Urine (*mutra*):** The Ayurvedic practitioner examines the colour and odour of your urine and you're asked how frequently you urinate. *Vata* types have frequent, clear, odourless urine; *pitta* types have small amounts of brown or deep yellow urine with a burnt odour; and *kapha* types have copious turbid, whitish urine with a stale smell.

- **Stools (*mala*):** The colour, consistency, and odour of your stool is considered. A normal healthy stool is firm and light brown in colour. *Vata* types have hard, dry stools that are grey in colour; *pitta* types have loose stools that are yellow, dark brown, or green in colour; and *kapha* types have slimy, pale stools containing mucus and bits of undigested food.

These eight examinations are combined with questions to enable the Ayurvedic practitioner to decide on the relative balance of the *doshas* for the person who may not be just one type but has more than one fighting for predominance.

The practitioner also takes into account other factors such as your age, vigour, mental state, and physical condition, as well as possible genetic and environmental factors, diet, and lifestyle. Analysis of dreams and astrological birth charts are also sometimes used to determine possible spirit, or karmic, influences.

After the Ayurvedic practitioner has determined the cause and stage of the disease and the nature of imbalance of the *doshas*, then an appropriate therapy can be selected.

Restoring Balance with Ayurvedic Therapies

Ayurveda aims to treat the whole person, not just the symptoms or disease. The key aim is to re-balance the *doshas* in the body, but secondary aims are to improve general health and vitality, strengthen digestive fire (*agni*), and promote longevity. The ultimate aim is to assist the person in following the three goals of life outlined in the *Vedas*: *dharma* (virtuous living), *artha* (prosperity), and *kama* (pleasure), which together may lead to the ultimate goal of *moksha* (spiritual liberation).

Ayurvedic healing includes the following:

- ✔ Medicinal treatment, or *ausadha* (using herbs and such)
- ✔ Cleansing and purifying techniques, or *panchakarma*
- ✔ Dietary therapy
- ✔ Lifestyle modification, or *pathya*
- ✔ Exercise (yoga) and massage therapy
- ✔ Meditation and other spiritual remedies

You might also use self-help techniques, such as personal hygiene, methods for enhancing fertility and virility, and rejuvenation techniques.

The physician, medical assistants, patients, and even the remedies themselves must all combine together effectively to obtain a cure.

These treatments are divided into three main types according to whether they're based on reasoning, the sacred, or character. Those based on reasoning are the medicinal treatments, the *panchakarma* cleansing and purification techniques, and the dietary and lifestyle advice. Those based on the sacred are the spiritual remedies such as reciting *mantras* (repeated words or phrases) or prayers, carrying out fasts, going on pilgrimages, or wearing sacred gemstones. Those based on character involve cultivating moral qualities and integrity and avoiding harmful influences such as alcohol, gambling, lying, cheating, and, in modern-day speak, 'sex, drugs, and rock and roll'!

The rest of this section describes these Ayurvedic therapies in more detail.

The four pillars

The ancient Ayurvedic physician Charaka wrote that four pillars determine successful therapy. The first is the physician, who must be knowledgeable and experienced and should also demonstrate physical cleanliness and purity of mind.

The second is the medicine, which should be grown, harvested, and prepared correctly to be effective – and, of course, prescribed correctly too.

The third is the medical attendant, who assists the physician in carrying out the therapies. They too should be knowledgeable, experienced, clean, and pure of mind, as well as compassionate and empathic with patients.

The fourth and final pillar is the patient, who has a duty to describe symptoms accurately, to follow the physician's instructions, and to be strongly motivated towards healing.

Ayurvedic medicines

Ayurvedic medicines are mainly made from plant material such as leaves, flowers, fruits, and spices but can also contain ground minerals and gemstones and animal products such as ghee (clarified butter), animal fats, beeswax, or honey.

The different plants and medicinal materials are classified according to their tastes, potencies, and 'ripening' effects (*vipaka*):

- ✔ Sweet, sour, salt, bitter, pungent, or astringent qualities
- ✔ Warming or cooling properties
- ✔ Post-digestive effects (the physical effects of their components after they've been digested in the body)
- ✔ Specific healing effects on the body (*prabhava*)

Herbs are cultivated and harvested carefully and then prescribed singly or combined together according to both ancient and modern formulae for maximum efficiency. They may be used dried or fresh and go through various processes, such as being ground, boiled, soaked, juiced, heated, and so on, to be made into medicines.

A cautionary tale

When I'm in India, I often visit the Ayurvedic pharmacies and am amazed at the range of products on offer. Few are in their raw state, as in the old-style traditional Chinese medicine pharmacies; most are carefully packaged, with extensive medical claims. Some aren't labelled in English and great care is needed here. Not all have gone through rigorous quality control and some contain contaminants and heavy metals such as lead, mercury, or arsenic.

A recent tragic case involved an Anglo-Indian woman who bought Ayurvedic remedies for weight loss while in India and took them extensively on returning to Britain. These medicines contained contaminants and she unfortunately died of liver failure before it was realised that it was these remedies that were making her ill.

Ayurvedic remedies sold in this country by responsible companies are carefully batch tested for correct ingredients and purity so that they're safe to take. However, not all distributors act this responsibly. Therefore, only take remedies from a reputable practitioner and supplier that specifies that they implement these checks and only take products clearly labelled in English showing that they've been batch tested.

The medicines may then be taken as pills (*vati*), powders (*churna*), pastes (*kalka*), juices (*svarasa*), decoctions (*kvatha*), or medicated oils (*tailas*). Herbal teas and rejuvenation elixirs are also popular over-the-counter remedies.

In general *pitta* remedies are cooling, *kapha* remedies are warming and help clear phlegm, and *vatta* remedies are calming. However, different combinations of tastes and properties are used according to individual balance.

The Panchakarma purification techniques

The *panchakarma* are five Ayurvedic techniques for cleansing and purifying the body and rebalancing the *doshas* that are used in both treatment and prevention of disease.

The body must be carefully prepared for these techniques. First, oil therapy (*snehana*) is used, whereby vegetable oils are taken orally, given as enemas, and/or massaged into the skin. This therapy helps to soften the skin and get rid of old waste matter that may have accumulated in your intestines. Second is sweating therapy (*svedana*) whereby the body is exposed to external heat from sweat baths or hot packs, or made to generate heat internally by means of exercises or swaddling in blankets. This sweating also helps to remove impurities from the body.

After the preparations are complete, the appropriate *panchakarma* can be selected:

- ✔ **Vamana:** The use of herbs, rock salt, and honey to induce vomiting in order to clear the digestive system and relieve mucus. It is often used for *kapha* conditions such as chest and nasal congestion as in bronchitis and rhinitis.

- ✔ **Virechana:** Involves drinking laxative and purgative herbs to cleanse the body. It is often used for *pitta* conditions such as fevers, intestinal worms, and skin diseases.

    Virechana is quite a rigorous therapy and isn't suitable for young children, the frail, or the elderly.

- ✔ **Vasti:** The use of enemas to cleanse the bowels. These are often used for *vata* conditions such as dry skin, irritable bowel, nervousness, and fatigue.

- ✔ **Nasya:** Nostril cleansing that involves inhaling medicinal oils, powders, or steam in order to relieve blocked noses, sinusitis, headaches, and nasal congestion, often signs of *kapha* imbalance.

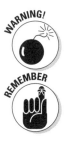

✔ **Raktamoskshana**: Blood-letting that uses leeches or surgical instruments to extract small amounts of blood, generate new blood cell production, and increase circulation. It is used for *rakta* (blood) disorders and *pitta* conditions such as boils, abscesses, and skin diseases.

Don't partake in the *raktamoskshana* therapy during pregnancy or if you suffer from anaemia.

Always follow *panchakarma* treatment with rest, appropriate dietary therapy, and any other relevant therapies. Such treatments must be done carefully and correctly by qualified practitioners; in India, they're usually only carried out in hospitals or clinical settings.

Ayurvedic dietary therapy

In Ayurveda, foods are classified in the same way as herbs, that is, according to their six *savours* or tastes, their energetic potencies of warming or cooling, and their post-digestive effects. Table 5-2 shows recommended foods and cooking methods for the three different *dosha* types.

Table 5-2	Dietary Therapy by Type	
Humour/Type	*Avoid*	*Okay to Eat/Drink*
Vata	Cold, raw, frozen and oily, fried foods as well as pungent, bitter, and astringent foods and drinks such as coffee.	Warm, cooked foods, especially steamed or grilled; sweet, sour, and salty foods such as sweet and dried fruits, onion (cooked), asparagus, carrots and other root vegetables, radishes (cooked), garlic, and dairy produce (in moderation).
Pitta	Hot, spicy, fried, pungent, sour, and salty foods, such as curried foods, pickles, and salted nuts.	Cool and raw or lightly steamed foods; sweet, bitter, and astringent foods; sweet and bitter vegetables; and items such as mint tea, salads, cucumber, oats, figs, rice, tofu, mushrooms, lentils, and ghee (clarified butter).
Kapha	Sweet, sour, phlegm-producing and salty foods including sugar and confectionary, dairy produce, and salt and salted foods such as crisps.	Light, dry, spicy, warm, and easily digestible foods with pungent, bitter, and astringent taste such as cranberries, fennel, aubergine, apples, lentils, chickpeas and other pulses, millet, couscous, and natural diuretics such as watermelon.

Ayurveda also advises that you eat food in moderation, chew slowly, and eat in a calm setting. This is especially important for *vatta* and *pitta* types. *Kapha* types need to eat little and often.

Lifestyle modification (pathya)

Ayurvedic practitioners recommend living according to the seasons (*rit-ucharya*). Doing so means wearing warm clothes and eating warm foods in cool or cold seasons, wearing cool clothes and eating cooling foods in warm or hot seasons, and drinking plenty of fluids in dry seasons. Cleanliness, regular habits, and sleep are regarded as important, and daily exercise, meditation, and offerings to Hindu gods are all encouraged.

Also recommended is that natural urges such as hunger, thirst, sneezing, yawning, and urination shouldn't be unnaturally suppressed and that good habits and virtues is cultivated. These good behaviours include telling the truth, being kind and generous, respecting your parents and teachers, and keeping good company. Harmful behaviours such as lying, cheating, envying, anger, and greed need to be overcome.

Vatta types need to try to slow down and keep to regular routines; *pitta* types need to try to keep cool, avoid stuffy environments, and wear natural fibres; and *kapha* types should vary their routine and incorporate new forms of stimulation and mental challenge into their lives.

Exercise and massage therapy

Ayurvedic medicine advises yoga exercises for keeping the body supple, the muscles toned, and for promoting mental concentration and calm. *Vata* types need to concentrate on gentle exercise and stationary yoga poses. *Pitta* types can take moderate exercise combining yoga poses with breathing exercises. *Kapha* types should take vigorous exercise combining aerobic exercise with yoga or doing energetic forms such as Ashtanga yoga.

Massage is done with the hands or feet or using heated linen pads. Different oils may be used to warm or cool the body according to *dosha* type. In *Marma* therapy, different points on the body, rather like the acupoints of acupuncture, are stimulated.

Meditation and other spiritual remedies

Yoga breathing exercises (*pranayama*), recitation of mantras, meditation and prayer are all encouraged to calm the mind, purify karma, and connect with the divine. *Vatta* types find sitting still hard, so can try walking meditation; *pitta* types can benefit from developing a regular seated meditation practice incorporating breathing techniques to calm the senses; and *kapha* types can benefit from active mantra chanting.

Deciding when to use Ayurvedic therapies

In India and Sri Lanka, Ayurvedic treatment is widely used for chronic conditions such as arthritis, joint pain, digestive problems, skin problems, and respiratory problems as well as for post-operative recovery, such as in the case of cardiac surgery and in the treatment of cancer.

If you're taking any form of Ayurvedic medicine and also Western medicine, always ensure that you advise both your Ayurvedic and orthodox medical practitioner in case of any potential interaction between the medicines.

Finding Out Whether Ayurvedic Medicine Works

A growing database of research into the therapeutic effect of Ayurvedic herbs and herbal formulae now exists, as well as some research on the therapeutic effects of yoga exercise. Unfortunately, however, even in India, only very limited good quality research has been carried out on Ayurvedic therapies in general. Therefore, its efficacy in treating various diseases remains largely clinically unproven, although of course it has been extensively tried and tested throughout centuries of use.

Some work on the effect of individual herbal remedies has been encouraging, such as the use of neem leaves to suppress head lice and other infections, Shatavari root to treat menopausal symptoms, Triphala (a mixture of three fruits) to treat constipation, Guggul for reducing cholesterol, Ashwagandha for treating stress and fatigue, and so on, but much of the evidence is anecdotal and more well-designed clinical trials are needed.

Finding a Practitioner of Ayurvedic Medicine

The practice of Ayurveda is not yet regulated in the UK, so currently anyone can call themselves an Ayurvedic practitioner. The regulation process is now beginning and university accredited training courses for practitioners have already been established. However, until proper regulation is in place, and given that some of the remedies used may potentially be toxic, take great care to check that your practitioner is well-trained and experienced and able to practice safely.

You can find practitioners in the UK via:

- **The Ayurvedic Practitioners Association** (www.apa.uk.com or phone 07983-124950). This association has established a new three-year full-time BSc course in Ayurveda (BSc Honours Complementary Health Sciences (Ayurveda)) with the University of Middlesex, plus a year of post-graduate clinical training and an optional MSc training.

- **The Ayurvedic Medical Association** (AMA UK). For details ring 0208-6576147 or 0208-6823876. Some of their members are Ayurvedic physicians who have completed a five-year course in India or Sri Lanka and have the initials BAMS: Bachelor of Ayurvedic Medicine and Surgery (India); or DAMS: Doctor of Ayurvedic Medicine and Surgery (Sri Lanka) after their names.

- **The Ayurvedic Company of Great Britain** (www.ayurvedagb.com or 0207-2246070). Their members may hold a Diploma in Ayurveda (Dipl. Ayu.) or a BA Hons Ayu from the Manipal Ayurvedic University of Europe (a joint venture between the Ayurvedic Company of Great Britain and Manipal University, India and formerly with Thames Valley University). This company has also established a British Ayurvedic Medical Council (BAMC) and a British Association of Accredited Ayurvedic Practitioners (BAAAP).

- **Maharishi Ayurveda** (www.maharishiayurveda.co.uk/practitioners.htm or via the Maharishi Ayurveda health centre on 01695-51008). Members are medical doctors who have also trained in the Maharishi Mahesh Yogi's Vedic Approach to Health.

In the US, practitioner details can be obtained from the National Ayurvedic Medical Association on www.ayurveda-nama.org

Chapter 6

Balancing Health with Tibetan Medicine

*I*n this chapter I introduce you to Tibetan medicine, which has been practised for more than 2,000 years. Its aim is to treat body, mind, and spirit in
order to bring about balance. Since the occupation of Tibet by China in 1959,
many exiled Tibetan physicians have settled in India and in the West, establishing Tibetan medical training and offering consultations.

I tell you about the Tibetan medical ideas about health and disease – and how
all diseases are thought to stem from one key source – and show you how
you can identify your 'type' according to the Tibetan system of 'humours',
which are thought to determine your physical, mental, and emotional health.

You'll find out about Tibetan medical therapies and also discover some
Tibetan medical healthcare tips that you may like to try out for yourself.

A (Very) Brief History of Tibetan Medicine

The origins of Tibetan medicine go back to native *Bon practitioners* in Tibet; shamans who used herbs and rituals to help heal people. Later, healing practices were more formalised, incorporating medical teachings from the Buddha from around 500 BC.

In the beginning all medical knowledge was passed on by word of mouth and along the way medical ideas from India, Persia, and China were added in. In the 18th century the Buddha's instructions were compiled into four great medical texts called the *rGyud bzhi* (pronounced 'gyu-zhee'), otherwise known as the Four Tantras. These texts are still used to teach Tibetan medicine and Tibetan physicians are able to quote long passages from it by heart.

In modern times public interest in Tibetan medicine has grown due to media attention for His Holiness the Dalai Lama, the leader of the Tibetan people and a Nobel Peace Prize Laureate, who is a great supporter of this system of medicine and also the attention attracted by celebrity Tibetan Buddhists such as Hollywood actors Richard Gere and Steven Seagal, which has led to increased media coverage for all things Tibetan.

The Medicine Buddha

Tibetan Medicine is integrally connected with the life philosophy and religion of Tibetan Buddhism. The origins of Buddhism date back to around the fifth century BC when the royal Prince Siddhartha from Lumbini, India, left his palace and family to seek spiritual enlightenment. He endured all kinds of extreme ascetic practices, such as lengthy fasting, but finally discovered a middle path of calm reflection and balance that led him to attain enlightenment under a Bodhi tree at the age of 35. From then on he was known as the Shakyamuni or Gautama Buddha and spent the next 45 years of his life teaching his philosophy of compassion, insight, and awareness, which are the foundations of Buddhism.

According to Buddhism anyone can become enlightened and so it is said that there were many Buddhas before the Guatama Buddha and there are also more to come.

Buddhism spread from India to other Asian countries and became the national religion in Tibet. According to legend, the Buddha also gave medical teachings and to do so he is said to have taken on the form of another Buddha, the Medicine Buddha known as Sangye Menchela. This Buddha is always coloured blue depicted holding a bowl of life-giving nectar in his hands and a myrobalam fruit symbolic of his ability to heal. The myrobalam tree grows in India and Tibet and its fruit is used in many Tibetan medicines even today. Traditionally this fruit is said to be able to cure all diseases and it is now known to be rich in certain valuable *antioxidants* (plant compounds that help to fight and prevent disease).

Tibetan physicians now practise in many major European cities and else-where around the world, including the US, Canada, Japan, Russia, and Australia. Many Tibetan physicians are also monks, and their colourful maroon-and-gold robes and cheerful, smiling faces are always eye-catching and memorable.

Modern pharmacological research, which has also looked at Tibetan herbs, has lent credence to this system of medicine, which is now increasingly popular in the West.

Grasping the idea behind Tibetan medicine

'Health through balance' is the central theme in Tibetan medicine. To be healthy, you need a balanced lifestyle, moderate behaviour, good diet, calm emotions, and spiritual health. An imbalance in any of these areas, such as constantly staying up late, eating badly or regularly getting angry, is thought to lead to disease. So the aim of diagnosis and treatment is to examine each of these areas, identify key imbalances, and then use remedies to restore balance and alleviate symptoms.

In this system all diseases are believed to have just one root cause – human ignorance. This concept comes from Tibetan Buddhism and it doesn't mean stupidity! Rather this concept means if we aren't enlightened we remain ignorant about the true nature of reality and are instead blinded by the illusions of the material world. This ignorance causes mental suffering and discontent, which in turn leads to physical imbalance and eventually, disease.

Understanding Tibetan medical concepts of health and disease

In Tibetan medical theory our human ignorance means that we suffer from three *poisons*; three types of negative thoughts that disturb our peace of mind. The three poisons are:

- ✔ **Attachment (or desire):** That is, strong desires for certain possessions, people, or states of being; for example, we long for a new house or car, we fall in love and become really attached to a person, or we constantly desire happiness.

- ✔ **Aversion (or hatred):** A dislike for certain things, individuals, or states of mind and a desire to avoid them; for example, we may dislike rain and grumble when the weather is bad, or we may dislike a particular person and seek to avoid them, or we may try to shy away from pain and unhappiness.

✔ **Confusion (or ignorance):** That is, indecision, mental lethargy, and listlessness; we are mentally confused, can't make up our minds about things and don't want to make the effort to wake up out of our ignorant state to enter an enlightened one.

According to Tibetan medicine these mental poisons also affect three humours that play a role in the physical body.

The three *humours* are seen as three types of energy that determine the function and make up of the body's organs and tissues. They are:

✔ *Loong* (pronounced *lu-ng*) – vital energy or 'wind'

✔ *Tripa* (pronounced *tree-pas*) – body heat or 'bile'

✔ *Peken* (pronounced *beh-gen*) – moisture and fluids or 'phlegm'

The three poisons and humours are closely connected. The poison of attachment or desire stirs up the wind humour; the poison of aversion or hatred gives rise to the bile humour; and the poison of confusion or ignorance aggravates the phlegm humour.

The humours are believed to circulate through the body via a network of subtle channels (similar to the *nadi* of Indian yoga or the meridians in traditional Chinese medicine). They're similar to the three *doshas* in Ayurveda (these are described in Chapter 5) and each has certain qualities and functions.

The wind humour

The wind humour is based in the abdomen and lower body and has the following qualities and functions in the body:

✔ The qualities of movement, lightness, and dryness

✔ Influences physical movement, respiration, thinking, digestion, and reproduction

✔ Helps regulate vitality, breathing, and mental clarity

The bile humour

The bile humour isn't the same as the Western idea of bile from the gall bladder. The 'bile' predominates in the centre of the body and its range of qualities and functions in the body include the following:

✔ The qualities of heat, lubrication, oiliness, and odour

✔ Controls hunger, thirst, complexion, and skin

✔ Affects digestion, vision, and temperament

The phlegm humour

The phlegm humour doesn't just refer to the gooey white stuff you sometimes find in your throat. This humour resides mainly in the upper body and its range of qualities and functions include the following:

✔ The qualities of coldness, heaviness, and stickiness

✔ Influences sleep, joint mobility, and mental awareness

✔ Affects digestion and excretion

According to Tibetan medical theory, when all three humours are balanced, good health results, but when any one humour predominates, disease occurs. Here are some examples of the kind of diseases linked to each humour:

✔ Typical wind diseases are joint pain and mental agitation.

✔ Typical bile diseases are digestive disorders, such as indigestion and gallstones.

✔ Typical phlegm diseases are joint stiffness and pain such as arthritis, chronic bloating, and diarrhoea.

The balance of the humours is said to determine your personal physical, mental, and emotional make-up as well as your predisposition to certain diseases. Your constitutional type is therefore described according to whichever humour or humours predominate in your body.

Determining Your Body Type According to Tibetan Medicine

You can determine your body type by completing the quiz below and after you know your type you can adjust your diet, lifestyle, and daily habits to help balance the humours and improve your health.

Taking the Tibetan medical humour quiz

To identify your body type according to Tibetan medicine, answer A, B, or C to each of the following questions:

1. What is your build?

    A. Slim, lean, hard to gain weight; very tall or short

    B. Medium build and height; may be quite muscular

    C. Heavy build, tendency to put on weight, may be short

2. What type of skin do you have?

    A. Dry, rough, and cool to touch

    B. Oily, smooth, and warm

    C. Pale, moist, or oily and cool

3. What are your nails like?

    A. Dry, brittle, and rough

    B. Strong, oily, and flexible

    C. Smooth, thick, and wide

4. What type of hair do you have?

    A. Fine, thin, flyaway, brittle

    B. Dry at the ends but greasy at the roots, or coloured, processed, or frizzy

    C. Normal to oily; sometimes lifeless and greasy

5. What does your tongue look like?

    A. Long and thin; pale with a clear coating

    B. Red-tipped with a greasy, yellow coating

    C. Full bodied with teeth marks and a thick, white coating

6. What type of appetite and digestion do you have?

    A. Irregular appetite and occasional digestive problems

    B. Good appetite, often hungry, regular digestion

    C. Steady appetite, slow eater, slow digestion

7. What is your temperament?

    A. Talkative, active, creative, imaginative, prone to anxiety

    B. Organised, industrious, impatient, irritable, determined

    C. Stable, calm, slow, thoughtful, possessive

8. What is your sleep like?

    A. Insomniac and wake often; little sleep needed and an early riser

    B. Hard to get to sleep and lots of dreams but wake energetic

    C. Deep and heavy; hard to wake up and still feel tired

9. Which do you dislike most?

    A. Draughts or hot and cold temperature fluctuations

    B. Hot conditions

    C. Cold and damp conditions

10. How do you feel when you have to make an important decision?

    A. Nervous but excited

    B. Decisive and confident

    C. Confused and undecided

Determining your type

To determine your personal humour make-up, add up the numbers of A, B, and C responses that you made for each of the quiz questions and see which you have the most of:

- **Mostly A responses:** *Loong*/**Wind type:** You're very active and able but tend to take on too much and are always in a rush. You may also suffer from headaches, joint aches and pains, and anxiety. You need to relax more and slow down the pace of your daily life.

- **Mostly B responses:** *Tripa*/**Bile type:** You're quick and intelligent but can also be impatient and irritable. You're dynamic and can make things happen but you don't suffer fools gladly. You may suffer from digestive problems and food-related headaches. You need to calm down and to strengthen your digestion.

- **Mostly C responses:** *Peken*/**Phlegm type:** You're stable and dependable and people love to confide in you! Your body is quite strong but you often feel tired and can be lethargic. Your digestion is slow and you have a tendency towards sugar cravings, bloating, weight gain, and water retention. You need to get things moving in your body, increase your vitality, and speed up your digestion.

Some people fall very clearly into one of the categories above. For others more than one type may play a role in your health. These are known as *combination types*. In the following section, I tell you some of Tibetan medicine's self-care recommendations for each type.

Helping Yourself with Tibetan Medicine Self-Care Approaches

After you've identified your Tibetan medicine body type according to the quiz, try following the Tibetan medicine self-care tips outlined below, designed to help rebalance the humours, and see how they make you feel.

✔ If you're predominantly a *Loong*/Wind type, try the following:

- Stop exhausting yourself. Learn to say 'No' and delegate more. Take steps to reduce stress and any sources of conflict in your life.

- Build some quiet times into your schedule when you can avoid noise and crowds. Talk less and make regular time just for you, to relax and indulge yourself.

- Cut down on stimulants like coffee, tea, colas, and sugar because these wind you up too much.

- Eat slowly and chew your food well and don't do anything else while eating.

- Limit your intake of cold or raw foods and increase your intake of warming foods such as soups, casseroles, and steamed vegetables. Root vegetables are particularly good for you because they help to nourish and ground you.

- Calm your mind and body with yoga, meditation, and deep breathing. Consider taking up an artistic hobby such as painting as an outlet for your creativity and imagination.

- Spend time in the loving company of close friends that nurture and support you.

✔ If you're predominantly a *Tripa*/Bile type, try the following:

- To improve your digestion, avoid saturated fats, rich foods, hot peppers, and spices.

- Cool yourself by eating lots of salad and raw or lightly steamed vegetables.

- Drink lots of good quality water (filtered if possible) every day.

- Avoid hot, stuffy environments and direct heat and keep out of the sun.

- Layer clothing so that you can keep cool and regulate body temperature.

- Take regular exercise, especially at the end of the day to release stress and tension and pave the way for a relaxed night's sleep.

- Practise patience and find how to overcome feelings of irritability or anger. Breathing exercises, relaxation training, and yoga can all help with this.

✔ If you're predominantly a *Peken*/Phlegm type, try the following:

- Eat little and often. Avoid dairy produce, refrigerated foods, oily foods, and saturated fats, which will slow you down further and make you feel heavy.

- Stabilise your blood sugar levels and reduce cravings by incorporating sunflower and pumpkin seeds in your diet and eating porridge for breakfast.

- Drink boiled water sprinkled with finely chopped fresh parsley to reduce water retention.

- Don't let yourself get stuck in a rut. Change your routine regularly, for example take a different route to work or do daily activities in a different order to stimulate your senses and overcome lethargy.

- Take regular, brisk exercise to increase vitality, speed up your metabolism, and improve digestion. Daily speed-walking is particularly good for you.

- Exercise your mind with mental challenges such as crosswords or mathematical puzzles.

- Sing your heart out, to the radio or in a choir, to energise your body.

Exploring Disease Types in Tibetan Medicine

In Tibetan medicine imbalances of the three *poisons* and the three *humours* are believed to lead to 84,000 different types of disease! To make these more manageable they have been classified into four categories:

- **Diseases due to early life:** These diseases start in infancy or childhood and are due to factors during conception, pregnancy, early feeding, and so on.

- **Diseases due to present lifestyle:** These diseases owe much to your bad habits such as late nights, drinking, smoking, junk food, sedentary lifestyle, stress, and so on.

- **Diseases due to past life:** These are diseases relating to the Buddhist idea of *karma*, the law of cause and effect and the belief in the concept of rebirth. According to this law it is said that actions in one life may produce a result in a subsequent life. Therefore, a disease in this life may be related to an action or experience in a past life.

- **Diseases due to spirit influence:** These diseases are thought to be due to the influence of some elemental forces or restless spirits ('ghosts' in the West).

Tibetan medicine believes four conditions influence disease. These are:

- **Diet:** You can't get away with eating loads of junk food forever without it starting to affect your body. Different types of foods are believed to have a direct effect on the balance of the different *humours*.

- **Behaviour:** Different lifestyle behaviours are also believed to influence the *humours* as mentioned earlier in this chapter. For example insufficient sleep is believed to aggravate the wind humour, too much sun exposure may aggravate bile, and too much lying around and doing nothing will make a phlegm condition worse.

- **Weather/season:** Climates and weather conditions affect the balance of the humours. For example, wind can stir up the wind humour, heat stirs up bile, and cold and damp aggravate phlegm.

- **Spirit:** This refers to your mental state. For example, agitation and worry are believed to aggravate the wind humour, irritation and frustration to disturb bile and indecision and confusion to contribute to a predominance of phlegm. The Tibetans are great believers in positive thinking and in dispelling negative thoughts, which may be why they're generally such smiley and happy people!

If these categories and conditions all sound too complicated to you, then you may like the way Tibetan medicine always boils things down to simple principles. This system of medicine also has two basic categories into which all diseases can be divided. They are:

- **Hot diseases:** Typified by redness, swelling, hot extremities, and acute pain.

- **Cold diseases:** Typified by coldness, stiffness, pallor, cold extremities, and chronic pain.

Restoring Balance with Tibetan Medicine Therapies

Tibetan medicine is currently used to treat a wide range of diseases including digestive problems, arthritis, late onset diabetes, headaches, fatigue, skin disorders, and respiratory problems. Tibetan physicians treat many thousands of patients with these health problems each year and there are large numbers of anecdotal reports of improvements but as yet little research evidence to prove effectiveness.

In order to restore the balance of the humours, Tibetan medicine uses five main types of therapy:

- **Dietary adjustment:** Dietary changes are fundamental to Tibetan medicine and are the first line of therapy. Eating correct amounts of food (not too much or too little) and adjusting the type of food you eat according to your constitutional type is essential. (Refer to the earlier section 'Helping Yourself with Tibetan Medicine Self-Care Approaches'.)

- **Behavioural change:** Making changes to your daily lifestyle and habits are the second line of treatment. Tibetan physicians advise regulating behaviour according to the humours so, for example, talkative wind types are advised to spend time quietly alone resting, while lethargic phlegm types are encouraged to get out of bed early and to get moving.

- **Medicines:** The main medicinal approach in Tibetan medicine is the use of herbal remedies. Plant roots, leaves, flowers, bark, fruits, minerals, and occasionally animal ingredients are all used and the formulae usually contain multiple ingredients. The remedies may be given in the form of pills, powders, decoctions or ointments.

- **Other therapies:** Tibetan physicians also use massage, bone-setting, and some acupuncture and moxibustion. The acupuncture and moxibustion techniques have mostly been adopted from Traditional Chinese Medicine (TCM) and quite recently incorporated into Tibetan medical practice (for more on TCM, see Chapter 4). However one technique unique to Tibetan medicine is Golden Needle therapy, which I describe in Chapter 9.

- **Religious rituals, prayers, dream analysis, and astrology:** Spiritual healing in Tibetan medicine is based on Tibetan Buddhist and Bon practices and can involve prayers and rituals by the physician and/or the patient. The Medicine Buddha also plays a role and his picture and mantra (a prayer saying his name) are often used to invoke healing. Sometimes dreams are investigated for healing signs and many doctors also study Tibetan medical astrology in order to be able to interpret disease and recommend appropriate cures. Many Tibetans also wear precious gems or talismans believed to help protect against disease.

Examining the Evidence for Tibetan Medicine

Research evidence for Tibetan medicine has concentrated mainly on specific herbal formulae. One of the most well-researched is the formula known as Padma 28 which has been trialled in Switzerland, Israel, and Denmark and been found to be effective for treating intermittent claudication (restricted circulation in the legs making walking painful and difficult), cardiac problems, and inflammation. (See www.swiss-inter.com/padma28e.htm for more information.)

A Californian study on Tibetan herbal medicine for breast cancer produced mixed results but had design flaws. Other studies have looked at Tibetan herbal medicine for various ailments, including diabetes, depression, and AIDS, and have yielded some promising results but more research is needed.

Research is currently being carried out at the Tibetan Medical and Astrological Institute (TMAI) in northern India (see www.men-tsee-khang.org for more information). It has also been stimulated in other countries following recent International congresses on Tibetan Medicine held in the US, Tibet, and Taiwan, and as a result more research studies are underway. (More information on these congresses and other aspects of Tibetan medicine is available at www.dharma-haven.org and www.tibetmed.org.)

The more esoteric aspects of Tibetan medicine such as prayer and chanting have not been scientifically evaluated.

Finding a Tibetan Medicine Physician

Full Tibetan medical training takes at least seven years and is currently only available in India, Nepal, and Tibet. Courses on or about Tibetan medicine are available in Europe but none fully qualify a person to practise as a Tibetan medical physician.

No regulation or professional association for Tibetan physicians currently exists in Europe although an International Association for Tibetan Physicians (IATP) is in the process of being established in the US. Several individual Tibetan physicians are members of European professional associations for herbal medicine or acupuncture and carry liability insurance for practising in Europe. Various Tibetan physicians are now resident and practising in different countries in Europe and also the US.

In the UK, the Tibet Foundation (Tel: 0207 930 6001; `www.tibet-foundation.org`) in London organises visits from highly experienced, qualified, and insured Tibetan physicians several times a year. They also sometimes have details of visits by Tibetan physicians to other countries.

Chapter 7

Exploring Japanese Medicine

*Y*ou may be a bit surprised to find a whole chapter devoted to Japanese medicine. Unlike its counterparts – Chinese, Ayurvedic, and Tibetan medicine – it is less well known; in fact many people think of Japanese medicine as a copy of Chinese medicine. Yet this notion is far from the truth. The Japanese excel at amalgamating and refining ideas and in the field of traditional medicine they absorbed ideas from China, Korea, India, Persia, and Europe, added some authentic ideas and influences of their own, and came up with some genuinely original therapies that are now popular all over the world. Ever heard of shiatsu, macrobiotics, Zen, or *kanpo*? These therapies all originated in Japan and in this chapter I introduce them to you and show you how they may be relevant to your health.

I must admit to some bias here, though. I had the pleasure of living, studying, and practising Asian medicine in Japan for five years and got to experience these Japanese therapies first hand and discovered just how beneficial they can be.

A (Very) Brief History of Japanese Medicine

Japanese medicine has its roots in the early native religion Shintoism, which is essentially a form of nature- and ancestor-worship that sees the world as inhabited by a myriad of deities and spirits. Neglect of these deities, or the influence of malevolent ones, was thought to be the root cause of disease and misfortune.

Amaterasu, the Sun Goddess

In Japanese mythology, two deities, Izanagi and Izanami, are said to have given birth to the physical world and all natural phenomena, including water, wind, and plant life. They represent the male and female principles (like the *yin* and *yang* of traditional Chinese medicine we discuss in Chapter 4). According to legend, the deities gave birth to the Sun Goddess, Amaterasu. Amaterasu came to be regarded as the supreme Shinto deity and protector for the Japanese race and was revered by ordinary people who prayed to her for sun and rain for their crops and for their general health and well-being.

Ancient treatments therefore involved offerings and appeasement rituals to important deities, exorcism of malevolent spirits, and ritual cleansing and bathing to atone for misdeeds and to purify the body. Herbs also played a part in rituals and healing and were used for cleansing the body inside and out. Even the earliest texts mention plants and fruits such as *kuzu* (arrowroot) and *momo* (peach) that could be used for healing.

Fast forward to the fifth and sixth centuries AD when physicians and monks from Korea and China first visited Japan. They brought new medical ideas and practices, including acupuncture and moxibustion, and introduced Buddhism. Later, in the 16th and 17th centuries, European missionaries arrived bringing knowledge of surgical techniques and Western medical practices. For a while all these approaches existed side by side and institutes of medicine and divination were established that taught European medicine alongside traditional practices such as acupuncture and moxibustion (for more on these check out Chapter 9), herbal medicine (find more in Chapter 11), and rituals for exorcism – a set-up that would be quite remarkable even today!

But the warlords of Japan were jumpy about foreigners getting too much influence so, at several times in Japan's history, they closed the doors to all outsiders. It is during these periods that Japanese medicine really came into its own as practitioners dived deep into their own resources and developed uniquely Japanese therapies.

Over the centuries these therapies have undergone constant development and innovation and now flourish in modern-day Japan, where traditional Japanese medicine and orthodox Western medicine exist quite comfortably side by side.

Deciphering Disease in Japanese Medicine

In Japanese tradition, disease is seen as linked to the following:

- ✔ Impurity
- ✔ Improper lifestyle
- ✔ Disruption in the flow of *ki* (vital energy)
- ✔ Spiritual influences

The impurity idea dates right back to those ancient traditions where diseases, wounds, menstruation, sexual intercourse, and bad lifestyle habits were regarded as impurities that required cleansing. As a result, even today, bathing and purging are central aspects of therapy and in fact cleanliness and communal bathing, such as at the wonderful natural *onsen* spa baths throughout Japan, is a national pastime.

Improper lifestyle habits refer to activities that conflict with living in harmony with the laws of nature. These habits include dressing inappropriately for the season, staying up late and getting inadequate sleep, eating unseasonable foods or over-eating, over-working and taking insufficient rest, staying indoors for long periods of time, excessive smoking or drinking, and excessive sexual contact. It is believed that these habits cause imbalance in the body, mind, and spirit and eventually result in disease.

Disruption of the flow of *ki*, or vital energy, in the body (this concept is identical to that of *qi* in Chinese medicine described in Chapter 4) is believed to be due to the influence of external pathogenic factors known as *ja-ki* (literally, evil energy). These factors are thought to be able to enter the body and disrupt body processes leading to chronic, weak, deficiency (*kyo*) conditions or acute, painful, excess (*jitsu*) ones. Disruption may also be caused by improper diet, stress, injury, environment, or even mental state. At any given time, *ki* energy may become depleted in a certain part of the body giving rise to an empty, or *kyo* state, while in another part of the body an accumulation or blockage of *ki* may exist leading to an excess, or *jitsu* condition. Yet *kyo* and *jitsu* co-exist with each other, just like *yin* and *yang* in Chinese medicine, and so in the body they represent a constantly changing state of balance within a unified whole.

The fulfilment of desires

Kyo and *jitsu* can be related to mental and emotional states and the fulfilment of needs and desires as well as to aspects of your physical body. So, for example, if you're hungry, this is an empty or *kyo* state with the desire or need for food. After you eat and become satiated, this is a *jitsu* state relating to fullness and the fulfilment of your desire.

The body always strives to maintain a balance between *kyo* and *jitsu* and a healthy person usually succeeds in achieving this. However, if things get too far out of balance, then the body can no longer cope, which is where Japanese therapies can be utilised to restore equilibrium.

 Spiritual influences are still taken into consideration in traditional medicine in modern-day Japan due to the widespread belief in karma and reincarnation. A belief in *karma* means accepting that every action you take, or every thought that you have, as well as your general conduct has an influence on your subsequent destiny, while a belief in reincarnation means believing in past and future lives.

Diseases are also thought to have a karmic cause, relating to a behaviour or experience in a past life. For such diseases it is believed that only spiritual remedies will help and therefore religious rituals, exorcism and prayer will be employed as therapy on the advice of priests or monks.

Understanding Your Health – the Japanese Way

In this section I show you how you can determine your own *kyo* (deficient) or *jitsu* (excess) balance by assessing yourself according to common characteristics associated with each. After you determine your basic type you can make simple changes to your diet, lifestyle, and daily habits to help restore balance in the body and improve your health.

Determining your type according to Japanese medicine

Go through both checklists in Table 7-1 answering yes or no to each of the questions. Then tally your totals for each checklist. The list with the most yes answers is your current type according to Japanese medicine.

Table 7-1	Figuring Out Your Type		
CHECKLIST A		*Yes*	*No*
Do you often feel tired or exhausted?			
Do you feel the cold easily?			
Do you suffer from mild aches or pains that feel better for warmth or pressure?			
Are you generally pale?			
Do you lack strength and muscle tone?			
Do you often feel mentally slow and forgetful?			
Do you often feel tired on waking?			
TOTAL 'YES'		___/7	
CHECKLIST B			
Do you often feel irritable and restless?			
Do you often feel hot?			
Do you suffer from acute pain and/or red and swollen joints?			
Do you experience stiffness and pain on pressure?			
Are you generally flushed or red-faced?			
Are you always on the go and constantly feeling hyped up?			
Do you find it hard to get to sleep and/or experience wakefulness during the night?			
TOTAL 'YES'		___/7	

Adopting self-care for your type

Now that you've added up your answers in each checklist and determined which type you scored most for, take a look at the descriptions below to see whether you're predominantly a *kyo* or *jitsu* type and what self-care practices you can adopt to support your body balance.

Deficiency (kyo) type

If most of your ticks are in Checklist A, then you are predominantly a *kyo* type. This means that you tend to be deficient in energy and may suffer from cold conditions, general weakness, fatigue, and impaired mental function to a greater or lesser degree.

According to Japanese medicine, deficient types may find the following self-care tips helpful to boost general vitality and protect against the health problems associated with deficiency:

- Keep yourself warm at all times.
- Wrap up well, taking care to keep your midriff, lower back, and feet covered.
- Avoid walking barefoot on cold floors.
- Avoid getting wet or sitting for long periods in damp or wet clothes.
- Eat lots of warming and easily digestible foods such as soups, casseroles, and steamed vegetables.
- Add warming spices such as cinnamon and ginger to your food and drinks.
- Chew your food well.
- Avoid intake of cold or iced foods and drinks.
- Avoid caffeine-based drinks such as coffee and colas and replace these with nourishing beverages such as dandelion coffee, ginseng tea, and ginger tea.
- Make sure that you drink six to eight glasses of water daily.
- Take some gentle exercise like walking every day.
- Do not overtire yourself.
- Get plenty of rest and sleep.
- Make sure you're comfortable and warm at night.
- Use ginger baths and compresses to warm your body.
- Avoid anxiety and worry and take steps to reduce your stress.

Excess (jitsu) type

If most of your ticks are in Checklist B, then you are predominantly a *jitsu* type. This means that you tend to have an excess of energy in particular parts of the body and may suffer from hot conditions, digestive problems, painful and stiff joints, irascibility, and impatience to a greater or lesser degree.

According to Japanese medicine, excess types may find the following self-care tips helpful to calm and cool things down, remove blockages, and protect against the health problems associated with excess.

- Keep yourself cool and avoid sitting in direct sun or hot, stuffy rooms.
- Wear clothing with thin layers of cotton or other natural fibres.

✔ Eat plenty of cooling foods such as salads and other raw foods.

✔ Avoid excessively spicy or over-hot foods.

✔ Avoid over-eating.

✔ Chew your food well.

✔ Avoid stimulants such as caffeine, alcohol, and sugar and avoid any recreational drugs.

✔ Drink six to eight glasses of water daily.

✔ Avoid sitting in any one place for extended periods. Get up and move about.

✔ Take regular, vigorous exercise.

✔ Practise deep breathing.

✔ Build appropriate relaxation into your daily routine.

✔ Work less, play more, and take regular breaks.

✔ Get adequate rest and sleep.

✔ Take short baths in warm, not hot, water, and add pouches of grated *daikon* (long white radish) and parsley to ease discomfort.

✔ Practise patience and tolerance.

Understanding Diagnosis in Japanese Medicine

Practitioners of Japanese medicine determine your *kyo* and *jitsu* and your overall health balance by means of four types of diagnosis (*shin*):

✔ Palpation (*Setsu-shin*)

✔ Observation (*Bo-shin*)

✔ Listening and smelling (*Bun-shin*)

✔ Questioning (*Mon-shin*)

Diagnosis by palpation (Setsu-shin)

With *Setsu-shin*, the practitioner takes pulses on each of your wrists and may also palpate your abdomen and specific points along the meridian channels

(channels of vital energy in the body – see Chapter 4 for the lowdown on these). As in traditional Chinese medicine, Japanese medicine recognises six pulses on each wrist, corresponding mainly to each of the major organs of the body. (Go to Chapters 2 and 4 to find out more about pulse taking.) In Japanese medicine, pulse taking has a slightly lighter touch than in Chinese medicine and the practitioner generally takes the pulses on both of your wrists at the same time, comparing the left and right sides of each pulse position with each other.

Abdominal palpation may also be used to determine the relative *kyo* and *jitsu* of all your internal organs. Master practitioner Shizuto Masunaga employed a unique form of *hara* (abdominal) diagnosis. This same form is used by many shiatsu practitioners and some acupuncturists today.

The practitioner palpates each area feeling for fullness (*jitsu*) or emptiness (*kyo*). A diagnosis for fullness occurs when the abdomen feels hard and often tender when pressed. In an emptiness diagnosis, the abdomen feels soft and fingers sink in without resistance.

Practitioners also often palpate along meridian lines. Again they are feeling for areas that are soft and sunken and that welcome pressure (*kyo*) or those that are hard and resistant and painful on pressure (*jitsu*). These points will form the basis of treatment in both Japanese acupuncture and massage, including *shiatsu*.

Diagnosis by observation (Bo-shin)

Bo-shin involves looking at the tongue and sometimes also the fingers, toes, ears, and face. The Japanese medicine practitioner examines the tongue to assess its colour, shape, and coating for information about the functioning of your internal organs (go to Chapter 2 for more details on tongue and face signs and what they can tell you about your health).

Micro-diagnosis, which involves the examination of an individual body part for information about the whole body, is also a speciality in Japanese medicine. Just as different parts of the tongue are said to correspond to various parts of the body, so too it is said to be possible to examine the hands, fingers, toes, face, ears, and so on for similar clues.

For example, in analysing the fingers and toes, redness, red spots, and the sensation of heat in a particular digit indicate a *jitsu* (excess) condition in the organ to which it corresponds, while pallor, white or brown spots, or sensations of coldness can indicate *kyo* (deficiency).

The practitioner may also take note of your gait, body size and proportions, skin, nails, hair, facial expressions, and even the colour of clothes that you're wearing as all can provide valuable clues to your current state of health.

Diagnosis by listening and smelling (Bun-shin)

Bun-shin diagnosis includes listening to the quality of your voice (loud, quiet, soft, grating, and so on), the sound of your breath (wheezy, rasping, noisy, quiet, and so on), and any gurgling sounds in the intestines that can indicate digestive problems or areas of blockage. A *Bun-shin* diagnosis also notices any type of body odour (bitter, pungent, sweet, and so on) or bad breath. In questioning, you are also likely to be asked about any type of odour associated with your urine and stools because this can also provide useful diagnostic information.

Diagnosis by questioning (Mon-shin)

Your Japanese medical practitioner is likely to ask you about everything from your taste in food, to your bowel and sleep habits, as well as the usual details of your symptoms and medical history. However, as with traditional Chinese medicine (TCM), some practitioners do not speak or ask you much at all, preferring to focus on observation and palpation to see what the body can communicate directly.

The body may reveal secrets you yourself are not yet aware of, such as signs of stress damage, even though you may be thinking that you are coping just fine, or early warning distress signs from a particular organ that you are cheerfully abusing, such as the lungs in smokers or the spleen and stomach in people who eat loads of sweets.

The four forms of diagnosis used in Japanese medicine are all closely linked to the correspondences of the Five Elements. Whiz over to Chapter 4 to see a full table outlining what these are and showing how you can make links, for example, between shouting and liver function, yellow skin and stomach function, and salty taste and the kidneys.

Once the Japanese practitioner has used these diagnostic skills to assess your health balance, then, with your practitioner, you can decide what form of treatment is the most suitable for you.

Restoring Balance with Japanese Therapies

Japanese therapies aim to purify, cleanse, and balance the body by expelling the pathogenic *ja-ki* (evil energy), balancing *kyo* and *jitsu*, and normalising the flow of *ki* vital energy and bodily functions. The overriding aim is to bring the body back into harmony with itself and back in tune with the cycles of the natural world.

The most widely used therapies are the following:

- Japanese acupuncture and moxibustion (warming therapy)
- *Kanpo* (herbal medicine)
- Japanese massage techniques (including *shiatsu* and *anma*)
- *Ampuku* (abdominal massage and therapy)
- Japanese manipulation techniques (including *honetsugi* (bone-setting) and *so-tai* (a gentle manipulation therapy))
- Cleansing hydrotherapies (*onsen* spa baths)
- Dietary therapy (using certain foods for their medicinal effects or following therapeutic diets)
- Japanese meditation practices such as Zen
- Spiritual medicine (prayer offerings, religious rituals, pilgrimages, and the like)

Alongside these therapies, practitioners are likely to give you a myriad of self-care recommendations related to your daily lifestyle (such as the ones mentioned in the section 'Adopting self-care for your type', earlier in this chapter).

Japanese acupuncture and moxibustion (warming therapy)

Japanese acupuncture is similar to the acupuncture practised in traditional Chinese medicine (TCM), but the needles are finer and the techniques more delicate and varied.

Insertion is generally painless and shallow. Sometimes the needle is just held against the skin without actually being inserted, or the skin is stimulated by the blunt edge of a small metal instrument. Fine metal rollers are also used to stimulate the meridian channels, especially in the treatment of children.

The selection of points is also a little different. Many different styles exist but in general fewer points are selected than in TCM and more use is made of the extraordinary meridians. (To read more about meridians and Japanese acupuncture, have a read of Chapters 4 and 9.)

The use of *ring needles*, which are worn for extended periods (also described in more detail in Chapter 9), is very popular as are tiny little magnets on plasters that can be worn for several days to stimulate circulation and ease pain.

Japanese acupuncturists also use a range of other associated techniques, which we discuss in the following sections.

Moxibustion

Moxibustion (also known as moxa) is a warming treatment that involves burning an aromatic herb, *Artemesia Vulgaris*, to increase circulation and stimulate the flow of *ki* (vital energy). In Japan, moxa applied directly to the skin is favoured, so fine moxa wool (the dried herb) is gently hand-rolled into tiny rice-grain-sized pieces and then placed directly on the skin, lit with a fine incense stick, and burnt down. The whole process is repeated several times on the same spot until the surrounding skin becomes red and warm.

During my Asian medical training in Japan, I spent many hours practising this technique, rolling the fine moxa wool into minute sausage shapes between the thumb and forefinger. Being speedy is handy when you have to repeat the treatment many times on various acupoints, often simultaneously. One of my teachers, Kitaoka-sensei, once demonstrated his swiftness across a set of six pairs of points on someone's back. With lightning speed he placed the moxa grains, lit them, put them out, and replaced them all in quick succession; by the time he got to the bottom pair on the lower back he was just in time to go back to the top pair by the neck as they burnt down and extinguished themselves. Watching him execute this skill was mesmerising, rather like watching an expert juggler in a circus!

The idea of the rice grain moxa is that it is used to warm and tonify the body when a person has a deficient (*kyo*) condition. The grains are placed repeatedly on the same point until the person starts to feel a sensation of heat. In Japanese medicine, since the moxa grains are so tiny, they are often allowed to burn right down to the skin. Doing so can produce tiny burn marks or blisters but is believed to be therapeutic by mobilising immune cell function. Actually, the marks disappear within a few days, leaving the skin unblemished.

In most people heat is felt after three to five moxa applications as the empty point becomes filled, but in some cases it can take much longer.

Cupping

Cupping is sometimes practised in Japanese medicine with round glass cups shaped like glass balls, which have an opening at one end. A lighted taper is placed inside to heat up the air inside the cup, which is then quickly placed on the skin. This process creates a vacuum, drawing up the skin into a bulge inside the cup and holding the cup in place. The effect is to stimulate circulation and the whole procedure is only mildly uncomfortable. However, cupping does leave small, red/purple rings on the skin, most famously seen on film star Gwyneth Paltrow's back, but these fade within a few days. The technique is particularly popular amongst elderly Japanese women with back pain, office workers with neck and shoulder pain, and young women with menstrual problems.

Blood-letting

Blood-letting involves a small incision being made in the skin with a fine three-edged needle and the removal of a few drops of blood. Usually this technique is used on the fingertips to relieve fever or on the upper back to relieve neck and shoulder pain. Blood-letting can be combined with cupping, and surgical gloves are used to prevent blood contact. The technique is used to remove blood stagnation and encourage fresh blood circulation.

ANECDOTE

Moxa for alcohol excess

The most moxa applications I have ever had to do was in the case of a young friend who had been disappointed in love and turned up at my Tokyo apartment just past midnight. He'd been on a bender, combining beer with huge amounts of Japanese whiskey and was in a terrible state. He staggered through the door, wailed something about his lost love, and then promptly passed out on the floor in a drunken stupor. I was unable to rouse him in any way. He was out cold and I was quite concerned. My partner, an acupuncturist, suggested moxa treatment and together we began lighting moxa grains on an emergency acupoint, used for alcohol poisoning, on the sole of the foot, taking one foot each and working in tandem. Almost one hour later, after nearly 100 applications to the same point the friend suddenly stirred, murmured something about feeling heat on his foot and then rolled over and slept soundly on the floor until the next morning. When he awoke he, remarkably, had no hangover and simply got up and went off to work. The moxa seemed to have restored him but they were unable to cure his broken heart!

The meaning of *kanpo*

The term *kanpo*, meaning 'the way of Han', is taken from an ancient Chinese herbal text called *Shang Han Lun*, written by a doctor, Zhang Zhong Jing, almost 2,000 years ago. Zhang has been nicknamed the Chinese Hippocrates because his prescriptions, herbal formulae, acupuncture, and lifestyle recommendations are still in use today.

Zhang is famous for having said, 'Even though doctors are not able to cure all diseases, they can discover the course of diseases by using certain theories, and guide themselves to treatment principles. If my book can help doctors do that, it would overwhelmingly satisfy my expectations by more than 50 per cent.' This humble sentiment has been more than met and we wonder how he would have felt if he'd known his ideas would endure for almost two millennia, inspiring countless practitioners and undoubtedly helping countless patients to this day.

Magnet therapy

Magnet therapy is very popular in Japan, with millions of tiny magnets on plasters being sold over the counter in pharmacies each year. These plasters are also quite widely used by Japanese acupuncturists, who place them on areas of stiffness and pain, to bring relief, or on acupoints, to balance the flow of energy within the meridian channels.

Kanpo (herbal medicine)

The Japanese herbal medicine tradition developed originally from Chinese texts but, like many of the therapies described earlier in this chapter, went through uniquely Japanese stages of refinement and development. Nowadays, in Japan, only medical doctors are legally allowed to practise *kanpo*, yet over the counter *kanpo* remedies for the general public are hugely popular.

Japanese formulae generally use fewer herbs than the Chinese ones and dried granular extracts are more commonly used than fresh herbal ingredients because they're convenient and easy to take.

Kanpo diagnosis is based on eight principles described below as four pairs of opposites:

- Determining if the person's symptoms are predominantly *kyo* (deficient) or *jitsu* (excess)
- Determining the stage of illness (chronic/acute)

✔ Ascertaining whether the disease is external and superficial or internal and deep

✔ Determining whether symptoms are predominantly hot or cold

The relative balance of the eight principles is diagnosed using the four methods of diagnosis described earlier in this chapter (palpation, including abdominal diagnosis; observation; listening and smelling; and questioning).

After the predominant underlying weakness, or *kyo*, has been identified, it can then be treated with appropriate medicinal herbs. This approach is almost the opposite to the Western medical one, which focuses on identifying and treating the invading germ, virus, or bacteria. In *kanpo*, the emphasis is on supporting the weak or vulnerable parts or systems of the body to prevent them from succumbing to invading pathogens.

Because *kanpo* medicine focuses on an individual's constitution and that person's particular response to the disease, the treatment for different people with the same disease, according to Western medicine, will often be different. So, for example, if five people were diagnosed with asthma, in Western medicine they may all be prescribed the same type of inhalant medication, yet, in *kanpo*, their herbal medicine prescriptions, while maybe having some ingredients in common, would probably all differ.

Most *kanpo* formulae have five to ten ingredients. They're usually made from plant ingredients including roots, bark, leaves, flowers, fruit, and fungi, although occasionally mineral or animal ingredients may be used. These ingredients are selected according to their individual effects on the body and also their combined effects with each other.

Kanpo herbal medicines are well researched and are regarded as safe to take, with virtually no side effects if prescribed and taken properly.

If you're pregnant, breast-feeding, or hoping to conceive you must always inform your practitioner or consult your GP before taking *kanpo* medicinal herbs.

You can take *kanpo* herbal medicines with Western medicine but ensure you're carefully monitored by qualified and experienced practitioners in case of interactions. Always inform your GP and herbal practitioner of any medicines and herbs that you're taking.

Japanese massage techniques (including shiatsu and anma)

Anma, *shiatsu*, and Western massage are the three most commonly practised types of massage in Japanese medicine nowadays. These three massage approaches have all been licensed as forms of therapy by the Japanese government since 1955. Although they share some similarities, their underlying theories and practice and their common usage today are quite different:

- ✔ *Anma* is used to treat general discomfort and to release tension or stress. This therapy is most commonly practised amongst blind practitioners in Japan or amongst *shiatsu* practitioners in the West.

- ✔ *Shiatsu*, based on meridian theory, is used for both diagnosis and treatment of a wide range of disorders. It has become a very successful and popular therapy in many Western countries. *Shiatsu* is also quite widely used for stress relief.

- ✔ Western massage is most widely used in the treatment of muscular and skeletal problems, often in medical settings.

Anma

Anma is the oldest of the massage traditions, having reportedly been brought over from China more than 1,500 years ago. It was once part of the mainstream of Japanese medicine but fell out of favour as Western massage approaches became more popular. *Anma* then became almost exclusively the preserve of blind massage practitioners. (Massage has long been an accepted occupation amongst blind people in Japan.) These practitioners kept the therapy alive and it is now once again popular in Japan and taught to sighted practitioners as well.

Anma is quite a vigorous form of massage designed more for therapy than for relaxation or pleasure. It involves gripping techniques where tense muscles are held and then released to ease muscle tension and promote blood circulation. *Anma* also involves direct stimulation of acupoints along the meridian channels using mainly the fingers, thumbs, knuckles, and sometimes the elbows. Pressure is applied quite firmly and deeply, and the treatment is carried out fully clothed with no oil being used.

Anma is ideal for treating tension-related ailments, muscular pain and stiffness, muscle strains, sports injuries, neck and shoulder problems, back problems, headaches, sinus problems, and so on.

Shiatsu

The term *shiatsu*, literally 'finger pressure', is a therapy that Tokujiro Namikoshi developed in the early 1900s, when he was just nine years old, using finger pressure massage to relieve his mother's painful rheumatism.

Namikoshi's *shiatsu* involves using the fingers, thumbs, and palms to apply pressure to the surfaces of the body in order to correct imbalances and promote health. Namikoshi believed that this type of therapy could stimulate the body's natural healing mechanisms.

Various other forms of *shiatsu* have been developed by other Japanese masters over the years. One of the most well known is *Zen-shiatsu*, developed by the great master practitioner, Shizuto Masunaga, which also employs the knees and elbows to apply firmer pressure and uses stretches to balance and realign the body.

Shiatsu can be performed through clothing or directly onto the skin. As *shiatsu* is a form of pressure therapy, oil isn't used.

Western massage

Western massage was introduced to Japan by visiting European doctors in the early 1900s, and is based on Western anatomy and physiology. This massage involves vigorous kneading, grasping, and rubbing techniques designed to stimulate the sympathetic nervous system and release muscle tension. Most moves are directed from the extremities towards the heart in order to promote the return of circulating blood to the heart. Western massage is performed directly onto the skin and oil may be used.

Ampuku (abdominal massage and therapy)

Ampuku therapy is diagnosis and therapy of the abdomen. As an ancient massage technique *ampuku* was banned during the American occupation of Japan after the Second World War but has enjoyed a revival, primarily amongst shiatsu practitioners in recent years.

The *hara* – your body's energetic powerhouse

The *hara* refers to the lower part of the abdomen between the navel and the pelvic bone. The word *hara* literally means belly; in Japan this area is believed to be the centre of energy in the body. Its central point is the *tanden* (known as the *dantien* in Chinese), an acupoint located an inch and a half below the navel on the mid-line of the body. This point is known as 'the sea of *ki*' as it is said that the *ki* (vital energy) of the body generates there and then radiates throughout the body as a whole. This point is also held to be the centre of gravity in the body.

In the Japanese tradition, good health and well-being are believed to be connected to having a strong *hara*. If your *hara* is strong, you stand tall; have a good posture; are calm, clear, and confident; and are able to ward off disease. A strong *hara* is also said to give you indomitable will-power that can be directed towards any activity that you undertake. In martial arts, the person with the strong *hara* is easily able to vanquish an opponent, even if they appear physically larger or stronger. The strong *hara* gives inner power that is believed to come from a renewable energy source that can be cultivated and utilised as necessary.

In *ampuku*, the practitioner generally kneels beside you, as you lie on a mattress on the floor, and then gently probes the abdomen with the fingers to identify areas of *kyo* (deficiency) and *jitsu* (excess).

The hands are then used to balance these areas and to stimulate circulation within the abdominal area. This technique is believed to work on both a physical level (stimulating blood and lymph circulation) and also on an energetic level since the abdomen is the seat of the *hara* – said to be the energetic powerhouse of the body.

Ampuku treatment is believed to access and mobilise this powerhouse, enabling vital energy to circulate freely to areas of need in the body. It is on this basis that *ampuku* actually claims to be able to heal specific diseases rather than to simply offer massage for relaxation. In Japan, some practitioners still exist who practise solely *ampuku*, both diagnosing and treating through the abdomen alone.

In the West, *ampuku* is mainly incorporated as part of *shiatsu* therapy.

Japanese manipulation techniques

Various forms of home-developed manipulation therapies are practised in Japan, though osteopathy and chiropractic, popular in Europe, are rarely found. The most common manipulation therapies are the following:

- ✔ **Honetsugi:** This therapy, literally meaning 'bone-setting', deals with sprains, strains, fractures, and dislocations and helps restore full movement and correct alignment to the joints.

- ✔ **Sei-tai:** This therapy aims to facilitate structural realignment by bringing the body back to order. It involves gentle manipulations and soft-tissue work applied to the spine and joints, together with stimulation of acupoints with direct finger pressure. The idea is to correct postural imbalances, restore normal movement and alignment to the spine and joints, activate the body's natural healing mechanism, and increase the vital energy supply to the internal organs. Nutritional and lifestyle advice may also be given.

- ✔ **So-tai:** This bodywork system was developed by Dr Keizo Hashimoto, who found that his medical training didn't enable him to heal patients with joint and pain problems effectively. He studied acupuncture and *sei-tai* and then came up with the idea of 'reverse motion treatment' whereby the body is moved in the direction in which it feels most comfortable in order to release tension in the opposite side.

  Dr Hashimoto also advocated that the treatment of joint pains should not be seen in isolation and should be combined with healthy breathing, eating, thinking, movement, and environment. There must be something in his approach for he lived to a healthy 96 years himself!

Releasing neck pain with *So-tai*

Following the principle of 'reverse motion treatment' you first turn your head slowly to the left and right sides to see which moves more easily and which is stiff and/or painful. Then, instead of trying to increase the movement on the stiff/painful side, you first turn to the comfortable side. If this was your right side, you would turn your head fully to the right, stretching your neck muscles and looking over your right shoulder. At the same time you offer some resistance to this turn by placing your right hand against your right cheek and trying to push it back to the forwards position.

This resistance tricks the muscle into working harder and helps to release tension in the muscle in the opposite side. You then slowly release the hand and turn the neck back to the left side. Hey presto! – you should now find that you can turn farther to the left than before and with less discomfort.

This simple principle can be applied to other joints of the body and it really works! When I trained in *So-tai*, my teacher asked someone with severe neck restriction to come to the front for a demonstration. The woman had awakened with a stiff neck, was unable to turn to the left-hand side, and was in considerable discomfort. The teacher adopted the approach outlined above, standing behind the woman and placing one of her hands on the woman's left shoulder and using the other to resist her turn to the right. She repeated this movement twice, each time asking the woman to return her head to the front. On the final release she asked the woman to turn her head to the left and there were gasps from the practitioner audience because she was suddenly able to look right over her left shoulder!

Japanese hydrotherapy

In Japan, bathing is a daily ritual and visiting mineral spa baths is a national pastime. The idea is that bathing can help ward off disease and different types of mineral waters at the various *onsen* spa baths around the country (of which more than a thousand exist) are highly prized for their particular healing properties. Spa baths may be hot or cold and the minerals they contain, such as sulphur and iron, are believed to help relieve arthritic, joint, and other health problems.

In the home, ingredients are sometimes added to baths for medicinal purposes. For example, you can add sliced ginger or mandarin orange peel to baths (usually dangled over the edge tied in a muslin pouch) to increase circulation and warm the body in winter and to prevent colds and flu. You can easily try out this practice for yourself!

Japanese dietary therapy

In Japan, it has long been believed that eating seasonal, fresh food in balanced combinations of colour and origin (that is, combining food from land, sea, and mountain in a single dish) is essential for health. Even ancient texts have detailed descriptions and diagrams of foods that are good to eat and which sorts of foods go well together or should not be combined.

One pioneering army doctor in the 1870s, Dr Sagen Ishizuka, spent many years identifying different types of food cures for various diseases and identified the importance of acid/alkaline balance in the body.

Dr Sagen Ishizuka's ideas were further developed by one of his students, George Ohsawa, into a system known as macrobiotics (taken from the Greek *macro* meaning 'big' and *bio* meaning 'life') that has become popular in the West.

In this system, foods are classified according to the traditional Chinese medicine (TCM) principles of *yin* (cooling foods such as lettuce and cucumber) and *yang* (warming foods such as ginger). In a macrobiotic diet it is recommended that a balance of the two are consumed, with an emphasis on whole grains, vegetables, seaweeds, and so on, and that no dairy produce, refined sugar, chemicals, preservatives, or hot spices are consumed. An emphasis is also placed on alkaline-forming foods because it is believed that acidity contributes to many diseases such as arthritis and joint pain, acid regurgitation and digestive imbalance.

Spiritual medicine

In Japan, meditation, pilgrimages, ritual offerings and prayers are also seen as an aspect of personal healthcare. The idea of appeasing the gods still exists, even amongst people who are not particularly religious, and various gods within Buddhism are linked to health and healing. These include Yakushi, the medicine Buddha; Nikko-Bosatsu, god of sunshine and good health; and Fukurokuju, one of the seven gods of good fortune, who is the god of health and fitness. It is believed that praying and making offerings to these deities can help prevent or cure disease.

Several traditions of spiritual or energetic healing also exist in Japan involving such practices as the laying on of hands. The most well known in the West is Reiki healing. (Take a look at Chapter 20 for details on this therapy.)

Deciding When to Use Japanese Therapies

Many Japanese people use traditional therapies alongside orthodox Western medical treatment. Typically, the traditional therapies are preferred for chronic ailments such as arthritis, back pain, digestive imbalance, or general malaise, and Western medicine, as practised in state-of-the-art Japanese hospitals, is used for acute and serious conditions such as heart attack or ulcers. However, a cross-over also exists between the two.

When I lived and practised Asian medicine in Japan, I encountered many patients who used Western medicine for a diagnosis and treatment and then also visited an acupuncturist, *kanpo* (herbal) specialist, or *shiatsu* or massage practitioner for either alternative or adjunct help. For example, people diagnosed with high cholesterol, gallstones, or non-insulin dependent diabetes would often have acupuncture or herbal treatment in an attempt to improve their condition and sometimes in order to avoid medication or surgery.

In the West, the most commonly used Japanese therapies are *shiatsu* (mostly for relaxation but also for pain relief and relief from common ailments), acupuncture (for almost any kind of ailment but often for pain, menstrual problems, digestive problems, urinary problems, and headaches), and *kanpo* (again for almost any condition but often for asthma and other respiratory complaints, skin problems, and more).

Exploring the Evidence for Japanese Medicine

In Japan, a considerable amount of research has been carried out on *kanpo* herbal medicine and acupuncture, although a lot of this work is in Japanese journals and not yet readily accessible to Western readers. Other Japanese medical approaches such as moxibustion, *shiatsu*, and some of the other massage or manipulation therapies have little research evidence to support them.

Various trials in recent years have demonstrated the effectiveness of *kanpo* herbal medicine for conditions such as asthma, eczema, menstrual problems, and digestive disorders.

It appears that Japanese-style acupuncture may also help various conditions including pain relief, arthritis, migraines, headaches, and insomnia but it is hard to evaluate this research without being fluent in Japanese. Some research has also been carried out on Japanese acupuncture in France and America but it is quite limited and more is needed.

Finding a Practitioner of Japanese Medicine

To find a Japanese-style acupuncturist (who may also practise Japanese moxibustion, cupping, and other therapies), contact acupuncturists via the professional acupuncture associations (you can find these towards the end of Chapter 9) and ask if they practise Japanese-style acupuncture. Increasing numbers of Western trained acupuncturists are now training in this approach.

You can contact *kanpo* herbal medicine practitioners via the Register of Chinese Herbal Medicine (www.rchm.co.uk) or the British Kanpo Association at the Kailash Centre, 7 New Court Street, London NW8 7AA (Tel: 020 7722 3939).

To find a *shiatsu* practitioner (who may also practise Japanese massage and manipulation therapies such as *anma*, *ampuku*, and *so-tai*), contact the Shiatsu Society (Tel: 0845 130 4560; www.shiatsu.org), the Zen Shiatsu Society (www.zen-shiatsu-society.co.uk), or Shiatsu International (Tel: 01787 880 005; www.shiatsu-international.com). No professional regulatory requirements currently exist for practitioners of *shiatsu*, but the General Shiatsu Council (GSC) is in the process of establishing a unified regulatory body for this therapy.

You can find international *sei-tai* practitioners at: www.imoto-seitai.com/english/ideology/index.html

For more information on macrobiotics and details of practitioners, contact the Macrobiotic Association of Great Britain (www.macrobiotics.org.uk).

Chapter 8

Dipping Your Toes into Nature Cure

*N*ature Cure, also known as Natural Therapeutics or Natural Hygiene, dates back to the health wisdom of Hippocrates in ancient Greece. However, Nature Cure had its heyday from the late 19th to the mid-20th centuries and also led to the development of what is known today as naturopathy (for more about naturopathy have a look at Chapter 13).

In this chapter, I introduce you to some of the great Nature Cure pioneers and their simple but astoundingly effective cures using only water, air, sun, and natural foods.

You'll find out about Nature Cure approaches that are still popular today and examine evidence for their effectiveness. I also give you some tips on where you can go to experience Nature Cure for yourself.

What Is Nature Cure?

The renowned practitioner Henry Lindlahr once described Nature Cure as 'a complete revolution in the art and science of living'. He argued that it wasn't so much a system of medicine to be imposed on the body as a way of living healthily and 'the application of common sense and reasoning to the solution of the problems of health, disease, and cure'.

Nature Cure involves methods for promoting health and preventing disease using natural resources such as water, sunlight, fresh air, and natural *dietetics* (the use of unadulterated and fresh wholefoods). This approach to health also suggests that disease can be resolved without any need for drugs, surgery, pills, or potions. Instead, advocates of Nature Cure believe that by following a natural, healthy lifestyle with wholesome, fresh food, fresh water, plenty of exercise and fresh air, a calm and positive mind, and a moral and ethical mind-set, most ill health can be prevented or eased.

Nature Cure's roots are in the keen observation and imitation of nature by ordinary people. In the 19th and early 20th centuries, Nature Cure was heralded as a return to nature and even a 'new gospel of health'. This approach was seen as an alternative to the somewhat primitive and barbaric medical practices of the time and as an antidote to 'sinful' habits such as drinking and smoking. One practitioner described Nature Cure as designed to 'free humanity from the destructive influences of alcoholism, meat-eating, dope and tobacco habits, drug-poisoning, vaccination, surgical mutilation, vivisection, and other abuses practised in the name of science'!

Initially Nature Cure practitioners faced huge opposition from the medical establishment but gradually some doctors started to adopt their practices and took them on to greater prominence and acceptance, especially in the US, Europe, and India.

A (Very) Brief History of Nature Cure

The founder of Nature Cure was a farmer, Vincent Priessnitz, who lived in Gräfenberg, in the Silesian mountains, then part of Austria, in the early 19th century. He became known as the 'Water Doctor' after developing cold water cures that were so successful people travelled from far and wide to receive them.

Priessnitz's successful cures led eventually to the foundation of a large water cure *sanitarium* (derived from the Latin *sanitas* and meaning 'a place dedicated to health') in his home town. Treatments there involved cold water therapy, including immersion in natural streams; outdoor exercise; mountain air; and wholesome, simple country fare based on black bread, vegetables, and fresh milk from cows fed on nutritious mountain grasses.

Origins of the cold water cure

Vincent Priessnitz once crushed his finger while working on his family's small farm and spontaneously stuck it in a nearby cold stream. He was amazed at how this quickly relieved the pain and reduced the swelling and bruising. He remembered this when, in 1819, he was knocked down by a carriage and severely injured. His doctor told him he would not recover from his injuries, which included many broken ribs and damaged limbs. However, Priessnitz was determined to get well as his family depended on him to work the farm since his father had gone blind.

Treatment with hot compresses just increased his pain and discomfort so instead he made cold water compresses for his injuries and these brought immediate relief. To everyone's surprise, with regular applications, he recovered quickly and was soon able to work the farm again.

Word soon spread about this cure and of Priessnitz's cures for other local people. Before long both rich and poor were travelling from far and wide to be treated by him and he eventually devoted himself full-time to this work, building the first Water Cure Establishment in 1826.

Other great Nature Cure pioneers and their innovations, which are still in use today have included:

- **Johannes Schroth,** an Austrian waggoner, famous for creating a 'dry' food diet and fasting regime known as the Schroth cure.

- **Father Sebastian Kneipp,** a Bavarian Catholic priest, who devised herbal and water cures and therapeutic herbal teas.

- **Dr Heinrich Lahmann,** a German physician, who devised outdoor exercise regimes and was one of the first to emphasise the importance of mineral intake and the dangers of eating excess salt.

- **Ignaz Von Peckzely**, a Hungarian doctor, who developed a form of eye diagnosis that later became iridology (for more about iridology, check out Chapter 13 on naturopathy).

- **Louis Kuhne** who devised a method of facial diagnosis and a regime of sun, steam, water, and sitz baths (see the 'Hydrotherapy' section, later in this chapter, for more on these), together with a vegetarian diet.

- **Arnold Rickli** who advocated *heliotherapy* (sunlight therapy) and created the first Light and Air Institution in Austria, in 1848.

- **Dr James C. Jackson** and **Dr John H. Kellogg**, who spread Nature Cure ideas in the US and created the first breakfast cereals!

Granula, granola, and the Kellogg cornflake

Dr James Caleb Jackson had his life and health saved by a Nature Cure practitioner and went on to found the Jackson Sanitarium in Dansville, New York, advocating 'Health by Right Living' – water, rest, exercise, diet, and psychotherapy. He also invented the first dry breakfast cereal, in 1863, called Granula and made from toasted, dried, and crumbled graham flour grains (a mixture of white flour, wheat bran, and wheat germ invented by Sylvester Graham), soaked overnight.

Dr John Harvey Kellogg set up Battle Creek Sanitarium, focusing on vegetarian diet, exercise, and regular enemas, and his work was made into the film *The Road to Wellville*.

John Kellogg invented the cornflake and set up a wholegrain food company with his brother, Will. However, they later parted ways because Will wanted to add sugar to the cereal whereas John wanted to remain true to Nature Cure's health food principles and avoid sugar. However it was Will's sugar-coated cereal company that became the most successful and which survives as the global Kellogg's food company today.

✔ **Dr Henry Lindlahr**, whose Nature Cure books became bestsellers in the US and Europe and are still in print today.

✔ **Stanley Lieff** who promoted Nature Cure through his Health for All magazine in the UK and opened a health farm in 1925 on the site of what is now the famous Champney's health resort.

✔ **Dr Alfred Vogel** who championed nature cures in Switzerland and whose remedies and health books are now sold all over the world. (You can read more about him in Chapter 13).

✔ **Dr Bernard Jensen**, perhaps the most well-known and influential Nature Cure practitioner who popularised iridology, opened various Nature Cure Sanitariums and training institutions in the US from the 1950s, and authored over 200 natural healthcare publications. He lived healthily and actively to the age of 91.

Deciphering Disease in Nature Cure

According to Nature Cure, disease is due to violation of the laws of nature; that is, improper eating, drinking, working, resting, breathing, and thinking, as well as inappropriate moral, social, and sexual conduct.

People are said to violate these laws for four reasons:

- **Indifference:** We don't care about eating the wrong things, avoiding exercise and the possible harmful effects on our body.

- **Ignorance:** We lack knowledge about the effects of poor diet, lack of exercise, immoral actions, and so on on the body, mind, and spirit.

- **Self-indulgence:** We're concerned only with our immediate pleasure and satisfaction and don't consider the long-term consequences.

- **Lack of self-control:** We simply don't know when to say 'enough' and to stop drinking, eating, and so on.

Violation of these natural laws is thought to have three main effects on the body:

- Lowered vitality

- Abnormal composition of blood and other body fluids, including lymph (the nearly colourless fluid that bathes body cells and flows through the lymphatic vessels)

- Accumulation of waste matter, morbid materials, and poisons in the body, leading to disruption of normal functions

Acute disease is seen as Nature's attempt at cleansing and healing the body, and is described as a 'healing crisis', which the body can overcome if correct habits and lifestyle are adopted alongside Nature Cures.

Chronic disease is where the body has gone beyond the point of 'healing crisis', and is thought to be associated with an over-accumulation of toxins and a level of dysfunction that causes significant damage to the body.

Diagnosis in Nature Cure

Nature Cure practitioners are interested in the study of the whole rather than just the parts, so they investigate the functioning of your whole body, mind, and emotions and not just your particular symptoms. They want to understand your overall lifestyle, habits, and mental attitude to understand how these are affecting your health. Diagnosis is made on the basis of some or all the following:

- **Dietary analysis:** The practitioner investigates what foods and beverages you eat and drink; how you prepare them; and where, when, and how you eat them.

Natural hygiene

In the US in the mid to late 19th century, some practitioners started to downplay the Nature Cure water cures and instead developed the *Hygienic movement* (the word comes from Hygeia, the Greek goddess of health). They were against the idea of seeking 'cures' and instead wanted to focus on the 'scientific application of the principles of Nature in the preservation and restoration of health'. Natural hygienists, as they came to be known, don't agree with the use of any remedies (including homeopathic remedies or herbs), manipulations or medicines (except for certain diseases such as diabetes), or surgery (except in the case of accidents and injuries). Instead, their emphasis is on educating patients in the correct use of food, fasting, water, air, light, exercise, rest, sleep, appropriate clothing and environment, and emotional health in order to provide the essentials for health.

Today natural hygiene's main promoter has been Dr Herbert Shelton. Natural hygiene practitioners currently exist in the US, Australia, India, and the UK, and many are members of the International Natural Hygiene Society.

- ✔ **Questioning about lifestyle habits:** The practitioner asks about your exercise, leisure, and sleep habits, as well as your exposure to fresh air and natural sunlight. Bowel habits will also be of interest!

- ✔ **Face and tongue diagnosis:** The practitioner analyses your facial patterns and expressions and your tongue to look for clues about the underlying causes of your disease. For example, a sallow, spotty skin and thickly coated tongue would be seen as a sign of accumulated waste matter in the intestines.

- ✔ **Observation:** The practitioner carefully observes your posture and gait to determine your overall structural balance and alignment, and may examine nails, skin and hair for signs of health.

- ✔ **Iridology:** The practitioner examines the iris of your eye using a special magnifying glass or eye inspection equipment to identify signs of imbalance or dysfunction.

- ✔ **Manipulation:** The practitioner moves your limbs and spine to test the range of movement of your joints and the alignment of your bones.

Restoring Health with Nature Cure

Nature Cure focuses on cleansing the body, removing accumulated waste matter and toxins, and improving overall vitality. Other important aims are to improve nutritional status through good eating practices and to 'restore the spirit' by boosting confidence, stimulating hope, and encouraging self-empowerment and self-help.

Nature Cure approaches, designed to awaken the body's self-healing ability include:

- **Return to nature:** Regular and appropriate eating, drinking, fasting, breathing, bathing, clothing, working, resting, sleeping, thinking, moral life, sexual life, and social life.

- **Elementary remedies:** The use of water, air, and sunlight for their therapeutic benefits.

- **Natural remedies:** The use of natural, nutrient-rich foods for health and healing, and sometimes also herbal and homeopathic remedies.

- **Mechanical remedies:** Using exercise, massage, and manipulation therapy.

- **Mental and spiritual remedies:** Relaxation, constructive thought, prayer, and meditation.

Nature Cure dietary therapy

Nature Cure recommends eating a simple, wholesome, unadulterated diet based on seasonal and fresh fruit and vegetables, lightly cooked, with the addition of protein from, for example, seeds, nuts, and whole grains. Here are some more specific Nature Cure recommendations for your diet:

- **Eat a vegetarian diet.** This is strongly recommended because it is alkaline in nature and rich in mineral salts and fibre (the chewy bits in vegetables, fruit, and whole grains), thereby assisting elimination and cleansing of the body. Green, leafy, and juicy vegetables, such as lettuce and watercress, are regarded as especially beneficial.

- **Consume raw and living foods.** These foods, such as sprouted grains, are packed with live enzymes and seen as especially nutritious.

- **Use simple dressings.** Plain lemon juice or olive oil are preferred to sugary and salty salad dressings.

- **Consider milk.** Milk, live yoghurt, whey products, and buttermilk were all originally recommended by Nature Cure practitioners (but not blue and other strong cheeses). Milk was seen as 'the only perfect natural food combination in existence' and was believed to be an ideal food for growth and repair. However, at that time milk came from grass-fed cattle living a natural existence in unspoilt meadows and on mountainsides. The animals weren't fed artificial foodstuffs, nor kept indoors, nor given cocktails of antibiotics, growth hormones, and other drugs as they sometimes are today. In addition, the milk was unpasteurised and therefore contained many live enzymes and *pro-biotic bacteria* (healthy bacteria for the intestines). It was therefore quite different from most milk on the market today.

Nowadays, Nature Cure practitioners are more likely to recommend plant milks such as oat, rice, soya, almond, and coconut milks instead of dairy milk, because they no longer consider dairy milk to be such a healthy food. This recommendation is partly because of concerns about modern dairy farming practices, as outlined above, and also because dairy intolerance now appears to be quite common, and in response to concerns about the possible links between dairy consumption and osteoporosis and certain cancers (for more on this read Professor Jane Plant's excellent books *Your Life in Your Hands: Understanding, Preventing and Overcoming Breast Cancer* and *Understanding, Preventing and Overcoming Osteoporosis* (Virgin Books)).

✔ **Ditch the coffee, tea, alcohol, tobacco, and other stimulants.** These are seen as toxic and fatiguing. Nature Cure advises replacing these with vegetable and fruit juices, herbal teas, dandelion coffee, and water. Fresh water plus lemon juice is regarded as the best drink for first thing in the morning, and prune or fig juice is recommended for sluggish bowels or constipation.

✔ **Stop the sugar.** Sugar and artificial sweeteners are considered deadly and putrefying and to be avoided at all costs. Nature Cure recommends using raw, enzyme-rich honey, unrefined maple syrup, and fresh and dried fruits as natural sweeteners instead.

✔ **Take your grains whole.** Because of the importance of chewing and saliva production and the higher levels of nutrients and fibre, whole grains (brown foods) are considered much better than refined white foods.

✔ **Go nuts!** Nuts (used sparingly) and seeds provide good nutrition. Pulses (beans, lentils, and so on) can also be good but use them in moderation because too many can cause digestive gas.

✔ **Restrict your salt and pepper.** Nature Cure practitioners recommend you add only vegetable or seaweed salts in cooking.

✔ **Avoid animal fats.** Olives are much better for you than sausage fry-ups or burgers.

✔ **Eat organic.** This advice is a recent addition. Nature Cure practitioners always recommend eating food that is as unadulterated as possible and pesticide-free.

Finding out about fasting

Fasting isn't so much about starving as about giving the digestive system a rest and cleansing the intestines of hardened waste matter that has built up over the years. In Nature Cure, fasts may be short (a day) or long (from several days to a few weeks). The length of time is never decided upon beforehand but adjusted according to your body's reaction and how you feel. Sometimes certain foods or drink are included. In the case of long fasts, water, vegetable or fruit juice, or vegetable broths may be used, and regular enemas (the introduction of liquid into the bowels by means of a tube to cleanse them) are essential to aid the cleansing process.

Any sort of long fast needs always to be carried out under careful supervision from an experienced practitioner because fasting can be dangerous if done incorrectly. Never use fasting as a method of dieting.

The most important part of the fast is breaking it correctly. If you rush back to jam doughnuts, burgers, and beers, then all benefits from the fast are lost and you may experience harmful after-effects. Break the fast gradually, beginning with liquids (vegetable and fruit juices) followed by small amounts of easily digestible foods. At the end of a successful therapeutic fast, you feel renewed vigour and have loads of energy.

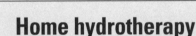

Home hydrotherapy

You can create your own hydrotherapy at home by making a warm, or cool, salt water bath.

For a warm-water bath, first fill your bath with warm water (37°C). Then add 300 to 1,000 grammes of salt rock crystals (available from health food shops) and dissolve. Next, drink a glass of water and then soak in the bath for up to 20 minutes. Do *not* exceed this time and don't use any soap or shampoos. Then get out and allow your body to dry naturally or rub yourself dry with a small, coarse towel. Don't apply any body creams or lotions. Drink another glass of water and then wrap yourself in a clean towel or cotton bathrobe and rest on your bed for 30 to 60 minutes. If necessary, cover up with blankets to keep warm.

Minerals and trace elements from the rock crystals are absorbed through your skin while you soak, and impurities are passed out of the body into the water and onto the towel. Wash your towel and clean the bath afterwards to

remove these impurities. At the end of the bath, you may feel initial tiredness but this is soon replaced with renewed vigour after your rest.

Alternatively, you can do the same treatment using cool water. For this, first fill the bath a quarter full with hot water into which you dissolve the rock salts. Then fill the bath to the normal level with cool water and repeat as above.

It is essential you do not allow yourself to get chilled using the cool bath and do not stay in it for longer than 15 minutes at a time. If you feel chilled at any time, get out at once and wrap yourself in a warm towel. If you find the cool water bathing difficult, just start with short soaks of a few minutes and gradually build up to the full 15 minutes over time, as your body adjusts.

Cold water baths are not advised for young children, the frail, or the elderly, or for anyone with high blood pressure or heart or kidney problems.

Hydrotherapy: The wonders of water cure

Water has always been seen in Nature Cure as the most potent remedy for both cleansing and healing. Water treatments may be internal, as in enemas, where water is used to flush out the colon, or external in the form of baths, compresses, or jets.

The baths may be hot, warm, cool, or cold and may involve full body or only partial immersion as in hip baths, where only the hips are placed in water in a specially shaped bath, like a seat, or sitz baths where the hips are in one part of the bath with hot water while the feet are in the other part with cold water. You change positions several times to alternate the hot and cold water on the hips and feet.

You can make compresses by soaking a towel in hot or cold water and then wringing it out and placing it on the affected part of your body. Hot compresses dilate the blood vessels and increase circulation, easing stiffness, while cold compresses restrict blood flow and help to reduce swelling and inflammation.

High-powered water jets are sometimes used to stimulate circulation. I vividly remember experiencing the Scottish version of this when I stayed at Tyringham, the renowned and, sadly, now defunct Nature Cure and naturo-pathic centre in England. I was asked to stand naked in a tiled area with my back to the therapist and to grasp two metal rails on the walls. I soon found out why, for she proceeded to direct two jets of high-powered, ice-cold water all over the back of my body! The force of these icy jets simply took my breath away but afterwards I felt completely invigorated.

Electrotherapy

Some early Nature Cure practitioners, notably John Harvey Kellogg, Dr Otis Carroll, and Harold Dick, pioneered the use of *constitutional hydrotherapy*, which involves applying moist pads with a small electrical current to stimu-late the skin while also using hot and cold water compresses.

Using an electrical current was found to produce much better results, in a shorter time, than spending two to four hours with alternating hot and cold baths, showers, or infusions, as was normal custom in Nature Cure clinics in the mid-1900s. Electrical stimulation was believed to increase white blood cell count, stimulate cellular activity, and facilitate elimination of toxins. This technique is now only practised by a few naturopaths.

Taking a sun bath

To practise heliotherapy, find a quiet, secluded place, then remove your clothes. (You may wish to wear a sun hat and swimwear to protect delicate skin.) Next, expose your skin to sunlight for 5 to 10 minutes, then go in the shade for 30 minutes, and then repeat this sequence. This practice is known as *skin gymnastics*.

Avoid overexposure to the sun and don't allow your skin to burn. Sip cool water while resting in shade. At the end of your sun bath, splash your body with cold water or take a cool shower. Allow your skin to dry naturally or pat it dry.

Heliotherapy: The healing power of the sun

Nowadays we have become very cautious about sun exposure, with good reason, because we know much more about the depletion of the earth's ozone layer and the risks of skin cancer. However, some controlled sunlight exposure is still important for everybody to allow the body to manufacture Vitamin D, essential for healthy, strong bones.

Nature Cure heliotherapy involves careful, limited skin exposure to the sun's rays at times when they're not at their peak (that is, avoiding the midday sun).

Heliotherapy not only encourages Vitamin D formation, it is also believed to stimulate circulation, increase oxygen metabolism in the skin cells, and help stop the spread of infections. (Exposing cuts or wounds to sunlight for short periods can also speed up healing.)

Air baths

The air bath was once described by Nature Cure practitioner Gordon Pitcairn-Knowles as 'one of the best safeguards against the troubles that most commonly assail us'. Our skin can get very little air exposure during autumn and winter months, when we're covered with layers of clothing, yet it still needs it.

Air baths are said to improve skin tone, stimulate circulation, improve temperature regulation, and increase your resistance to draughts, colds, and temperature changes.

TIP

Taking an air bath

To take an air bath, stand naked in a room at home or in your garden, and walk around exposing your skin to different air flows and temperatures. You can also do light exercises or skin brushing with a dry loofah or soft, natural bristle brush, from the feet up towards the heart, if you wish (for more about skin brushing, see the description in Chapter 13). Continue walking around for five to ten minutes but don't let yourself get cold.

The best time to take an air bath is first thing in the morning upon waking. Air baths are also beneficial for the bed-ridden and can be performed by just pulling back the covers and turning onto front, back, and side positions.

At the end of the air bath, rub your body vigorously with your hands and then take a cool or warm shower and dress in comfortable clothing made from natural fibres.

Other Nature Cure therapies

A sampling of other Nature Cure therapies includes herbal and homeopathic remedies; gymnastics, massage, and manipulation; and self-care.

Herbal and homeopathic remedies

Many Nature Cure practitioners have also been trained in herbalism or homeopathy, so herbal and homeopathic remedies as well as biochemical tissue salts are often featured in Nature Cure programmes.

Gymnastics, massage, and manipulation

Many early Nature Cure practitioners also trained in osteopathy or chiropractics, so some of these therapies' manipulations and massage treatments are often incorporated into Nature Cure (for more about these treatments, see Chapters 14 and 15 on osteopathy and chiropractics).

Self-care in Nature Cure

Nature Cure recommends keeping regular hours for sleep, with the hours between 10 p.m. and 2 a.m. being regarded as the most important. Old Nature Cure books say these hours are significant because the earth is farthest from the sun at this time. Breathing exercises, wearing clothes made from natural fibres, positive thinking, prayer, meditation, and moderate social and sexual activity are all seen as important, too.

Schüssler's biochemical tissue salts

A German physician trained in homeopathy, Wilhelm Schüssler came up with the idea toward the end of the 19th century that 12 tissue salts formed the basis of all cellular activity in the body. He disregarded the hundred or so homeopathic remedies already created by that time by Dr Samuel Hahnemann, the founder of homeopathy, and instead claimed that his 12 homeopathically prepared tissue salts were all that the body required for healing.

His 12 salts are available in tablet form over the counter in health food shops and chemists and can be taken singly or in combination, according to the ailment. The 12 salts are:

- **Calcarea phosphorica:** Made from calcium phosphate
- **Calcarea sulphurica:** Made from calcium sulphate
- **Ferrum phosphoricum:** Made from iron phosphate
- **Silicea:** Made from silicon dioxide
- **Chloride of potassium:** Made from potassium chloride
- **Kali phosphoricum:** Made from potassium phosphate
- **Kali sulphuricum:** Made from potassium sulphate
- **Magnesia phosphorica:** Made from magnesium phosphate
- **Calcarea fluorica:** Made from calcium fluoride
- **Natrum muriaticum:** Made from sodium chloride (table salt)
- **Natrum phosphoricum:** Made from sodium phosphate
- **Natrum sulphuricum:** Made from sodium sulphate

Finding Out if Nature Cure Works

Most of the evidence to support Nature Cure is anecdotal, based on all the cures apparently achieved in Nature Cure sanitariums during the hundreds of years that they've been operating. Little modern research has focused on Nature Cure therapies other than hydrotherapy. Some studies appear to confirm the benefits of hot and cold water treatments for conditions such as varicose veins and arthritis. Hydrotherapy has also been shown to be useful in the treatment of sports injuries.

Modern day research on Vitamin D has confirmed that a minimum of 15 to 20 minutes exposure to moderate sunlight is essential to stimulate Vitamin D production in the body; this vitamin plays a role in ensuring strong and healthy bones. These findings appear to support the Nature Cure advocacy of heliotherapy (controlled sun exposure).

Modern nutritional research also supports many of the concepts underlying Nature Cure's dietary approach, with its emphasis on an essentially natural diet of whole grains, fresh fruit, and vegetables. This approach to diet can be translated today as recommendations for additive-free, unprocessed, and organic food, and we now know that whole grains are much richer in essential B vitamins, fibre, and other nutrients than their refined equivalents.

Other Nature Cure approaches, such as fasting and enemas, lack a scientific evidence base and many medics do not support their use.

Deciding When to Use Nature Cure Therapies

Nature Cure has traditionally been seen as especially beneficial for joint, digestive, circulatory and respiratory disorders, weight problems, and skin diseases, and is widely used for these conditions in modern Nature Clinics in Europe and India. However, little research proves the effectiveness of Nature Cure approaches for these conditions.

Only practise certain Nature Cure techniques, such as fasting and enemas, under the careful supervision of a Nature Cure practitioner, naturopath, or trained staff at a Nature Cure establishment.

Finding a Practitioner of Nature Cure

Many practitioners of Nature Cure now call themselves naturopaths and are members of naturopathic professional bodies (go to the end of Chapter 13 to see a list of these and how to find a naturopath).

Natural hygienists can be located via the International Natural Hygiene Society (INHS) at www.naturalhygienesociety.org. Many of these practitioners also offer fasting retreats.

One of the best ways to experience Nature Cure is to visit a Nature Cure establishment. These exist in Europe, the US, India, and Australasia and you can locate them via the Internet.

My own personal favourites are Elaine Bruce's Living Foods Centre in the UK (www.livingfoods.co.uk) and The Ann Wigmore Natural Health Institute in Puerto Rico (www.annwigmore.org), which run on Nature Cure principles. I have also visited the fantastic Viva Mayr Centre in Austria (www.viva-mayr.com). In the US I have heard good reports about the Arthritis Nature Cure Centre in Colorado, (www.arthritis-nature-cure.com) although I have never visited it myself.

Part III
Using Popular Complementary Therapies

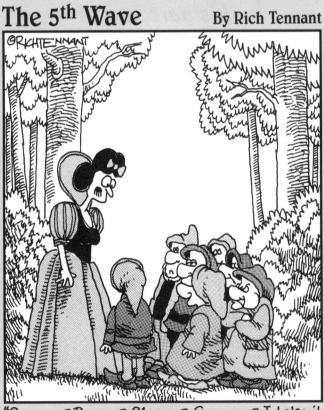

The 5th Wave   By Rich Tennant

"Sneezy? Dopey? Sleepy? Grumpy? I take it
no one here's ever heard of homeopathy?"

In this part . . .

*A*cupuncture, herbal medicine, homeopathy, nutritional medicine, and naturopathy are major complementary medicines that have taken the West by storm. In this part I dispel the myths, explain how each therapy works, and advise on how to find safe and effective practitioners.

What are you waiting for? Dive right in . . .

Chapter 9

Getting to the Point of Acupuncture

*N*ot too long ago acupuncture was considered weird and wacky by Westerners – a strange and maybe painful practice used by ancients and oddballs in the Far East. However in recent times this notion has been thoroughly disproved and acupuncture now takes pride of place in many hospitals and complementary medicine clinics throughout the Western world.

In this chapter I introduce you to modern acupuncture practice, describe the different types of acupuncture instruments and techniques used, and let you know what kind of ailments may be helped by this safe and effective therapy. I also explain why your acupuncturist may spend quite a bit of time gazing at your face and tongue, holding onto your wrist, and asking questions about your digestion and bowel movements.

On the way I answer the acupuncture questions that I'm most often asked, such as 'Does it hurt?' 'Is it safe?' 'Do I have to undress?' and 'How will I know if it's working?'

Finally, I tell you how to ensure that your acupuncturist is properly trained and competent and not using you for darts practice!

Finding Out about Acupuncture

Acupuncture involves the insertion of fine needles into different parts of your body to balance and to heal. This ancient practice has existed in the Far East for over 2,000 years and is now one of the most popular forms of complementary medicine in the West.

Some people are scared of needles and think that acupuncture is painful but when it is done properly acupuncture doesn't hurt and can actually be quite comfortable. My patients have often fallen asleep during treatment because they feel so relaxed! I describe alternatives to needles later on in this chapter.

The needles used for acupuncture are nothing like the big needles you see in syringes or horror films! Acupuncture needles are very fine and are inserted quickly, painlessly, and often shallowly into the skin, by hand or with the use of a small guide tube.

A (very) brief history of acupuncture

Acupuncture is believed to have originated in China around 2,500 years ago and began as a treatment with stone needles. Later bronze, gold and silver needles were developed and today all needles used are single use and most are made from sterilised stainless steel.

Acupuncture has its roots in Daoist philosophy, which essentially emphasises the concept of balance, the unity in all life, and the power of nature and the natural order of things.

Acupuncture was first described in the ancient Chinese text *The Yellow Emperor's Classic of Internal Medicine* thought to have been written around 300 BC. This text comprises of discussions between the legendary Yellow Emperor and his physician on health and disease.

Acupuncture thrived in China until the 17th and 18th centuries when the arrival of Western missionaries led to the introduction of Western medicine. This in turn, led to a decline in acupuncture practice, especially in cities, until it was revived as part of Chairman Mao's Cultural Revolution in the 1960s and 1970s. Since that time it has been part of mainstream medicine in China.

Acupuncture was first brought to Europe by missionaries in the 19th century but it was not until the 1950s that serious study and practice of it began. The historic visit to China by US President Richard Nixon in 1972 opened the eyes of the world to Chinese culture and paved the way for acupuncture study amongst US practitioners.

Acupuncture today

Acupuncture is now widely practised in most European countries, the US, Australasia and India. In the UK alone there are now over 2,500 acupuncturists while in China there are estimated to be over 50,000!

In Western countries acupuncture training now lasts for three or four years and many countries have laws governing its practice.

Understanding How Acupuncture Works

According to acupuncture theory health is dependent on the flow of vital energy, known as *qi* or *chi* (pronounced *chee*) in Chinese and *ki* (*kee*) in Japanese. This energy is said to flow through a network of invisible channels, known as *meridians*, that are believed to course the whole body. These channels have various key points along them, known as *acupoints*, into which acupuncture needles can be inserted to redirect and rebalance the flow of '*qi*'.

The meridians have never been proven scientifically although some work has suggested that they are electrical channels, which can be mapped quite precisely and that acupoints may be identified by changes in the electrical response of the skin (see Chapter 22 on Energy Medicine for more on this). However, this work remains controversial.

The power of qi

The Chinese character for *qi* is nowadays often seen as a design image in literature about acupuncture, on clothing, bags, martial arts logos, and so on (see the figure below). The actual character is made up of parts that represent the physical energy obtained from food (the central part of the character developed from drawings of a stalk of rice) and non-physical energy from air, space, and heaven (the wavy lines at the top of the character representing the flow of air or water). So next time you notice this design you can tell everyone that it actually represents the uniting of physical and heavenly energy to produce powerful vitality!

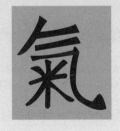

Acupuncturists believe that improved flow of *qi*, triggered by needle stimulation, pressure, or heat treatments can improve circulation and enhance internal organ and body system function, although this has not yet been fully proven scientifically.

Twelve main *meridians*, mostly corresponding with specific internal organs, contain over 365 acupoints. Some of these are classified as major points, believed to directly influence various physical systems and organs, while others are considered more minor and have a less specific effect.

Modern research has suggested that acupuncture can produce a whole series of measurable effects on the body, including the following:

- Releasing of feel-good chemicals in the brain, known as endorphins
- Speeding up of cell repair and renewal
- Lowering of blood pressure
- Blocking of pain pathways
- Stimulating the nervous system
- Reducing inflammation

On the basis of this research, some people believe that acupuncture works by promoting biochemical changes that facilitate healing.

Other researchers have tried to measure energetic changes that may result from acupuncture, using a technique called *Kirlian photography* (see Chapter 22 for more on this). These photos suggest that acupuncture may produce energetic changes in the body, however, although the pictures are intriguing and beautiful, this technique is not widely accepted by doctors or scientists.

So no one is really sure exactly *how* acupuncture works and yet it does appear to be effective for certain types of health problems.

Exploring Different Types of Acupuncture

Styles of acupuncture vary according to the country where they were developed or the master acupuncturist who developed them.

Japanese acupuncture

The main features of Japanese acupuncture are the following:

- Acupuncturists use very fine needles, insertion is usually shallow, and sometimes the needle is just touched against the skin and not inserted at all. Great emphasis is placed on making the acupuncture treatment painless. Basically, if it hurts, Japanese clients won't be back!

✔ Tubes, called *shinkan*, are a clever invention by Japanese acupuncturists to make needling genuinely painless. The needle is placed in a narrow tube before insertion. Your skin receptors are so busy feeling the soft, rounded edge of the tube they're unable to feel the needle that is then popped in through the middle. These guide tubes are used by many Western and Chinese acupuncturists.

✔ Acupuncturists use many individual, specialist techniques. Examples are *Ippon hari*, or 'One Needle Acupuncture', where just one needle in a single point constitutes the entire acupuncture treatment; and *ryodoraku*, a type of acupuncture using electrical stimulation of acupuncture needles, especially for pain relief.

Chinese acupuncture

The main features of Chinese acupuncture are the following:

✔ Needles are usually slightly thicker than Japanese needles and inserted directly by hand.

✔ Chinese practitioners aim to achieve *de qi*, a needling sensation often felt as tingling, heat, or a dull ache when the needles are inserted. Many argue that acupuncture only works when this sensation is obtained and, when I was learning acupuncture in China, some of my patients used to grab the needle handles and gyrate them themselves in order to increase sensation for this reason! In contrast, patients in Japan and the West tend to prefer more subtle and gentle techniques.

✔ The teaching and practise of acupuncture has been more standardised in China than in Japan. You get pretty much the same sort of treatment wherever you go and whoever gives the treatment.

Tibetan Golden Needle therapy

In Tibetan medicine, no specific tradition of acupuncture exists but Tibetans have a special technique known as the Golden Needle. A thick needle made of gold is placed against the skin at the top of the head, in the exact centre of the scalp. The precise point is found by drawing one piece of string from the top of one ear to the other and another piece of string from the nose tip along the mid-line over to the back of the neck. The point is where the two pieces of string intersect.

The needle is held against the skin, but not inserted, at this point and a ball of moxa wool, the dried herb mugwort, is placed around the top of the needle and lit. As it burns, heat travels down the shaft of the needle, as gold is a good conductor of heat. The point on the scalp is then heated and this heat is said to have an invigorating effect on the whole body. Gold needles are hard to sterilise so they're not used to pierce the skin but are used as conductors on the surface of the skin.

Korean acupuncture

Special features of Korean acupuncture are the following:

- ✔ The use of copper needles with coiled wire handles.

- ✔ The emphasis on hand acupuncture. Korean practitioners have developed detailed charts of hand acupuncture points that can be used for treating the whole body.

Western acupuncture

In the West, the following acupuncture techniques are common:

- ✔ Chinese acupuncture techniques are widely practised because this was the first type of acupuncture introduced to Europe by Jesuits and missionary doctors in the 19th century. Many Chinese acupuncturists also now live and practise in the West.

- ✔ Japanese acupuncture techniques have been introduced more recently and are rapidly gaining in popularity amongst Western-trained acupuncturists.

- ✔ New forms of acupuncture are being developed, such as Trigger Point acupuncture, which involves direct manipulation at points of muscular tightness, used for the relief of pain in the US and Europe.

Other types of acupuncture

Specialties within acupuncture practice include the following:

- ✔ **Scalp acupuncture:** Long, fine needles are inserted into, and across, specific regions of your scalp that are believed to correspond with specific body organs and systems

- ✔ **Auricular acupuncture:** Small needles are inserted into ear acupoints, or seeds are taped in place over these points, believed to correspond to each area of your body according to a system of micro-diagnosis whereby individual parts of your body, such as the ear are believed to map your body as a whole.

- ✔ **Facial acupuncture:** Fine needles are inserted in your face and thought to stimulate collagen and enhance your skin tone and appearance.

- ✔ **Electro-acupuncture:** Electrical stimulation of the points is used by connecting the acupuncture needles to an electrical circuit. This technique is often used for pain relief.

Discovering Whom and What Acupuncture Is Good For

Acupuncture is nowadays commonly used for a wide range of ailments. Acupuncture is generally used to treat pain, relieve common ailments, and promote general health. Typical conditions treated by acupuncturists include:

- Asthma
- Headaches
- Migraines
- Menstrual pains
- Digestive problems
- Back and neck pain and sports injuries
- Joint problems
- Urinary problems
- High blood pressure
- Diabetes
- Heart and circulation problems
- Endocrine (hormonal) disorders
- Childhood disorders
- Drug addiction and alcoholism

Acupuncture is increasingly being used by a range of health professionals including doctors, nurses, midwives, dentists, physiotherapists, osteopaths, chiropractors and vets in different medical settings, such as the following:

- Midwives may use acupuncture for the relief of pregnancy symptoms, such as morning sickness, and as an aid during labour.
- Physiotherapists, nurses, and doctors are increasingly using acupuncture in the treatment of pain.
- Certain operations have been carried out incorporating acupuncture anaesthesia.
- Dentists sometimes use acupuncture instead of local anaesthetic to reduce pain and discomfort during dental treatment.

Prevention and the Chinese physicians of old

In ancient China, families paid their acupuncturist to keep them well. If someone became sick, treatment was free until they recovered. Acupuncturists to the Emperor, or high-ranking officials, were under even more pressure – if the Emperor or official didn't recover, the penalties were severe; in some cases the physician was even put to death!

More and more people nowadays are having acupuncture as a preventive form of treatment believing it will enhance their health and help prevent illness, although there is no direct evidence to support this idea.

Evidence that it works

Many trials in different countries have been carried out to investigate the effectiveness of acupuncture and there is a growing body of research evidence to support its use. Studies have demonstrated its effectiveness for back and neck pain, nausea (particularly postoperative) and dental problems. There are also some encouraging studies to support its use for treating headaches, hay fever, osteoarthritis, fibromyalgia, prostate problems, anxiety and depression, labour pain, and bed-wetting and in several studies acupuncture has been shown to be more effective than placebo, normally some sort of fake acupuncture. However, not all studies have given positive results and more good research is needed.

You can obtain good acupuncture research summaries from the Acupuncture Research Resource Centre (www.acupunctureresearch.org.uk) and in the Cochrane Reviews (www.cochrane.org/reviews). Other studies can be found in the NHS Complementary and Alternative Medicine Specialist Library (www.library.nhs.uk/cam).

You can find additional research evidence for acupuncture at one of the societies dedicated to acupuncture research: The Foundation for Traditional Chinese Medicine (www.ftcm.org.uk), the Oriental Medicine Research Trust (www.omresearch.org), and the Society for Acupuncture Research (www.acupunctureresearch.org).

When not to use acupuncture

Don't use acupuncture for the following conditions:

✔ **Rapidly infectious conditions:** For example, acupuncture alone does not cure a severe viral chest infection or stop the spread of measles.

Treating children

Even infants and small children can benefit from acupuncture. Paediatric acupuncturists specialise in treating really young patients with very gentle and non-scary techniques.

These acupuncturists may do away with needles altogether and just use tiny rollers or pressure devices to gently stimulate the acupoints and meridian pathways. Or pressure may simply be applied with the fingertips (read more about acupressure in Chapter 17).

If needles are used, they're usually tiny and very fine and often they're only placed lightly in the skin and then withdrawn rather than being left in – a sensible idea in the case of wriggly children!

✔ **Serious terminal illnesses, such as cancerous tumours:** Acupuncture may be used to relieve nausea from chemotherapy, or to ease pain associated with cancer, but no evidence shows it can cure cancer.

✔ **Very acute conditions:** For example, something more than acupuncture is needed if a person suffers a heart attack or has a raging fever.

Acupuncture may still be able to play a role in such conditions, relieving or reducing symptoms and aiding recovery, but you need to seek medical advice first.

Certain points are forbidden for use during pregnancy because they can induce labour. Always let your acupuncturist know if you are, or think that you may be, pregnant so that these points can be avoided.

What to Expect in a Typical Consultation

Acupuncture consultations usually start with the practitioner asking you questions about your health and examining you using some form of Asian diagnosis. You may also have been asked to complete a health questionnaire beforehand.

Questioning

The acupuncturist will ask you about your current symptoms, medical history, diet, and lifestyle and may also include detailed questions about your taste preferences, toilet habits, sleep patterns and mind and emotions. All these bits of information are relevant to acupuncture diagnosis, especially in terms of Traditional Chinese Medicine's (TCM) Five Element system (see Chapter 4). Your practitioner isn't just being nosy or peculiar; this information is used to create a holistic picture of you and your health and to formulate an accurate diagnosis.

Diagnostic methods

Your acupuncturist may use the following types of diagnoses:

- **Pulse-taking:** Don't be surprised when your practitioner uses three fingers on each wrist to measure your pulse! In TCM, the pulse is felt at six different positions and at more than one depth on each of your wrists. Acupuncturists claim that pulse-taking can give valuable information about the functioning of your internal organs. (Take a look at Chapter 2 for more about these amazing pulses.)

  The pulse-taking may take a few minutes as the practitioner feels for different pulse 'qualities' in each position. Different amounts of pressure are applied with the fingertips to feel the pulses at different depths in your skin.

- **Tongue diagnosis:** Your acupuncturist will ask you to stick your tongue out and will investigate its shape, colour, coatings, and movement. Tongue signs can reveal a lot about your inner state of health and can even give away that you're suffering a hangover from the night before. To read more about what the tongue can reveal, take a look at Chapter 2.

- **Abdominal diagnosis:** Your practitioner may ask you to lie down on the treatment couch and then start gently prodding your belly. Areas of tenderness or discomfort can give clues about meridian blockages or inner organ imbalance. Check out the *ampuku* therapy section in Chapter 7 for more details.

- **Facial diagnosis:** Your acupuncturist may be trained in facial diagnosis, in which case be prepared to be stared at as your face and skin are checked for signs and blemishes that may indicate problems with specific internal organs. (You can find more about this in Chapter 2.)

- **Other diagnosis:** The sound of your voice, your breathing patterns, your posture, and even the colour of clothing that you are wearing may also play a part in your examination if the acupuncturist is using Five Element diagnosis. Have a look at the Five Element table of correspondences in Chapter 4 to find out more about this fascinating system.

Having acupuncture

After the acupuncturist has made the diagnosis of the underlying cause of your condition, or imbalance, points are selected to help rebalance the body and restore *qi* flow. As you lie on a couch needles are gently inserted and then you may be left alone to relax with them in for 15 minutes or so and to allow them to take effect. Many people find this period of relaxation very beneficial and some even doze off!

Getting the needles

Acupuncture needles come in various different lengths and thicknesses and are made from different types of materials. Here are some key facts:

- ✔ Acupuncture needles are made of different types of metal, usually stainless steel, silver, or copper and occasionally gold.

- ✔ Stainless steel needles are for general use while silver, copper, and gold needles are used more for particular types of tonifying treatment such as in the case of arthritis or rejuvenating facial acupuncture.

- ✔ Needles also vary in thickness and length. The finest are as thin as a hair while the thickest are almost like darning needles (these are very rarely used!). Most Western acupuncturists use the finest needles that they can so that you won't feel any discomfort.

- ✔ The shortest needles are just half an inch (1–1½cm) in length, including the handle,

while the longest are about 6 inches (around 15cm). The shortest needles are used for the face and ears while the longest ones are used for the buttocks or for *threading*, a treatment used in China, where several acupuncture points are linked together, but rarely practised by Western acupuncturists.

- ✔ The most commonly used needles are 1½ to 2 inches long (4–5cm) and only the tips are usually inserted into your skin.

- ✔ Needles can also come in the form of tiny, circular studs, known as *ring needles*. These needles consist of a tiny piece of circular wire with a fine tip that is gently pressed into your skin. This wire is then covered with a plaster and can remain in place for several days providing gentle, ongoing stimulation to an acupuncture point.

Needles of differing length and thickness may be used (see the nearby side bar for more on the needles).

All needles used in the West are single use, sterilised and disposable and sealed in individual blister packs so that there is no risk whatsoever of getting any kind of virus or infection from acupuncture treatment. This practice means that only new needles, manufactured to high standards of quality and hygiene, will be used on you during acupuncture treatments.

During the treatment your needles may be checked several times to observe the changes in *qi* sensation around the needle, or to manipulate the needle for greater effect. Sometimes other treatments are also be used while the needles are inserted (see under 'Other types of treatment').

The acupuncturist may also re-check your pulse during the treatment to note changes in quality.

Noble needles

In ancient Japan, needles were all handmade by great craftsmen, and the needle maker was held in higher esteem than the acupuncturist, being regarded as the more skilled person. Today, needles are generally mass-produced by machine and the handmade needles have all but died out. Increased emphasis on hygiene and safety in order to prevent any transmission of disease via acupuncture needles created this situation.

Sometimes treatment is divided into two parts, with the needles first being inserted in the back of the body, while you lie on your front and then, after removal and you have turned over, they may be inserted in the front of your body. At other times, just one side or part of the body may be treated.

If you're left alone, take care not to wriggle or move about as you may dislodge the needles – with painful consequences! Many practices have an alarm bell by the treatment table to call for help if you need it.

Go to the toilet before you have acupuncture and make sure that you're in a comfortable position before treatment commences so that you'll be able to relax and not need to get up after the needles have been inserted.

At the end of your treatment the needles are gently removed and disposed of carefully using specially designed waste containers. Sealed 'sharps' containers are used for the disposal of acupuncture needles. Your practitioner simply drops used needles in through a small slit in the container and when full it is taken away to be destroyed at high temperatures, separate from other waste.

Other types of treatment

Acupuncturists may also use other therapies, such as moxibustion, cupping, acupressure, and/or massage:

- ✔ **Moxibustion:** Also known as *moxa,* this warming treatment involves burning an aromatic herb, *Artemesia Vulgaris,* on your skin or on the needle top. The moxa also comes in rolls that can be waved to and fro over the problem area to warm it. Moxa treatment is believed to increase your circulation and stimulate the flow of *qi* and is often used to treat weakness and debility, muscle ache and back pain. It is now becoming less commonly used because of the smoke and strong aroma that it produces although different types of smokeless moxa now exist.

✔ **Cupping:** This treatment involves placing metal or glass suction cups (that have had a lighted taper inside) on cold or painful parts of your body, to create a vacuum. The cup grips tightly onto your skin and this is thought to increase circulation and move the *qi* in the area where it is placed. Cupping is thought to be particularly helpful for back pain, shoulder pain, and menstrual problems.

✔ **Blood-letting:** Not as blood-thirsty as it sounds, this ancient practice involves making a tiny incision in your skin with a very fine 3-edged pricking needle. A few drops of blood are then removed by gently squeezing the surrounding skin or using cupping to draw the blood out. This technique is said to improve blood circulation and ease swelling and pain. Blood-letting is still used in the East, for example in the treatment of pain or fever, but is rarer in the West because of concern about disease transmission via the handling of live blood.

✔ **Plum blossom needle therapy:** This therapy involves using a small hammer with a round head containing five or more small needle points. The hammer is tapped lightly onto your skin for a stimulant effect. This therapy is sometimes used on the scalp to stimulate hair growth.

✔ **Massage:** Different types of massage may be used in combination with acupuncture, but perhaps the most common are *Tui Na* and *Shiatsu* (check out Chapter 17 for more about both of these).

Finding yourself at the end of the treatment

Once the needles, and any cups or moxa, have been removed you can get up slowly. Drinking a glass of water is a good idea and you may also find that you need to go to the toilet.

You may feel relaxed and quite sleepy after treatment or you may feel revitalised and energetic. How you feel can depend on a number of factors including the type of ailment you are suffering from, your underlying health, and the type of treatment received.

After acupuncture treatment, try to take things easy and avoid stresses and strains that may reduce the benefits. Getting an early night is also a good idea, as research has suggested that acupuncture treatment continues to have some effect on the body for at least 24 hours. People often sleep well the evening of their acupuncture treatment!

Duration and frequency

Acupuncture sessions generally last from 20 minutes to an hour, but can be as long as 90 minutes if massage or other treatment, like cupping, is also incorporated.

A course of five or ten treatments is common. These may initially be at weekly intervals and then become less frequent when the treatment starts to take effect and your symptoms improve.

Knowing Whether Your Acupuncture Is Working

The success of your acupuncture depends on the skill of your acupuncturist and on the response of your body. Certain signs can help you to know whether the acupuncture is working or not, for example:

- ✔ Don't expect immediate results. Sometimes symptoms get worse before they get better.

- ✔ Discuss with your acupuncturist what changes you can expect and after what length of time.

- ✔ Typically, symptoms start to decrease in severity and duration after a few treatments.

- ✔ As the course of treatments goes on, you may become symptom-free for longer periods of time and may be able to have longer gaps between treatments.

- ✔ If you have no improvement after ten treatments, acupuncture may not be effective for your condition and you may need to consider another form of therapy. Discuss this situation with your practitioner.

Common Questions about Acupuncture Treatment

Here are some questions I am often asked about acupuncture treatment:

- ✔ **Will it hurt?** It shouldn't if you're relaxed and your acupuncturist is proficient. If you tense up and worry, you're going to feel more. So breathe, relax, and enjoy your acupuncture treatment.

✔ **Is it safe?** Acupuncturists that are members of one of the professional associations are required to observe a Code of Safe Practice, with hygiene and safety standards approved by the Department of Health. Check that your acupuncturist is a member of one of these organisations to ensure that you receive safe acupuncture.

✔ **Do I have to take my clothes off?** Usually you just need to remove outer garments so that the acupuncturist can get to the relevant acupoints. In China, patients often keep *all* their clothes on and I vividly remember struggling to push up layer after layer of clothing just to get to simple knee or elbow points. Well, it was –20°C outside at the height of the Beijing winter and the local people liked to wrap up warm!

✔ **Will I be lying down or sitting up?** Treatment is usually given while you lie down comfortably on a treatment couch. Sometimes treatment is given while you're sitting up in a chair. This practice is common in China, where I have seen up to 20 people being treated simultaneously on rows of chairs! It is less common in the West.

✔ **How many needles will I have?** As few as one or two, or as many as 20 or more, depending on the type of treatment and the type of problem.

✔ **What happens if I'm scared of needles?** If you're nervous, using either no needles (using acupressure/finger tip pressure therapy instead) or just a small number of needles with only light stimulation is usually possible. Most acupuncturists are sympathetic and willing to help you get accustomed to the acupuncture process and release your fear.

✔ **Can I still donate blood after I have had acupuncture?** If you've been treated by a member of the BAcC or the BMAS, (see 'Finding a good acupuncturist' below) you're eligible to donate blood through the National Blood Service. Members of these organisations are covered by safety codes that ensure safe acupuncture practice and prevention of the spread of infectious diseases.

Very occasionally a person feels faint during treatment. Faintness is more likely if the person is sitting up or nervous about having acupuncture for the first time. If you feel faint, let your acupuncturist know immediately so that he or she can remove needles if necessary and prevent you from actually fainting. Lying down usually alleviates this feeling.

How not to practise acupuncture! A Chinese tale

I can't resist a chuckle to myself as I write this warning about fainting for it reminds me of a demonstration I witnessed in a hospital in China many years ago. A senior acupuncture doctor had rather pompously got together a whole group of foreign practitioners and dignitaries for a demonstration of his acupuncture skills. He pulled in an elderly farm worker, announcing that with just one needle he could free the man of his back pain and enable him to stand up straight. (The poor man was bent over double with a back strain and pain.) The acupuncturist took his needle and without further preparation or warning firmly inserted it into the groove above the man's lip, where he stood. The man was so taken aback that he promptly fainted and crumpled to the floor in a heap. We were all hurriedly ushered out of the room, both concerned for the man and trying to stifle our laughter at this 'expert' demonstration. Fortunately the elderly man recovered quickly and by the time we were allowed back in the room he too was smiling broadly and claiming that he felt much better. Rest assured that this type of practise isn't the norm!

Finding a good acupuncturist

At the moment, anyone can call themselves an acupuncturist in the UK, but this situation will change very soon as professional registration, which will protect the title, is underway.

The majority of UK trained acupuncturists are members of either the British Acupuncture Council (BAcC) (www.acupuncture.org.uk) or the British Medical Acupuncture Society (BMAS) (www.medical-acupuncture.co.uk). Both of these operate a members' directory.

Many Chinese acupuncturists in the UK, who have trained in China and come to practise in the UK, belong to the Association of Traditional Chinese Medicine (www.atcm.co.uk).

Look for the letters after the person's name to check that they're a member of one of these reputable bodies:

- ✔ **MBAcC, member of the British Acupuncture Council:** Most members are not medical practitioners but all have undergone at least three years of full-time or part-time equivalent study.

- ✔ **MBMAS, member of the British Medical Acupuncture Society:** All members are medically qualified or belong to professions allied to medicine, such as nursing. Most have only taken a short course in acupuncture, such as the BMAS four- or five-day Foundation Course, but some have completed a full training in acupuncture at an acupuncture college.

In most European countries, other than the UK and the Netherlands, you have to be a medical doctor to be allowed to legally practise acupuncture.

In the US, an acupuncture licensing board and a national acupuncture council exist and the practice of acupuncture is regulated state by state. Many acupuncturists are members of the American Association of Oriental Medicine (Tel: 00 1916 443 4770; www.aaom.org) while medically qualified practitioners belong to the American Academy of Medical Acupuncture (Tel: 00 1323 937 5514; www.medicalacupuncture.org).

In Australia acupuncturists can be located via the Australian Acupuncture and Chinese Medicine Association Ltd. (www.acupuncture.org.au).

Other ways you can find a good acupuncturist include:

✔ Asking friends, family, and colleagues for personal recommendations.

✔ Asking local sports and leisure clubs if they provide acupuncture.

✔ Asking your GP for a referral.

Questioning your acupuncturist

You may like to consider asking your practitioner about the following:

✔ Ask about qualifications. Normally practitioners are happy to provide details of their training and qualifications.

✔ Check that your practitioner is fully covered by indemnity and liability insurance designed to cover you in case of any accident or inappropriate treatment.

✔ Ask your practitioner about their experience in treating your particular ailment and their usual degree of success!

✔ Also ask about fees and likely frequency and duration of treatment.

Counting the cost of acupuncture

Typical fees are £25 to £55 for an initial acupuncture consultation but may be more in prominent practices in city centres or with very experienced practitioners. First consultations typically last for 30 to 90 minutes and normally includes medical history taking, and pulse and tongue diagnosis. Follow-up treatments are often shorter and may cost less.

Sometimes just one or two treatments are all that are needed, such as for certain types of pain relief, but often a course of treatment, typically ten treatments, is given.

Some acupuncturists work in GP practices and NHS clinics. Ask your doctor if you can be referred to an acupuncturist on the NHS. In such cases the treatment is usually free, although you may have a long wait for an appointment.

Some private health insurances cover acupuncture treatment. You may need to be referred by your doctor in order to claim. Check with your provider for advice.

Some acupuncturists offer concessions on courses of treatments, or for those on benefits, or with real financial need. Ask your acupuncturist for details.

Acupuncture safety tips

To reassure yourself that you're receiving acupuncture in a safe environment, consider the following issues:

- ✔ Check that your acupuncturist uses all new, disposable needles from sealed blister packs that are opened in front of you.
- ✔ Re-usable stainless steel needles sterilised in an autoclave (sterilising device) are no longer deemed acceptable.
- ✔ The treatment room should be clean and ideally have a washable floor, or a washable mat under the treatment couch, and a basin for hand washing.
- ✔ The practice should display a Health and Safety certificate showing that it has met the requirements for safe acupuncture practise.
- ✔ All used needles should be disposed of immediately after use into a 'sharps' container specially designed for the purpose.

Ensuring satisfaction

If you're disappointed or otherwise dissatisfied with your acupuncture treatment, try the following:

- ✔ Talk things over with your practitioner.
- ✔ Contact their professional body to make a formal complaint.

Helping Yourself with Acupuncture

Over-the-counter acupuncture devices and equipment are big business in the East and are becoming so in the West. If you want to give yourself a bit of stimulation, you can buy the following:

✔ **Acupuncture rollers:** These are hand-held metal rollers that you run along meridian lines on the skin. Rather like pastry cutters, these are said to stimulate the flow of *qi*.

✔ **Ring needles:** These are tiny, metal, press-stud needles in the shape of a small ring with a needle tip in the centre. They come in boxes, with each ring needle on an individual square plaster to stick them onto the skin. Charts give you common acupoints used for a range of ailments. The ring needles are stuck on appropriate points and left in place for several days.

✔ **Moxa rolls:** You can buy moxa ready rolled into cigar-shaped rolls for easy home use. You can light the rolls and pass them over areas of the body that feel cold or painful, to warm them and increase circulation. Watch out for fire hazard! Moxa rolls and cones can continue to burn for some time, so dispose of them in cold water to make sure that you extinguish all embers. Keep the room well ventilated too, and purchase smokeless moxa rolls.

You can purchase any of the above from any Asian medical supplier such as AcuMedic (Tel: 020 7388 6704; www.acumedic.com).

Chapter 10

Homing In on Homeopathy

*H*omeopathy is one of the most widely practised, yet also one of the most controversial, forms of complementary medicine. This system of medicine is based on the principle of 'like cures like' and uses minute doses of substances that would *cause* symptoms in a healthy person, to *treat* those same symptoms in a sick person.

For more than 200 years, homeopathic medicines have successfully been used in Europe, India, the US, and elsewhere to treat a wide range of ailments and their popularity continues today. Homeopathy is now practised by many doctors, nurses, dentists, and vets as well as those trained specifically in homeopathy, and over-the-counter homeopathic remedies are big sellers in pharmacies and health food shops.

However, controversy rages because the substances used in homeopathic remedies are so diluted that no molecules of the original plant, mineral, or animal substance remain. For this reason, critics argue that homeopathic medicines cannot possibly be having any effect other than as a *placebo* – that is, the effects are all in the mind of users. Also, research evidence showing positive effects for homeopathy is very limited and no one knows exactly how it works.

In this chapter, you discover the roots of homeopathy and look at the type of ailments it seems to help. I also examine ideas about how it may work and give you a bird's-eye view of what happens in a homeopathic consultation. Finally, I give you some tips on how you may like to use homeopathy yourself.

Finding Out about Homeopathy

The term homeopathy was coined by Dr Samuel Hahnemann from the Greek words *homoios*, meaning 'similar', and *pathos*, meaning 'suffering'. Hahnemann based his therapy on the following principles:

- ✔ **The Law of Similars:** Hahnemann believed that the effects of a substance on a healthy person could be identified by a system of *proving* (see the later section 'A (very) brief history of homeopathy') and then used to treat the same symptoms in a sick person. This Law was revised by later homeopaths to the Law of Sameness, or the Doctrine of Isopathy, whereby a disease may be cured by diluted preparations of itself.

- ✔ **Infinitesimality:** Hahnemann experimented with diluting substances to remove their toxicity and vigorously shaking them between dilutions, which he believed released their healing power. He concluded, controversially, that the more diluted a substance was, the more potent the remedy became. This is also known as the *Principle of Minimum Dose*.

- ✔ **Individualisation:** Hahnemann considered each person to be unique according to their own complex physical, mental, and emotional make-up and believed that the whole person, and all their symptoms, needed to be treated, not only their disease and disease-related symptoms.

Homeopathic remedies are made from highly diluted plant, mineral, human, and animal substances and even poisons and are believed to work by somehow triggering the person's natural healing ability. *Sarcodes* are remedies prepared from healthy animal or human tissue or organs (for example, the remedy thyroidinum is prepared from a specimen of thyroid tissue). *Nosodes* are preparations made from diseased or pathological specimens.

A (very) brief history of homeopathy

The idea of like curing like has existed in medicine since ancient Greek times, when it was mentioned by the great physician Hippocrates. It has also been featured in folk medicine through the ages. However, the inspired work of a German doctor, Samuel Hahnemann, in the late 18th century, led to homeopathy being developed into a comprehensive system of medicine.

Hahnemann practised medicine for many years but gradually became disillusioned with the barbaric practices that were common at the time. He gave up his practice and concentrated on translating medical texts from various sources in his search for a more natural, yet effective system of medicine. The works of the renowned Scottish physician William Cullen and the great Swiss alchemist Paracelsus seem to have given him the clues he was looking for.

Poison and a case of cinchona bark

In Cullen's great *Materia Medica,* Hahnemann read about the use of a bark, from the Peruvian cinchona tree, to treat malaria. Now we know that this bark is effective against malarial fever because of its quinine content but at the time Cullen claimed it was because of the bark's bitterness. Hahnemann found this claim hard to accept since other bitter substances did not ease malaria. So he got some of the bark, which had become quite a common medicine in Europe at the time, and tried it on himself for two weeks. To his surprise he started to develop fever-like symptoms that mimicked malaria (some people have since suggested that he may have been allergic to the bark!). This outcome gave him the idea that more diseases may be cured by substances that could produce disease-like symptoms in the body.

Hahnemann wanted to try out various medicines of the day to see their effect on healthy bodies but realised doing so would be difficult with substances such as arsenic and mercury – common medicinal substances at the time but also known to be poisonous.

The great Swiss physician and alchemist Paracelsus had already suggested that it was 'the dose that makes the poison' and so Hahnemann hit on the idea of dissolving the substance in water or alcohol and then repeatedly diluting it until little of the original harmful substance was left, in order to make it safe. He also added a process of *succussion* – vigorous shaking between dilutions – which he believed somehow released the healing energy of the substance, although no scientific verification for this exists.

After experiencing malaria-like symptoms with cinchona bark, Hahnemann started testing out other substances – a system he called *proving* – using himself and other healthy volunteers. He carefully observed the symptoms that were produced in the healthy subjects and then tried using the same substances on sick people with similar symptoms.

Hahnemann found that large amounts of a substance sometimes made symptoms worse and so he started to experiment with increased dilutions. To his surprise, the more diluted a substance was, the more potent it seemed to become as a remedy. He later called this concept the Law of Potentisation and, as he and others experimented by making ever greater dilutions, he noted that, even beyond the point where technically none of the original substance was left, the remedy could still have therapeutic effects.

Hahnemann started to practise again using his homeopathy, and his gentle, effective style of treatment rapidly gained popularity. He carried on testing out more and more substances by 'proving' and wrote his findings up in a series of voluminous books. His ideas soon began to spread around Europe and farther afield. In England his system of medicine soon became the treatment of choice for the upper classes and even enjoyed royal patronage, as it still does today. German doctors also took his therapy to America and India, where it is now used by more than 300,000 practitioners!

Grasping the idea behind homeopathy

Homeopathy is based on nine basic principles. The key principle is Hahnemann's *Law of Similars* described in the earlier section 'Finding Out about Homeopathy'. Other important principles include:

1. **The miasms,** which are three basic patterns of disease that underlie all human suffering – skin conditions, inflammatory conditions, and degenerative conditions (see the later section 'Exploring miasms' for more).

2. **Proving,** which means that the profile of a remedy can be identified by giving it to volunteers and then recording all mental, physical, and emotional symptoms experienced.

3. **The totality of symptoms** – that the whole person needs to be treated, not just the disease. All symptoms are regarded as important, not only the disease-specific ones.

4. **Hering's law of direction of cure,** which homeopath Constantine Hering added in the 1800s. This law suggests that cure moves in a predictable order: downwards and outwards, from the most important organs or body systems to the lesser ones; from the mental to the emotional to the physical; and from the most recent symptoms to the oldest ones. Homeopaths use observation of this process to determine if a remedy appears to be working or needs to be adjusted.

5. **Vital force** or an inherent 'life force' that governs health and disease. This concept has been likened to that of *Qi* in acupuncture. A weak vital force leads to disease. Hahnemann believed that homeopathic remedies could somehow stimulate the vital force.

6. **The single remedy,** a principle of classical homeopathy, advocates using only one remedy at a time according to its proving. However, many homeopaths now use combination remedies (known as *complex homeopathy*). Classical homeopaths disapprove of this practice arguing that combined remedies have never been subject to provings so their effects are unknown.

7. **Potentisation,** which is the belief that diluting and succussing remedies gives them their power.

8. **Susceptibility,** the principle that each person is different and responds best to different potencies of remedies.

Choosing the remedy

For homeopathy to work, you need to use the right remedy. The remedy is selected according to a *repertory* (a huge guidebook on the profiles for different remedies) compiled from provings. Many homeopaths use large repertory books but some also now rely on computerised repertories.

Homeopathic potencies

Homeopathic potencies are described by means of numbers and letters, such as 30c.

The Roman numerals X (10), L (50), C (100), and M (1,000) refer to the number of parts of water or alcohol that one part of the original substance, or *mother tincture*, is diluted in. The numbers refer to how many times each drop has been taken from one volume and added to another.

The Roman numeral C indicates the Centesimal Scale, evolved by Hahnemann and using 1 in 100 dilutions, while the Roman numeral X represents the Decimal Scale, evolved by Constantine Hering and using 1 in 10 dilutions.

Potencies range from low potencies of 1x, 3x, 3c, 6x, 30x, and 30c and so on, through mid potencies of 200c, to high potencies such as 1m, 10m, and 50m (a 1/50,000 dilution). Remember, the more diluted the mixture, the higher the potency.

These low and high potencies are often misunderstood to mean weaker or stronger remedies but potency relates to the action of the remedy rather than its strength.

If the symptoms abate and the person's general condition improves, then the selected remedy has been correct. If no improvement is noted, then an alternative remedy may be chosen.

Selecting the potency

The potency of the remedy depends on the number of times it has been diluted and succussed.

Factors that determine the choice of potency include the person's pattern of symptoms; their susceptibility to the remedy as determined by the homeopath; the nature and severity of their disease; and their age, constitution, temperament, and vitality. The potency may be increased over time.

Lower potencies are generally taken every few hours for a few days while higher ones are taken much less frequently, often just once in a week.

Determining constitutional types

Dr James Tyler Kent was responsible for developing remedies for what he called *constitutional types* of patients. This idea was further developed by his student Margaret Tyler and in modern times by the well-known Greek homeopath George Vithoulkas.

According to this concept many different constitutional types exist, characterised by different physical, mental, and emotional traits. Each type is associated with a particular remedy, and named after it, but other remedies may also be prescribed for different types too.

Making homeopathic remedies

First the raw, natural material for the remedy is obtained from plant, mineral, human, or animal sources (nowadays, other more esoteric sources may also be used such as sunlight and holy water). The material is then chopped or ground and left to soak in a mixture, usually of 90 per cent alcohol and 10 per cent distilled water, for 2 to 4 weeks. Every now and then, the mixture is shaken to encourage the materials to dissolve in the liquid. When ready, this liquid is strained and bottled and is now known as the *mother tincture*. A single drop of this tincture is taken and added to 99 drops of alcohol or water and then shaken or knocked rapidly against the hand or other hard but elastic surface (this process is called *succussion*). For each step of the dilution process, Hahnemann recommended that the liquid be succussed ten times. Succussion is a laborious process, so one of his followers, General Korsakov, invented a machine to carry out this process and modern versions of this machine are used today.

A dilution of 1 part per 100 is known as a *1C potency*. If one drop of this solution is taken and added to 99 parts water or alcohol, this becomes a *2C potency*. It is now 1 part in 10,000. If this process is done six times you get a solution with a *6C potency*, which is commonly sold in shops. This means the medicine has been diluted a million, million times, the equivalent to a drop of water in 20 swimming pools. If the medicine is diluted to a *15C potency*, this is the equivalent of a million, million, million, million, million times dilution, less than one drop in all the world's oceans. When you get to *30C potencies* (Hahnemann's preferred level of dilution), you're talking about astronomical levels of dilution. Yet the weaker the dilution, the stronger the medicine is considered to be, as long as it is succussed between each successive dilution.

The diluted liquid is then bottled; or applied to sugar- or lactose-based tablets; *pillules* (tiny, rounded pills); sucrose granules, which are then dried and packaged; or it can be added to ointments and creams.

Some examples of common homeopathic constitutional types are:

- ✔ **The Pulsatilla Type** is typically caring and kind and has a strong desire to be liked and accepted. They can be tearful and temperamental. This type is easily run down and may suffer frequent colds and flu.

- ✔ **The Nux Vomica Type** is typically highly competitive, hard working, strongly driven, and ambitious. Such people often suffer from overwork, stress, irritability, and impatience.

- ✔ **The Silica Type** is usually diligent and conscientious but lacking in confidence and often rather frail and prone to colds.

- ✔ **The Graphites Type** is prone to indecision and may be rather bulky physically and generally lazy, both mentally and physically. This type also has a tendency to suffer from skin problems.

- ✔ **The Lycopodium Type** is often outwardly successful but hides deep insecurity within. This type often suffers from digestive complaints.

Exploring miasms

Hahnemann was also concerned with the problem of curing chronic diseases and after 30 years of practise he identified three *miasms* that he believed were the basis for all disease in later life.

The word miasm comes from a Greek word meaning 'infection' or 'stain'. Hahnemann used the word to refer to an inherited condition, a trace of a former illness, or a toxicity, passed on subtly from generation to generation and predisposing an individual to certain types of disease. The three miasms that he identified were:

- ✔ **The psoric** is the most fundamental miasm and is associated with 'the itch' and scabies. The psoric miasm is said to underlie any skin condition, especially itchy ones.

- ✔ **The sycotic** is linked to the venereal disease gonorrhoea, and inflammatory conditions.

- ✔ **The syphilitic** is linked to the venereal disease syphilis and degenerative conditions.

Some homeopaths believe that the miasms may be combined; for example, a combination of the psoric and the sycotic is known as the *tubercular miasm*, linked to tuberculosis, while others believe that this is a separate miasm in its own right.

Developing nosodes

Hahnemann developed *nosode* remedies (from the Greek word *nosos*, meaning disease) from diseased matter in sick humans (such as discharges of pus or mucus) in order to treat these miasms. This sounds disgusting but the multiple dilutions meant these toxic substances were rendered harmless. So, for example, psoric miasms were treated with the remedy *Psorinum*, derived directly from infected scabies cells.

Homeopathic immunisation?

Nosodes (remedies made from diseased matter) are used by some homeopaths for homeopathic immunisation against childhood diseases, or for treating animals, but this practise is very controversial and there's no evidence that it works. For example, at certain boarding kennels nosodes have been given to healthy dogs during a distemper outbreak in an attempt to protect them against the disease but there is no way of knowing if this was effective or not. More controversially, some parents have chosen to give their children homeopathic nosodes in place of actual immunisations. This practice has been severely criticised in medical circles because no evidence exists to show that the nosodes can protect against childhood diseases. Many homeopaths also disagree with this practice.

Hahnemann believed that the nosodes could help to clear patterns of inherited illness and toxicity. However, he also sensibly advocated good hygiene, healthy diet, fresh air, and exercise as important for health, too!

Homeopathy today

Homeopathy is not yet fully regulated in the UK, although moves are well underway to create a single register under the auspices of the Council for Organisations Registering Homeopaths (CORH) as a step towards this.

Most homeopaths are registered with one of the two main professional bodies (see the later section, 'Finding a Good Homeopath') and a New Registering and Regulatory Body (NRRB) is also being established.

New rules established in 2006 for the labelling of homeopathic products mean that therapeutic indications, such as 'for colds' or 'for chilblains', can now be displayed on over-the-counter homeopathic remedies as a useful guide for buyers.

In Europe and in India, homeopathy has continued to flourish, with several million consultations taking place each year. In the US homeopathy suffered a decline as orthodox medicine and modern pharmaceuticals became more prominent. Homeopathy is now becoming popular again, with remedies sold in many pharmacies and drug stores. However, practising laws vary from state to state and in many places you have to be a medical doctor to practise homeopathy.

Exploring Different Types of Homeopathy

Several different homeopathic approaches are in use today, including, among others, classical, complex, and clinical.

✔ **Classical homeopathy:** *Classical homeopathy* is based on the original work of Hahnemann. Followers of this approach prefer to use just one remedy at a time at a single potency. They believe that the real art is to identify the single, best remedy and potency for the person and then to carefully observe its effects, making adjustments as necessary. The advantage of this approach is that it is easier to determine the effects of any specific remedy.

✔ **Complex homeopathy:** *Complex homeopathy* involves combinations of more than one remedy, sometimes at different potencies, and may also involve some herbal medicine. This form of homeopathy developed out of the work of 20th-century practitioners such as Swiss naturopath Alfred Vogel and German medical homeopath Dr Hans-Heinrich Reckeweg, who called his system homotoxicology, referring to the importance of toxins underlying disease. He believed that the body could select the most appropriate remedy and potency from complex formulae to deactivate and remove toxins.

✔ **Clinical homeopathy:** This approach, advocated by the medical doctor Douglas Borland, focuses on specific remedies for individual diseases and is usually referred to as *therapeutic homeopathy/prescribing*.

✔ **Dr Schüssler's Tissue Salts:** Dr Wilhelm Schüssler, (sometimes also spelt Schuessler) a homeopathic physician, was an early follower of Hahnemann who initially used the full range of homeopathic remedies but later became convinced that most disease was linked to imbalance of minerals within the body's cells. In 1872, he developed homeopathic remedies for 12 of the most common, essential mineral tissue salts found in the body using a dilution ratio of just 1:9 rather than the usual 1:99. This ratio means that the remedies do contain minute amounts of the actual mineral substance and so are part homeopathic and part micro-nutrient. Rather than treating like with like, these remedies are designed to enable the cell to rectify its imbalance. Schüssler Tissue Salts are now widely available in health food shops and are also available in combination formulae.

✔ **Animal homeopathy:** Increasing numbers of vets are now using homeopathic prescribing in the treatment of animals. The remedies, potencies, and so on are selected in the same way as for humans, with consideration given to the animal's temperament and behaviour as well as their symptoms. Typical treatments are for infertility in cattle, infectious diseases in pigs, salmonella in chickens, and Cushing's disease in horses and dogs, although the efficacy of these treatments still remains largely unproven.

Understanding How It Works

Hahnemann believed that the process of dilution and *succussion* (vigorous shaking) somehow left an imprint of the substance that could trigger healing in the body.

The placebo effect

The placebo effect is an improvement in health that is not due to actual treatment. For example, people who get better while on a doctor's waiting list, without actually being seen or treated, are said to have been cured by the placebo of being on the waiting list rather than any medicine. Similarly, critics suggest that homeopathy works because psychologically people feel better after taking a pill even though the pill contains no measurable active substances.

Several studies that compare the effects of giving homeopathic remedies to giving identical pills or tablets that have not been homeopathically treated have yielded similar results, leading at least one researcher to conclude that 'homeopathy is little better than placebo'. However, a quite recent large-scale analysis of many trials combined suggested that the overall effect of homeopathy *was* greater than placebo. Both types of studies have been criticised and so the controversy currently still rages and further investigation is needed.

Modern-day homeopaths believe that this process somehow creates a vibrational or electrochemical pattern that is somehow then conveyed through water in the body direct to the cells.

Huge excitement was generated in 1988, when French researcher Jacques Benveniste published his work in the renowned journal, *Nature*, suggesting that water could hold a memory of the substances with which it came in contact. His work on tiny cells suggested that a substance could still produce noticeable effects on the live cells even when hugely diluted.

However, Benveniste's work was later discredited on the grounds that errors had occurred in data collection and analysis of results and his results could not be repeated elsewhere. Subsequently some laboratories do claim to have repeated his results but this has not yet been proven. Benveniste maintained to his death that his work could become a landmark finding of the 21st century and many of his supporters continue his work today.

Dr Masaru Emoto from Japan, who has developed a photographic technique for imaging water crystals, also claims that water may be able to carry a memory, but again his work remains controversial and unproven. Sceptics remain entirely unconvinced that water can have such a memory or that homeopathy can have any effect whatsoever other than placebo.

All this controversy means that many medics and scientists still reject homeopathy outright, while those who do accept it admit that they have no idea how it really works.

Discovering Whom and What Homeopathy Is Good For

Homeopaths claim that their remedies can bring about some sort of improvement for most ailments. Most homeopaths treat everyone from babies to the elderly and are used to dealing with both acute (recent, more severe) conditions and chronic (more long-lasting and often less severe) ones.

A typical cross-section of ailments treated by homeopaths includes hay fever, colds and flu, infant problems such as teething and colic, skin problems such as eczema and psoriasis, respiratory conditions such as asthma and coughs, digestive problems, joint problems such as rheumatism and arthritis, anxiety and depression, fevers, headaches, and chronic fatigue.

What's the evidence that it works?

Several large-scale studies, where data is pooled from different research trials, have concluded that homeopathy isn't effective. These include studies at the Peninsular Medical School in Exeter by Professor Ezard Ernst and his colleagues, such as one that looked at studies of osteoarthritis being treated by homeopathy, and concluded that overall it was ineffective.

Some individual trials have shown positive results for homeopathy. These include three trials at the Glasgow Homeopathic Hospital by Dr David Reilly, which suggested that homeopathy could ease hay fever, and a study by Professor George Lewith and his colleagues at Southampton University, which showed that homeopathy could reduce allergic reactions to the house dust mite in asthma sufferers. Other trials have suggested homeopathy may help treat glue ear, infant diarrhoea, vertigo, premenstrual syndrome, asthma, and chronic fatigue – to name but a few conditions – as well as boost immune function in people that are HIV-positive. Some animal studies have also been encouraging.

Some large-scale trials have also yielded encouraging results. For example, a huge study at the Bristol Homeopathic Hospital reported that more than 70 per cent of 6,500 patients surveyed said that they noted improvements from their homeopathic treatment.

However, many studies have been criticised for design flaws and many have yielded negative or conflicting results so more good research is needed.

Homeopathic ABC

My son Michael was a very healthy baby, born at home. I had a fantastic pregnancy and an easy labour using only the homeopathic remedy *Arnica* to ease discomfort during the labour and no other drugs or remedies of any kind. I recovered quickly and baby Michael thrived until one day, aged about 7 months, he suddenly developed a bright red patch on the side of his cheek and became irritable and upset. He already had a few teeth and teething had been uneventful, so I wasn't too worried and thought this was probably just a slightly more difficult one. However, as the day wore on he became increasingly clingy and listless, wanting to be carried all the time, and I began to get concerned. I called a homeopathic colleague, who

kindly came round to see him. She prescribed the childhood combination remedy ABC (Aconite, Belladonna, and Chamomilla) for Michael and the transformation was remarkable. Having been clingy and discomforted for nearly 10 hours, within 30 minutes of taking the remedy he was smiling happily and crawling about vigorously as usual with no sign of discomfort or of the redness on his cheek. He slept well that night and the next morning a beautiful new tooth started to peek through his gums but he didn't even seem to notice it. I used this combination remedy often thereafter when he had difficulty teething and found it to be a really useful childhood ABC!

For more on homeopathy research, look at the research pages on the Society of Homeopath's site (www.homeopathy-soh.org), the British Homeopathic Association (www.trusthomeopathy.org/case/res_toc.html) or the NHS Complementary and Alternative Medicine Specialist Library (www.library.nhs.uk/cam).

When not to use homeopathy

Homeopathy is held to be entirely safe and non-toxic because of the level of dilution of the remedies; therefore it is not considered to have any contra-indications and can be used by anyone. However, using inappropriate remedies may trigger mild symptoms as the remedy 'proves' itself, that is, it may bring on symptoms in an otherwise healthy person. Stopping the remedy should bring quick relief.

What to Expect in a Typical Consultation

Your first consultation with a homeopath is likely to be quite lengthy. The homeopath usually starts by asking you questions about your health and your life.

Questioning

The questions asked by homeopaths are sometimes surprising, as they seem so wide-ranging. They're likely to cover not only your symptoms but also your general mood, diet, lifestyle, preferences, fears, and so on. The homeopath will also be interested in how you react to different types of weather or other environmental changes, how you feel at different times of the day, and more.

Diagnosis

Diagnosis is based not only on your current symptoms but also your physical, mental, emotional, and even spiritual state. Your answers to questions will be used to build up a picture of your constitutional type, and of the best remedy and potency for you.

Written repertories will be consulted to check the appropriate remedy and may lead to further questioning to whittle down different alternatives. Increasingly, homeopaths are also using computer programs that enable them to rapidly check through the more than 2,000 remedies now available. The homeopath may also examine you or take account of other signs by doing the following:

- ✔ Listening to the tone of your voice
- ✔ Examining your skin tone and complexion
- ✔ Checking for any specific odours
- ✔ Observing your facial expressions and posture

The homeopath also aims to identify or rule out any serious underlying disease that may require medical referral.

Treatment

The homeopath should explain your proposed treatment plan and give you precise instructions on how to take the remedy. Follow these instructions carefully. Sometimes the remedy is labelled, but some homeopaths prefer to give the remedy 'blind' and only tell you what it was after you've taken it.

The chosen remedy, or combination of remedies, is usually made up on the spot and then given to you, or else sent on to you shortly afterwards.

Remedies are often given as pills or tablets made from a lactose base. If you are intolerant to lactose (found in dairy products), inform your homeopath, who can then give you non-lactose remedies (usually made from fruit sugar) as an alternative. Sometimes powders, creams, or liquids may be given.

Taking homeopathic remedies

Never handle homeopathic remedies. Tip them direct from the cap of the dispenser into your mouth or transfer them via a spoon. Once in the mouth, allow the remedy to dissolve gradually.

Homeopathic remedies are considered so subtle and sensitive, you're generally advised to take them 20 minutes before, or at least an hour or so after, food, rather than with food. Also avoid taking them anywhere near consumption of coffee, tea, peppermint (including in toothpaste and mouthwashes – most homeopaths recommend that you use herbal, non-mint toothpaste while taking homeopathic remedies), or cigarettes. Other strong smells or substances are also thought to interfere with the remedies, including menthol, camphor, eucalyptus (these are often found in cold remedies), and aromatherapy oils. Don't use these substances at the same time as homeopathy and don't store them near homeopathic tablets.

Store homeopathic tablets in a cool, dark place away from any other substances with strong odours.

If you're flying, try to avoid putting your remedy through the x-ray scanners. Many airports will allow homeopathy to be hand-checked but you *must* also carry a prescription from your homeopath or a receipt from your homeopathic supplier as verification. With current tighter restrictions on hand luggage, homeopathic medicines may not always be permitted – check with your airline before flying. You may have to check them in your main baggage.

Remember to always tell your homeopath if you're taking any other medicines, supplements, or remedies, and about any recent dental treatment, in case these may interfere with the chosen remedy.

Your homeopath may also give you some general lifestyle and dietary advice.

Knowing what to expect once you start treatment

After taking your remedy, you may start to notice some changes. Sometimes people feel almost immediate improvement and just continue to feel better as treatment goes on. Other times, symptoms may appear to get slightly worse before they get better. This is regarded by homeopaths as a *healing crisis*, which normally passes quickly.

If you have any severe increase in symptoms or any other outcome that you're worried about, consult your homeopath as soon as possible. If symptoms are just mild, you may want to make a note of them to discuss with your homeopath at your next appointment.

Knowing how long to continue taking the remedy

Your homeopath will give you precise instructions for taking your remedy and you need to follow these carefully. In general, remedies are only taken for a short time and dosage is decreased or stopped as symptoms improve.

Duration and frequency

Your first consultation with a homeopath usually lasts between one and two hours. Subsequent visits are shorter, usually 30 minutes or so. You'll probably be asked to have one or two of these shorter follow-up visits to check that the remedy is working and to make any necessary adjustments to the remedy being taken.

Knowing Whether Your Homeopathy Treatment Is Working

You may experience immediate benefits from a homeopathic remedy or you may experience a mild flare-up of symptoms and feel more tired than usual. These effects should pass in a day or so and improvements should be noticeable. Be patient and allow the remedy to work its course.

If you experience a significant deterioration in your symptoms, or a marked fever, contact your homeopath for advice.

Ask your homeopath what improvements you can realistically expect over what sort of timescale. For best results, carefully follow the directions for taking the remedy and the diet and lifestyle advice given by your homeopath.

If you have no improvement after a course of treatment, then it may be that the right remedy has not been selected for your ailment or that homeopathy may not be effective for your condition. Discuss this situation with your practitioner.

Here are some common questions that I'm often asked about homeopathy:

- **Are homeopathic remedies safe?** Yes, because they're so diluted, homeopathic remedies do not normally have any toxicity or side effects, so pregnant women and babies can take them. Reported side effects are extremely rare.

- **Can I treat myself with homeopathic remedies?** Yes, many people keep homeopathic remedies in their first aid cupboard at home and use them for common minor ailments such as bruises, cuts, colds and flu. Many health centres and colleges also run courses on self-use homeopathy where you can learn more (see, for example, www.revital.com).

If you have any serious complaint or medical concern, always seek the advice of a qualified health professional.

- **How often do I take the remedies?** How often you take the remedies depends on your general health and the type of health problem that you're trying to rectify. For acute conditions, such as a new bruise being treated with the remedy Arnica, the remedy may be taken every 15 minutes, every 30 minutes, every hour, or every two hours, according to the severity of the symptoms or the recommendation from your practitioner. For chronic conditions, the remedy is usually taken three to six times a day. Once the remedy starts to work you normally tail off its use and it is only re-used if symptoms recur. You usually take nosodes only once (refer to the earlier section 'Developing nosodes').

Most homeopaths strongly caution against self-prescribing of nosodes because they consider them to have very potent effects on the body.

- **Does it matter if I drink coffee while taking homeopathic remedies?** The potency of homeopathic remedies may be affected by strong tastes and odours. Try to cut out, or reduce intake of items such as coffee, tea, and mint while on homeopathic remedies and at least to take them one hour before or after the remedy. Good alternatives are herbal teas, dandelion coffee, juices, smoothies, and good old-fashioned water!

- **Do the remedies taste bad?** No, most have a mildly sweet taste.

- **Can I take other medication at the same time?** Yes, homeopathic remedies can be taken at the same time as most medicines but do inform your homeopath of what you are currently taking.

Finding a Good Homeopath

Most qualified homeopaths in the UK are members of one of the following:

✔ **Society of Homeopaths** (Tel: 0845 450 6611; `www.homeopathy-soh.org`): This is the largest organisation registering professional homeopaths in the UK. All its members have undergone a three-year full-time, or four-year part-time, training approved by the Society. Not all members are also medically qualified. The Society regulates standards of training and practice and has a complaints procedure for the public. It also operates a directory of registered practitioners. Members have the letters RSHom or FSHom after their names.

✔ **British Homeopathic Association and the Faculty of Homeopathy** (Tel: 0870 444 3950; `www.trusthomeopathy.org/trust/tru_sea.html`): This organisation has more than 1,300 members worldwide. All are medically qualified or from disciplines allied to medicine (such as nurses, midwives, dentists, pharmacists, podiatrists, and vets). Full members have the letters FFHom (Fellow of the Faculty of Homeopathy) or MFHom (Member of the Faculty) after their names. Those with a basic level of training are designated as LFHom (Med). The Association operates a Code of Ethics and complaints procedure and a member directory.

In the UK you can see a homeopath on the NHS. Five homeopathic hospitals – in Bristol, Glasgow, Liverpool, London, and Tunbridge Wells – were incorporated into the NHS when it was set up. Your GP can refer you to one of these hospitals. Many health insurance companies also cover homeopathic treatment.

In the US, laws about the practice of homeopathy vary from state to state. Take a look at the National Center for Homeopathy (Tel: 00 1 703 548 7790; `www.homeopathic.org`).

You can find homeopathic associations in other countries (for example, India, Australia, and New Zealand) at `www.homeopathyhome.com`

Other ways of finding a homeopath are to:

✔ Ask friends, family, and colleagues for personal recommendations.

✔ Consider visiting the teaching clinics at homeopathy colleges. All students practise under close supervision from experienced practitioners and fees are low compared to private practice.

To find a homeopathic vet, contact the British Association of Homeopathic Veterinary Surgeons (BAHVS) (Tel: 01367 718115; `www.bahvs.com`) for a list of vets trained in homeopathy. A few have gained the Faculty of Homeopathy's veterinary qualifications VetMFHom or VetFFHom.

Questions to ask your homeopath

You may want to ask your homeopath about the following:

- ✓ **Qualifications:** Most practitioners are happy to give details of their training and qualifications.
- ✓ **Insurance:** Members of professional associations must have appropriate indemnity insurance.
- ✓ **Experience:** Ask your practitioner about their experience in treating your particular ailment and their usual degree of success.
- ✓ **Treatment:** Ask about the likely frequency of consultations that you may need and the costs involved.

Counting the cost of homeopathy

Initial homeopathy consultations usually cost around £40 to £100, while follow-up sessions are in the region of £20 to £45. NHS homeopathic hospital treatment, by referral from your GP, is free.

Some homeopaths offer concessions for infants, retired persons, or those on benefits. Ask your homeopath for details.

Gaining satisfaction

If you're dissatisfied with your treatment, first talk things over with your practitioner. If you think that the practitioner has been negligent or unethical in any way, then contact their professional body and go through the formal complaints procedure.

Chapter 11

Unearthing Herbal Medicine

In This Chapter

▶ Finding out about different types of herbal medicine

▶ Understanding how it works

▶ Discovering what herbal medicine can be good for

▶ Knowing what to expect in a typical consultation

▶ Knowing how to find a safe and effective herbalist

*H*erbal medicine is the oldest and most widely used form of medicine in the world today. All ancient cultures and folk medicine traditions used herbal remedies and even today around 80 per cent of the world's population are said to use plants as their main form of medicine.

Many common Western medical drugs are actually based on plants, and modern research has enabled the active ingredients of different medicinal plants to be isolated so that we can have a better understanding of how they work in the body.

Herbalists specialising in Western medical herbs, or herbs from other traditions, such as the Chinese, Ayurvedic, Tibetan, and Japanese herbal medicine systems, are now quite widespread in the Western world.

In this chapter, I delve briefly into the history of herbal medicine and also consider how it is practised today. I take a look at different types of herbal medicine, discuss what herbal medicine is used for, and consider the evidence for its effectiveness.

I tell you what a typical herbal medicine consultation is like and I end with some tips on how you can make your own herbal remedies.

Finding Out about Herbal Medicine

Herbal medicine is the use of plant materials to prevent and treat disease. Various parts of the plant may be used such as the root, berries, bark, leaves, and flowers, and these may be made into ointments, tinctures, teas, creams, powders, and pills.

You can obtain herbal remedies over the counter, make them up at home, or have them prescribed by a professional herbalist. Herbal remedies and herbal medicine consultations are hugely popular and to protect the public various steps are underway to regulate both herbal medicine as a profession and herbal remedies sold to the public.

Since herbal medicine is so widespread, and the predominant form of medicine in many parts of the world, some argue that it should not even be regarded as a form of complementary medicine at all, but rather a type of mainstream medicine. In addition, in some countries such as Japan you have to be medically qualified in order to prescribe herbs. However, in the UK, US, Australia, and some other countries herbal medicine has the status of a complementary therapy and it is therefore included as such in this book.

A (very) brief history of herbal medicine

All ancient cultures and their peoples evolved some sort of herbal medicine using local plants for health and healing. The ancient Greeks, Egyptians, Persians, Chinese, Indians, Tibetans, and Native Americans are all known to have made good use of herbs. Several of these cultures also developed comprehensive *materia medica*, ancient texts outlining different plants and their medicinal uses, which are used even today. Herbal know-how was developed initially using trial and error and then formulations were refined as knowledge grew. Travelling physicians and monks also played an important role in the development of herbal medicine as they grew plants, experimented with remedies, and took news of different herbal cures between countries and cultures.

In the Middle Ages, several individuals in religious settings made detailed studies of plants and used them to treat both their religious community and the lay communities in their locality. Hildegard of Bingen, for example, a German girl who was sent to join a religious community from the age of eight after having a series of mystical visions, rose to head her religious community and wrote many accounts of the healing properties of plants.

Others didn't fare as well and many wise women who'd mastered the use of herbs as medicines are believed to have been burnt at the stake as witches because of their so-called powers.

The Doctrine of Signatures: Secret signs of plants

The Doctrine of Signatures is an idea that became widespread in the 17th-century based on a religious belief in the unity of all things in nature. The idea is believed to have originated from a young German shoemaker, Jakob Böhme, who was shown in a vision the design of God's creation, which involved a divine imprint on all living things just waiting to be revealed. The alchemist Paracelsus expanded this idea and suggested that close observation of the colour and form of plants could give vital signs as to their medical use. For example, a plant with yellow flowers or sap may be used to treat jaundice, while one with a leaf the same shape as the liver may be used to treat liver diseases. Paracelsus called this idea the Doctrine of Signatures and published a book describing many plants, their signatures, and possible medicinal uses. This concept can also be found in some Native cultures, and is an attractive idea that sometimes turned out to be correct but often was not and is nowadays generally disregarded.

The invention of the printing press in the 15th-century meant that herbal knowledge could be spread more widely, and pioneers such as the alchemist Paracelsus and later the 17th-century botanist and physician Nicholas Culpeper wrote herbal texts that had a profound impact on the theory and practice of herbal medicine. Paracelsus travelled widely, picking up tips on medicinal remedies and compiling them into various texts outlining the medicinal properties of different plants. He was also responsible for popularising the idea of the 'Doctrine of Signatures'.

Nicholas Culpeper, an English physician, botanist, herbalist, and astrologer, was against many of the barbaric practices and high fees charged by most doctors in his day. Having married into a wealthy family he was able to treat many patients for free and he also firmly believed in empowering people to treat themselves. He published a low-cost pamphlet on herbal medicinal cures, which became a bestseller, much to the anger of many of his greedy physician colleagues! He also wrote a large number of academic texts on herbs and their healing properties, which are still used as a valuable reference by herbalists today.

With scientific advances in the 18th-century, herbal medicine began to fall out of favour, and by the 20th-century, with the development of medicinal drugs such as penicillin (used to treat infections) and insulin (used to treat diabetes), herbal medicine had been relegated to a side note in mainstream medical practice. Laboratory work was increasingly used to isolate individual ingredients from plants and to test their medicinal effects. As a result many compounds have been isolated and reproduced synthetically to form modern pharmaceuticals. For example, the compound digoxin, extracted from foxglove (*Digitalis purpurea*), was isolated and used to make heart medications, and extracts of salicylic acid from willow bark (*Salix alba*) to make aspirin.

Modern scientific work on plants has also increased the sophistication of knowledge and training in the therapeutic use of plants and today herbalism has come back into prominence as a major healthcare profession.

Herbal medicine today

In the UK, herbal medicine is currently going through a process of voluntary regulation. Until this regulation is completed, anyone can call themselves a herbalist, so check details of your herbalist's training and experience. British medical herbalists and phytotherapists have normally undergone lengthy training and are members of a reputable professional association that controls standards of training and practice (see the later section 'Finding a Good Medical Herbalist or Phytotherapist'). In the US, no formal register of herbalists exists and laws regulating the practice of herbal medicine vary from state to state.

Herbal medicine is hugely popular in other countries around the world, from the African countries, to South America, to Australasia, and is recognised by the World Health Organisation (WHO) as an important system of medicine.

Many modern herbalists now use herbs from more than one tradition around the world.

Grasping the idea behind herbal medicine

The world has around 422,000 different species of flowering plants (as estimated by plant conservationist Dr David Bramwell), of which only a tiny proportion has been investigated scientifically for their medicinal properties. Yet it is known, from those that have been investigated, that plants contain a great variety of active ingredients that can have powerful effects on different body systems or individual organs. For example, some may have a general relaxant or stimulant effect while others can specifically alter heart rate, lower blood pressure, induce vomiting, alter liver function, and so on. Their effects may also be different when used singly or in combination with other plants.

In herbalism, the idea is to use plants to stimulate the body's natural healing ability and restore balance. Herbalists need to have a comprehensive understanding of the constituents of different plants, the appropriate uses of different herbal formulations, the effects of different plants and herbal formulations on the body, their role in the treatment of different diseases, and also possible interactions of different herbs with each other or with standard medicinal drugs.

Herbalists generally believe in the *Theory of Synergy*, that is, that the whole plant has a more potent therapeutic effect than individual ingredients of the plant in isolation. The Theory of Synergy thus relates to the idea of the perfection inherent in nature. For example, the plant meadowsweet contains salicylic acid, which is the basis for the drug aspirin (willow bark also contains this compound). Salicylic acid or aspirin taken in isolation can trigger stomach irritation or even bleeding. Yet meadowsweet also contains mucilaginous compounds, that is, compounds that form a mucous-like coating to soothe and protect internal tissues. Thus use of the whole plant can counteract the possible harmful effect of salicylic acid taken on its own.

Another example of the Theory of Synergy is the use of pharmaceutical diuretics (drugs designed to get rid of water retention by stimulating urination) compared to herbal ones. Diuretic drugs can cause a loss of the mineral potassium in the body, which has to then be replaced with potassium supplements. In contrast, dandelion leaves, used by herbalists, have a strong diuretic effect but also contain potassium thus preventing any lowering of potassium levels.

Exploring Different Types of Herbal Medicine

The main types of herbal medicine practised currently in the West are: Western, Chinese, Japanese, Tibetan, and Ayurvedic herbal medicine.

Western herbal medicine

Western herbal medicine has its roots in the Greek and Roman medical traditions and also incorporates influences from other cultures including the Native American tradition. (The herb Echinacea, for example, mentioned later in this chapter as an immune booster, was a centuries-old Native American herbal remedy that was gifted by a tribal chief to the naturopath Alfred Vogel, who brought its seeds to Europe for cultivation. Read more about this story in Chapter 13 on naturopathy.) Western herbal medicine is based on herbs that grow freely in Europe and America, many of which have now been extensively researched. Some are common garden herbs such as parsley (a diuretic that helps ease water retention) or camomile (for easing tension and aiding relaxation). However, some Western herbalists also now use herbs from other parts of the world.

Chinese herbal medicine

Herbal medicine is a branch of the thousands of years old system of Traditional Chinese Medicine (TCM). Based on ancient texts such as the *Shang Han Lun* (*The Discussion of Cold-induced Disorders*), several hundred different types of plant materials, as well as some non-plant ingredients (such as animal products or minerals) form the basis of Chinese herbal formulae. Often, several herbs are combined in one formula and the herbs are generally given in their raw form to be made into teas, or in the form of herbal pills. Formulae are designed to rebalance the *yin* and *yang* in the body and the Five Elements (for more about these, see Chapter 4) and are tailored directly to the patient, often based on ancient formulae.

Japanese herbal medicine

The Japanese herbal medicine tradition, known as *kanpo*, is based on the same principles as Chinese herbal medicine but aims to identify and treat the overall constitution, or *sho*, of the patient. This tradition also generally uses smaller numbers of ingredients than Chinese herbal formulae and the herbs are usually given in the form of fine powders. For more about *kanpo*, check out Chapter 7.

Tibetan herbal medicine

In Tibetan herbal medicine, the roots, leaves, flowers, bark, and fruits of plants are mainly used together, sometimes with crushed minerals and gemstones and very occasionally with animal products. Formulae are based on the centuries-old medical texts, the 'Four Tantras', called the *rGyud bzhi* (pronounced 'gyu-zhee'), and usually contain a number of ingredients. The aim is to balance the Three Humours of wind, bile, and phlegm. The remedies are usually given as pills or ointments, but sometimes decoctions or powders are used. Many include the plant myrobalam (*Terminalia chebula*), which, according to the Tibetan medical texts, is said to help cure all diseases.

Precious Pills are a highly prized special form of Tibetan herbal medicine. These contain extracts from gemstones such as lapis lazuli and are identified by the different colours of silk in which they are wrapped. Herbs are classified according to various properties such as 'warming' or 'cooling' and are carefully harvested and prepared according to the seasons and their inherent properties. For example, warming herbs may be dried in the sun to increase their warming properties while cooling herbs are prepared in cool shade. For more on Tibetan medicine, take a peek at Chapter 6.

Ayurvedic herbal medicine

Ayurvedic herbal medicines are used to balance the *doshas* (humours) that make up the three constitutional types of *vata* (wind), *pitta* (choler or bile), and *kapha* (phlegm). The medicines are made from plant materials such as leaves, flowers, and fruits, and may also contain spices, ground minerals and gemstones, animal fats (including *ghee*, or clarified butter), beeswax, and honey. Different plants are classified according to their tastes, potencies, and effects on the body. The herbs may be prescribed individually or in combinations and are usually given in the form of pills, powders, teas, oils, or decoctions. For more on Ayurvedic medicine, have a look at Chapter 5.

Discovering Whom and What Herbal Medicine Is Good For

Herbal medicine is used for a wide range of disorders amongst people of any age group. Common conditions treated by herbalists include the following:

- ✔ Eczema
- ✔ Asthma and other respiratory problems
- ✔ Digestive problems
- ✔ Migraine and headaches
- ✔ Joint problems
- ✔ Urinary problems
- ✔ Circulatory problems
- ✔ Menstrual and menopausal imbalance
- ✔ Insomnia
- ✔ Anxiety

Evidence that it works

Studies around the world have demonstrated the effectiveness of herbal medicine for a wide range of conditions. New regulations on herbal products in some countries (which mean that medical claims for individual herbal products have to be backed by scientific evidence) have also provided added impetus for research work.

Here are just a few of the individual herbs that now have a good body of evidence to support their use for different conditions.

- ✔ **Echinacea:** Shown to boost white blood cell count and support immune function.

- ✔ **Garlic:** Proved to lower 'bad' (low density lipoprotein) cholesterol (see Chapter 12 for more about this) and shown to be effective in reducing the severity and duration of colds and flu.

- ✔ **Ginger:** Found to help prevent or reduce travel sickness, morning sickness, and nausea associated with chemotherapy.

- ✔ **Ginkgo biloba:** Found to improve memory and blood circulation.

- ✔ **Hawthorn:** Shown to support circulation and heart function.

- ✔ **Peppermint:** Found to ease digestive irritation.

- ✔ **Saw palmetto:** May play a role in preventing prostate enlargement.

- ✔ **St John's Wort:** An effective anti-depressant. In Germany it is said that doctors prescribe this more often than anti-depressant medication to treat depression.

Other research has also investigated the use of specific herbal formulae such as Chinese herbal formulae used in the treatments of eczema and asthma. Much research has also been carried out on Japanese and Ayurvedic herbs.

You can find lots of good studies investigating the effectiveness of herbal medicine on the following Web sites:

- ✔ **Cochrane Library:** `www.cochrane.org/reviews/clibintro.htm`

- ✔ **NHS Complementary and Alternative Medicine Specialist Library:** `www.library.nhs.uk/cam`

- ✔ **PubMed:** `www.nlm.nih.gov/nccam/camonpubmed.html`

- ✔ **American Botanical Council:** `www.herbalgram.org`

When not to use herbal medicine

Just because herbs are natural doesn't necessarily mean that they're safe. Some herbs, such as belladonna, are poisonous, while others can have potent interactions with standard medicines. For example, ginkgo biloba, which has a blood-thinning effect, should not be combined with other blood-thinning medication. Also, St John's Wort isn't recommended for use at the same time as anti-depressant medication or drugs for asthma or high blood pressure and has been found to interact with the contraceptive pill and make it less effective. However, if you're already taking one of these herbs and medications simultaneously don't simply stop taking the herb because this can cause dangerous increases in blood levels of the drug you're taking. Instead, consult your GP or a herbalist as soon as possible for advice.

Herbal medicines may also be contaminated, for example with heavy metals, or be unstandardised, meaning that they may contain little or no active ingredients. Unlicensed herbal medicines may also be labelled incorrectly or contain substitute plants or even pharmaceutical ingredients, such as steroids found in some Chinese 'herbal' creams for eczema.

Only buy or use herbal products from reputable practitioners and suppliers that clearly label their products and ensure that they meet industry and legislative standards for quality and safety. In the UK, regulated herbal products always have either a Product Licence (PL) number or a Traditional Herbal Registration (THR) number on the label, so look out for these.

Always ask your herbal practitioner or product supplier to give you products clearly labelled in English, including ingredients and dosage instructions.

Additional herbal safety advice, and warnings about particular products found to be unsafe, can be found on the Medicines and Healthcare products Regulatory Agency (MHRA) Web site at www.mhra.gov.uk.

Contra-indications for herbal medicines should also be carefully followed, for example, some aren't suitable for use during pregnancy, while others that may make you sleepy aren't suitable for use while driving or operating heavy machinery. Consuming alcohol or taking recreational drugs is also inadvisable while taking herbal medicine.

In the case of serious diseases such as cancer, insulin-dependent diabetes, epilepsy, and HIV infection, among others, herbal medicine may play a part in an overall health programme but is not a substitute for orthodox medical care.

Herbal medicines need to be used with care by:

- ✔ Pregnant or breastfeeding women
- ✔ Children
- ✔ The elderly

And herbal medicine needs to be avoided if you are:

- ✔ About to undergo surgery (since some herbal medicines may alter the effects of anaesthetics or drugs used in surgery).
- ✔ Suffering from liver disease, since some herbs may affect liver function or cause toxicity.

What to Expect in a Typical Consultation

A consultation with a herbalist normally starts with some general discussion about your health.

Questioning

Your herbalist will ask about your medical history and general health as well as your current symptoms. Usually you will also be asked questions about your general diet, lifestyle, emotional health, and stress levels.

Always remember to inform your practitioner if you're taking any form of medication, such as blood pressure medication or anti-depressants, or are on the contraceptive pill or hormone replacement since these medications may interact with herbs that the practitioner decides to recommend for you.

Diagnostic methods

Medical herbalists are also trained in standard forms of medical diagnosis and so may take your pulse, check your blood pressure, listen to your chest, and so on. Practitioners of Chinese, Ayurvedic, Tibetan, or Japanese herbal medicine may also use forms of Oriental or Asian medical diagnosis such as tongue, face, and Oriental pulse diagnosis (for more on these, check out the chapters in Part II of this book).

The herbalist then usually identifies a particular herb, or a combined herbal formula, to balance your body system(s) or organ(s) that have been identified as being imbalanced and diagnosed as underlying your current symptoms.

Your herbalist may also give you advice on diet and lifestyle.

Treating with herbal remedies

Herbal medicines may be taken in a variety of different ways. Here are some of the most common applications used by herbalists:

- ✔ **Creams:** Emulsifying wax is melted in a glass bowl over a pan of boiling water and finely chopped fresh or dried plant materials are added. Glycerine and water may also be added and the mixture slowly stirred and then strained through a press, cooled, and stored in glass jars. The cream can be applied directly to your body and is often used in the treatment of eczema or other skin conditions.

- ✔ **Decoctions:** The plant material is placed in a saucepan and covered with water, which is brought to a simmer and kept simmering until the liquid has reduced by about a third. It is strained and kept cool or refrigerated for use at regular intervals during the day. Decoctions may be used for many different conditions.

- ✔ **Herbal teas/infusions:** Plant ingredients such as bark, leaves, or flowers may be infused in boiled water, steeped for a few minutes, strained and drunk as a tea. These are also sometimes known as 'tisanes'. Infusions are weaker than decoctions but may be a useful part of treatment for mild ailments, for example camomile tea to relax at bedtime or peppermint tea to aid digestion.

- ✔ **Herbal oils:** Plant ingredients may be infused in hot or cold oil (usually olive, almond, or canola oils) and stored in dark glass bottles ready for use (many oils deteriorate when exposed to light). These may be used for massage purposes, for example oils based on arnica or silver birch for easing muscular and arthritic pain or sports injuries, or for culinary use.

- ✔ **Macerations:** These are the same as infusions (see above) except the plant materials are soaked in cold water and left overnight before being strained the following morning and then drunk. Some herbs such as valerian (for promoting relaxation and treating insomnia and anxiety) are better soaked in cool than hot water.

- ✔ **Ointments:** Lard, vegetable fat, and/or beeswax are melted in a pan or in a glass bowl over boiling water. Finely chopped dried or fresh herbs are added and left to steep for 10 to 15 minutes. The mixture is strained through a fine cloth and poured into dark, glass jars and allowed to cool and set before being sealed. Herbal ointments may be used for cuts, grazes, skin infections, joint and muscle problems, and more.

- **Poultices and compresses:** These are used to enable the body to absorb herbal compounds via the skin. A poultice is a moist paste of crushed fresh herbs applied directly to the skin or wrapped in gauze and held in place for an hour or so or even overnight. A compress involves soaking a clean piece of muslin, gauze, or cotton in a hot decoction or infusion and applying it to the affected area and replacing once cooled. Poultices and compresses are good for bruises, swellings, cramps, skin problems, and so on.

- **Syrups:** A herbal infusion is made and then unrefined sugar or honey is added, stirred, and boiled until the sugar or honey has dissolved and the liquid has become thick and syrupy. It is cooled and stored using corks or non-sealant lids to prevent the bottle exploding if the sugars ferment! Syrups are often used for coughs and other respiratory complaints.

- **Tablets and capsules:** Plant materials can be dried and made into pills or tablets, or powdered and used to fill capsules, and can then easily be taken at exact dosages at regular intervals.

- **Tinctures:** Plant material is soaked in alcohol in water for one to two weeks, to extract the active ingredients, and then strained (through muslin or using a specially designed press) and bottled in dark glass bottles. Herbal tinctures are used for many types of conditions.

Duration and frequency

The first session with a herbalist is usually around 60 minutes. Follow-ups – usually after two to four weeks – are generally 15 to 30 minutes.

Often only one or two sessions are needed for minor ailments, but if you have a long-standing problem, such as chronic eczema or asthma, then treatments spaced out over several months may be needed. Herbal treatment may be adjusted at each follow-up.

At the end of the treatment, you'll be told how, and how often, to take the herbal remedies given, and you'll be advised about any possible side effects.

Knowing Whether Your Herbal Medicine Treatment Is Working

Herbal medicines generally take some time to work. Most take at least a few days, and often longer, before they become fully effective in the body, although some are much more fast-acting. Occasionally, symptoms may flare up with herbal treatment before they get better but this effect isn't very common and should only be short lived if it does occur.

Here are some tips for when you're taking herbal medicine:

✔ If you experience a marked increase in the severity of your symptoms or any pain, nausea, or other side effect, always contact your herbalist, or doctor, as soon as possible to discuss these.

✔ Ask your herbalist what improvements you can realistically expect over what sort of timescale.

✔ For best results, follow the instructions for taking the herbal remedy exactly, as well as any other dietary or lifestyle advice given.

✔ If you have no improvement after a course of treatment, then your herbal medicine may need adjusting, so it's important to maintain follow-up with your practitioner. If, even after adjustment, you obtain no relief from your symptoms, then you may need to consider another form of therapy. Discuss this situation with your practitioner.

If you experience any significant adverse reaction to any herbal medicinal product, you should report it immediately using the Yellow Card system on www.mhra.gov.uk or on Phytonet at www.escop.com/phytonet.htm.

Common Questions about Herbal Medicine Treatment

Here are some questions that I'm often asked about herbal medicine:

✔ **Do they taste horrible?** Sometimes, yes! Some herbs are bitter but liquorice is often added to sweeten the taste. In the case of herbal infusions or decoctions, you can add a little honey to sweeten the taste if you want. Most are palatable or can be disguised in juice or food.

✔ **Can I expect any side effects?** Herbal medicines of good quality prescribed by a trained herbalist and taken correctly are normally be safe to take and cause no side effects.

✔ **How long will they take to work?** Herbal medicines aren't quick fixes and generally take longer to work than standard medications.

✔ **Can I make the remedies myself?** Some simple herbal remedies can be made for home use (see the nearby sidebar for an example), but medicinal prescriptions should only be prepared by a fully trained and experienced herbalist or produced by a reliable and reputable supplier.

Helping yourself with herbal medicine

You can have a lot of fun making your own herbal teas (also known as tisanes or infusions). Creating your own tea means you can use the freshest of ingredients for really great taste, plus there's no need to drink all the bleaching agents and chemicals that go into making fine, white tea bags. Here's how:

✔ Place a handful of fresh herb leaves, such as rosemary, thyme, basil, parsley, mint, or camomile flowers, or 1 to 2 teaspoons of the dried herb, in a tea pot.

✔ Add two mugfuls of freshly boiled water, stir, and steep for eight minutes.

✔ Strain and pour.

✔ If wished, add a teaspoon of honey to sweeten or a slice of lemon, lime, or fresh ginger for added 'zing'.

✔ If using the herb for medicinal purposes (such as peppermint to ease irritable bowel), then drink a cup of the herb tea three to five times daily.

✔ If wished, you can make up a large batch, and store it in a cool place and drink it throughout the day. Any liquid not consumed in 24 hours can be given to your house or garden plants.

Take a look at Chapter 26 for more ideas on home herbal use.

Finding a Good Herbalist

To find a qualified Western herbalist or phytotherapist in your area contact one of the following:

✔ The National Institute of Medical Herbalists (NIMH) (Tel: 01392 426 022; www.nimh.org.uk). Members have the letters MNIMH or FNIMH after their names.

✔ The College of Practitioners of Phytotherapy (Herbal Advice Line: 0906 802 0117; www.phytotherapists.org). Members have the letters MCPP after their names. Various types of herbalists are also listed on the Unified Register of Herbal Practitioners (www.urhp.com).

✔ The Association of Master Herbalists (www.associationofmaster herbalists.co.uk)

✔ The International Register of Consultant Herbalists and Homeopaths (IRCH) (Tel: 01792 655 886; www.irch.org)

You can find Chinese herbal practitioners via the Register of Chinese Herbal Medicine (RCHM) (www.rchm.co.uk). *Kanpo* practitioners can be contacted via the British Kanpo Association (Tel: 020 7722 3939). Tibetan physicians can be contacted via the Tibet Foundation (Tel: 0207 930 6001; www.tibet-foundation.org). For details of contact organisations for Ayurvedic physicians, see those listed at the end of Chapter 5 on Ayurvedic medicine.

You can find general information about European herbal practitioners and regulation on the Web site of the European Herbal and Traditional Medicine Practitioners Association (www.ehpa.eu).

In the US, where there's currently no national system regulating the practice of herbal medicine, you can contact practitioners via the American Herbalists Guild (www.americanherbalist.com), or via bodies representing different types of practitioners using herbal medicine. These include:

- ✔ The American Association of Naturopathic Physicians (Toll free: 00 1 866 538 2267; www.naturopathic.org). Naturopaths are trained to use botanical medicines.

- ✔ The American Association of Oriental Medicine (Toll free: 00 1 866 455 7999; www.aaom.org) or the Acupuncture and Oriental Medicine Alliance (www.aomalliance.org). These organisations include acupuncturists who may also practise Chinese herbal medicine, depending on the laws in different states.

- ✔ The National Ayurvedic Medical Association (Tel: 00 1800 669 8914; www.ayurveda-nama.org). Practitioners use Ayurvedic herbal medicine.

In Australia, you can contact practitioners via the National Herbalists Association of Australia (NHAA) (Tel: +61 (2) 8765 0071; www.nhaa.org.au).

Other ways of finding a herbalist include:

- ✔ Asking friends, family, and colleagues for personal recommendations.

- ✔ Asking your doctor for a referral (some have links to local practitioners or even a herbal practitioner in their surgery).

- ✔ Visiting the teaching clinics at herbal medicine colleges. All students practise under close supervision from experienced practitioners and fees are low compared to private practice.

Finding out more about the safe practice of herbal medicine

Lots more useful information about the safe practice of herbal medicine, and the regulation of herbal medicine practitioners, can be found via the following links:

- ✔ **British Herbal Medicine Association (BHMA):** www.bhma.info
- ✔ **Plant Medicine:** www.phytotherapy.info
- ✔ **European Scientific Cooperative on Phytotherapy (ESCOP):** www.escop.com
- ✔ **European Herbal Practitioners Association (EHPA):** www.ehpa.eu. This association represents around 2,000 European practitioners of Western, Chinese, Tibetan, Japanese, and Ayurvedic herbal medicine.
- ✔ **American Botanical Council (ABC):** www.herbalgram.org

Counting the cost of herbal medicine

Initial herbal medicine consultations can cost from £35 to £90, while follow-up sessions are in the region of £15 to £35. Herbal medicine treatments on the NHS are free but usually exclude the cost of the herbal medicines. Some private health insurance schemes cover herbal medicine treatment. Some herbalists offer concessions for retired persons or those on benefits. Ask for details.

Ensuring satisfaction

If you're dissatisfied with your treatment, first talk things over with your practitioner. If you think that the practitioner has been negligent, incompetent, or unethical in any way, contact their professional association, who should have a formal complaints procedure in place.

Chapter 12

Nibbling on Nutritional Therapy

. . . .

In This Chapter

▶ Finding out what nutritional therapy is all about

▶ Understanding how it works

▶ Discovering what nutritional therapy can be good for

▶ Knowing what to expect in a typical consultation

▶ Finding a safe and effective nutritional therapist

. . . .

*N*utritional therapy is all about what you consume and the effect that has on your health, both now and in the future. You may hanker for cream cakes and burgers but are they doing you any good? Are they setting you up for a range of health problems in your old age such as diabetes and heart disease? A nutrition practitioner can help steer you towards making healthy dietary choices to promote health and prevent disease.

No matter which complementary therapies you're interested in, diet and nutrition always play a part to a greater or lesser degree. You have to eat to live and what you eat affects your health. Many of the therapies incorporate general dietary advice while some have quite specific dietary approaches, which this chapter explores.

I take a look at the origins and key principles of nutritional therapy and how it's practised today, including the latest in nutritional diagnostic testing. I also chew over a few of the different types of diet that are currently used in therapy.

At the end of the chapter you'll find a few nutritional therapy tips for improving your diet and your health.

Finding Out about Nutritional Therapy

Nutritional therapists work by assessing your diet and nutritional status and investigating how any dietary imbalance or nutritional deficiencies or excesses may be affecting your health. To assess digestive health and pinpoint problem areas, they may use food diaries; dietary analyses; nutritional testing by means of blood, urine, saliva, or hair analysis; and allergy or food intolerance testing.

Treatment involves dietary change, sometimes food exclusion (as in the case of food allergies or intolerances), and sometimes the use of nutritional supplements. You may also be put on some sort of detox regime to cleanse your gut and strengthen the digestive system. Sometimes other therapies may also be used such as colonics, which uses water to flush the bowel clean.

Traditional medical systems such as Chinese, Ayurvedic and Tibetan medicine all have their own specific approaches to diet. Nutritional regimes have also always been central to Nature Cure and naturopathy (see Chapters 8 and 13).

Modern nutritional medicine has taken things a step further, by incorporating scientific advances concerning individual nutrients and their role in the body, and identifying specific food and nutrient programmes for individual diseases. A large body of research now exists to support this approach.

Scientific work has also led to a specific nutritional approach called *orthomolecular therapy*, which recommends the use of mega doses of certain vitamins and minerals to treat particular physical or psychological disorders.

The aim of all nutritional therapy is to use nutritional means to strengthen the digestive process, rid the body of any excess toxins, and rebalance nutrient status in order to promote healing and well-being.

Lifestyle, exercise, stress levels, emotional well-being, and medical history are also considered as part of the diagnosis and treatment.

Nutritional therapy is used for all types of people, of all ages, with a wide range of different conditions or diseases.

A (very) brief history of nutritional therapy

In this section I look first at the nutritional approaches in traditional medicine, then consider the Nature Cure and naturopathic approaches, and lastly introduce you to modern developments in the field of nutrition.

Exploring traditional medicine ideas about nutrition

The dietary approach in traditional medicine focuses on the 'energetics' of foods and their general effects on the body.

✔ In **Traditional Chinese Medicine (TCM),** foods are divided according to their *yin*, *yang*, or neutral properties, and food advice is based on identification of the balance of the Five Elements – water, wood, fire, earth, and metal – in a person. For example, if a person is diagnosed as having an imbalance of the wood element, associated with the liver and gall bladder, then raw foods, especially leafy greens and salads, would be recommended while a person with an imbalance of the earth element, associated with the spleen and stomach, would be advised to limit sweets and sugary foods and to eat easily digestible and warming foods such as casseroles and soups. (For more about this TCM dietary approach, check out Chapter 4.)

✔ In the ancient Indian medical tradition of **Ayurveda,** you're assessed according to the strength of your digestive 'fire' and the balance of the *doshas* that determine your constitutional type. Each type is associated with specific dietary recommendations. *Vata* (wind) types are advised to chew their food slowly and to eat mainly light, easily digestible foods while avoiding stimulants like coffee and sugar and also any cold or raw foods. On the other hand, *pitta* (choler or bile) types are advised to drink lots of water and to have cooling food and drinks such as raw food, salads, and mint tea while avoiding an excess of curries and spices. The *kapha'* (phlegm) types are advised to avoid mucus-producing 'phlegmy' foods such as ice cream, dairy products, and wheat, and to control their cravings for fatty and sugary foods. Instead they're encouraged to eat and drink natural diuretics, such as watermelon and parsley tea, to get rid of excess fluid in the body. (For more about the Ayurvedic approach to diet, nip over to Chapter 5.)

✔ In **Japanese medicine,** the emphasis is on eating seasonal, fresh food in the correct combinations. Foods are classified according to their *yin* (cooling) and *yang* (warming) properties as in TCM, and alkaline foods, such as green, leafy vegetables and seaweeds, are seen as particularly beneficial to health. (For more about the Japanese approach to diet, take a look at Chapter 7.)

✔ In **Tibetan medicine,** dietary change is regarded as the most important form of therapy in tackling disease. Dietary advice is based on your classification according to the balance of three *humours* in the body. The approach is similar to the *dosha* system in Ayurveda but some of the dietary recommendations are specifically Tibetan.

Windy (*loong*) types are advised to eat nourishing foods such as *ma-sha* (soya beans), milk and butter from the female yak (known as a *dri*), and lamb dumplings (a type of *momo*) – if not vegetarian – to eat in a calm and quiet environment, and to take their time with a meal to aid digestion. They also need to avoid stimulants such as tea, coffee, and sugar. Bile (*tripa*) types need to eat lots of fresh and cooling foods and avoid mustard and other hot foods and spices and also an excess of Tibetan beer, known as *chang*. Phlegm (*peken*) types should avoid mucus-producing, cold foods like cold milk or ices and eat lots of warming foods such as clear broths that incorporate onions, garlic, and radish. (For more on the dietary treatments in Tibetan medicine, go to Chapter 6.)

Exploring Nature Cure and naturopathic ideas about nutrition

Nature Cure practitioners in the 19th and 20th centuries started looking at the constituents of individual foods and evolving the concept of 'food as medicine' for improving health and longevity and relieving disease.

- ✔ The **Nature Cure** approach to diet, advocated in Europe and the US, emphasised the benefits of a vegetarian diet combined with careful fasting to keep the colon cleansed. Raw and living foods, packed with live enzymes, were seen as particularly beneficial, as was milk, which at that time was unpasteurised and untreated and considered wholesome since it came from mountain grass-fed, free-range cattle that led natural lives. Whole grain, unrefined, and simple foods were considered the most nutritious and health-giving. (For more about this approach, take a look at Chapter 8.)

- ✔ The Nature Cure approach was incorporated into modern **naturopathic nutrition,** which uses dietary advice, healing foods, and sometimes nutritional supplementation to stimulate your body's natural healing ability and to address specific ailments by nutritional means. (For more about naturopathy, go to Chapter 13.)

Exploring modern ideas about nutrition

In the 20th and 21st centuries, the focus in nutritional medicine has been on identifying and investigating the role of individual nutrients. This work grew out of earlier discoveries that certain foods can help prevent and relieve particular diseases. For example, James Lind discovered that citrus fruit can ward off the disease of scurvy, characterised by bleeding gums, bruising, and eventually death, and suffered by sailors on long voyages without any fresh fruit or vegetables. However, he didn't know that scurvy was actually a nutritional deficiency disease.

That leap came later from the work of Polish biochemist Casimir Funk, living in London in the 1920s, who first suggested that tiny components of food may be vital for the maintenance of health. He called these *vital amines* (*vita* meaning life and *amines* meaning organic derivatives of ammonia), also known as *vitamines* and then later renamed as *vitamins*, when it was realised that he'd got the ammonia bit wrong!

Funk and British biochemist, Frederick Hopkins, went on to propose that diseases such as scurvy, rickets, beri-beri, and pellagra (take a look at Table 12-1 for the gory details) were actually nutrient deficiency diseases. This simple, yet earth-shattering, proposal was the beginning of the end for such diseases and the beginning of nutritional therapy as an important field of medicine.

Table 12-1   **Dietary Deficiency Diseases**

Vitamin Deficiency	Vitamin A (Retinol)	Vitamin B1 (Thiamin)	Vitamin B2 (Riboflavin)	Vitamin B3 (Niacin)	Folic Acid	Vitamin C	Vitamin D
Disease		*Beri-beri*		*Pellagra*	*Megablastic Anaemia*	*Scurvy*	*Rickets/ Osteomalacia*
Where?	Developing world, especially poorer countries in East Asia, Africa, India	China, Japan, Thailand, Philippines, Malaysia	Developing world	Africa, Central America	Developing world	Anywhere	Developing world
Who?	Children, pregnant women; in the West, occasionally fussy eaters, homeless, smokers, alcoholics, elderly	Children or adults that are malnourished, alcoholics, drug addicts	Alcoholics, smokers, tea and coffee drinkers, vegans	Anyone	Elderly, pregnant women, alcoholics, homeless, epileptics on medication, people with malabsorption problems, sometimes vegetarians/ vegans on limited diets	Ancient sailors, elderly, babies, smokers, food faddists who don't eat any fresh fruit or vegetables	Traditionally, sufferers were poor children in industrial cities made to work indoors or climb chimneys, those with lack of light exposure such as the elderly or sometimes devout Muslim women who stay fully covered whenever outside

(continued)

Table 12-1 *(continued)*

Vitamin Deficiency	*Vitamin A (Retinol)*	*Vitamin B1 (Thiamin)*	*Vitamin B2 (Riboflavin)*	*Vitamin B3 (Niacin)*	*Folic Acid*	*Vitamin C*	*Vitamin D*
Disease		*Beri-beri*		*Pellagra*	*Megablastic Anaemia*	*Scurvy*	*Rickets/ Osteomalacia*
Signs and symptoms	Acne, dandruff, cystitis, thrush, poor vision, night blindness, stunted growth, skin problems	Two types of beri-beri: **Dry** causes tingling, numbness in limbs, muscle weakness, paralysis; **Wet** causes swelling, water retention, heart and circulation problems	Cracks and sores in mouth and eyes, grit under eyelids, chapped skin, cataracts, hair loss, sluggishness, trembling	Itching skin (first sign), and then dermatitis, diarrhoea, dementia; skin becomes dark and scaly, made worse by light exposure; digestive problems, mental disorder	Retarded growth, weakness, vertigo, breathlessness, pallor, premature grey hair, sore and red tongue	Small red spots, bleeding gums, bruising, delayed wound healing, weakness, pain, anaemia	Weak bones, knock knees, bow legs, muscular weakness, respiratory infections, convulsions
Causes	Insufficient intake of Vitamin A or beta-carotene-rich foods or lack of enzymes for conversion of beta-carotene into retinol	Only eating white rice, stripped of Vitamin B1, easily destroyed by heat	Stable with heat but destroyed by UV light and irradiation	Maize-based diet; lack of milk and eggs; rich in the amino acid tryptophan, which can be converted into nicotinamide (a precursor for B3)	Insufficient folic acid-rich foods in diet, over-cooking foods	Insufficient fresh fruit and vegetables in the diet; poor cooking techniques that cause Vitamin C loss, such as over-boiling vegetables in lots of water or re-heating food	Lack of exposure to sunlight, dietary lack

Vitamin Deficiency	Vitamin A (Retinol)	Vitamin B1 (Thiamin)	Vitamin B2 (Riboflavin)	Vitamin B3 (Niacin)	Folic Acid	Vitamin C	Vitamin D
Disease		Beri-beri		Pellagra	Megablastic Anaemia	Scurvy	Rickets/Osteomalacia
End result?	Blindness and death due to diarrhoea and gastrointestinal disease	Heart failure and death	Often occurs together with beri-beri; people usually die of beri-beri before riboflavin deficiency is diagnosed	Death rate peaked in 1920s and 1930s, now common only in parts of South Africa	Premature birth, miscarriage, impaired protein synthesis, poor replacement of red blood cells	Death	Death (usually from respiratory infection)
Food sources	Egg yolk; fish; butter; offal (Vitamin A); all yellow, orange red, and dark green vegetables (beta-carotene)	Milk, offal pork, eggs, whole grains, fortified cereals	Marmite, lamb's liver, mushrooms, watercress, asparagus, bean sprouts, milk, mackerel	Beef, chicken, liver, fish, nuts, rice (niacin); milk, cheese, eggs (tryptophan)	Whole grains, bulgur wheat, chicken liver, kidney beans, chick peas, orange juice, green vegetables	Fresh fruit and vegetables, especially citrus fruits	Dairy produce, butter, fortified margarines and cereals, fatty fish (but most Vitamin D is produced in the body from sunlight exposure)

Nutrients in the news

Vitamins and minerals are not the only nutrients to have made headline news. Other hot topics in the field of nutrition have been the following:

✔ **Fibre:** Found in plant foods, fibre passes undigested through the body and is needed to promote regular bowel movements and maintain healthy cholesterol levels. *Soluble fibre*, found in oats, pulses, fruits, and vegetables, can help reduce low-density lipoprotein (LDL) (sometimes known as bad cholesterol) in the blood and balance blood sugar levels by slowing sugar absorption. *Insoluble fibre*, found mainly in cereals and whole grains, aids bowel movements and helps ward off hunger by making you feel full. Adults need a minimum of 25g of fibre in their diet every day.

✔ **Water:** Dehydration is a really common problem due to people not drinking enough water and drinking too many diuretic drinks such as coffee, tea, and colas, which cause your body to lose water. Around 70 per cent of your body is made up of water and it is essential for normal cellular function, for healthy digestion, circulation, excretion, brain function, and temperature regulation. Dehydration can cause impaired mental function; headaches; heart, kidney, liver, and gall bladder problems; and eventually death. You can get water from both foods (fruit, vegetables, grains, fish, meat, and so on) and drinks, but adults need 35ml fluid per kilogram of body weight from all these sources daily to stay healthy. For most people, this means around six to eight glasses of water daily sipped between meals or before meals (to prevent dilution of digestive juices). Tap water may be contaminated with heavy metals, pesticides, and other pollutants, so drinking filtered or glass-bottled water may be more beneficial for health.

Drinking an excess of water can be as dangerous as not drinking enough as it can seriously affect the sodium/potassium mineral balance in the body and cause kidney problems.

✔ **Antioxidants:** A lot of attention has been paid recently to the role of certain antioxidants, which are food substances that may help prevent damage and ageing in the body. Antioxidants include vitamins A, C, and E, carotenoids (substances such as beta-carotenes that give carrots and other vegetables their orange, red, yellow, and green colours and which the body can convert into Vitamin A), and the mineral selenium. Some studies suggest that these substances may help prevent diseases such as cancer, heart disease, and stroke and that they should be included in the diet daily in the form of fresh fruit and vegetables, nuts, and seeds.

✔ **Phyto-nutrients:** From the Greek word *phyto*, meaning 'plant', phyto-nutrients are biologically active plant compounds that give plants their colour, flavour, and smell, and which also have special health benefits. They are thought to protect the body against damage from free radicals (rogue particles that damage and destroy tissue) and a range of diseases including cancer and heart disease. Hundreds of phyto-nutrients have been identified in recent years and they include phyto-oestrogens, found in soya, red clover, cereals, pulses, nuts, and seeds, which are similar to human oestrogen and may help prevent menopausal symptoms and certain types of cancer; and glucosinolates, found in brassica vegetables such as broccoli and cabbage, which may protect against heart disease and cancer.

✔ **'Good' and 'bad' fats:** Saturated fatty acids – found mainly in animal fats – plus trans fats and hydrogenated fats created unnaturally during food processing have been linked to heart disease and cancer. However, polyunsaturated *essential fatty acids* found in vegetable oils, polyunsaturated margarine, nuts, and seeds (the omega 6s) and in oily fish, such as mackerel, salmon, trout, herring, sardines, and pilchards; fish oils; and some nuts and seeds (the omega 3s) have been found to be beneficial for health and to help maintain healthy heart, liver, and brain function.

✔ **Cholesterol:** Made in the body and obtained from the diet (liver, eggs, and meat) and needed for building and repair of cells. It is now known that both good and bad types of cholesterol exist. Low-density lipoproteins (LDL cholesterol), and very-low-density lipoproteins (VLDL cholesterol), known as bad cholesterols, increase in the body with diets high in saturated fats and lead to increased risk of blocked arteries and heart disease. On the other hand, high-density lipoproteins (HDL cholesterol), also known as good cholesterol, help remove excess cholesterol from the tissues and reduce the risk of cardiovascular problems.

Grasping the idea behind nutritional therapy

According to nutritional therapy, the underlying root cause of nutritional and digestive imbalances leading to diseases may be any, or a combination of, the following:

✔ Regular consumption of refined and processed foods, such as white bread, flour, pasta and rice, ready-meals, and so on, leading to a low intake of essential nutrients.

✔ Frequent intake of junk foods loaded with unhealthy fats, salt, sugar, and so on that may damage the internal organs.

✔ Modern vegetables having lower levels of nutrients due to impoverisation of the soil because of intensive farming practices.

✔ Inadequate fibre in the diet due to eating refined bread, pasta, cereals, and so on, leading to constipation.

✔ Dehydration due to low water intake and high intake of diuretics such as coffee and tea, which contribute to a loss of body fluids and slow down gut function.

✔ Lack of sufficient essential fatty acids, found in plant, nut, and seed oils and in oily fish, to soothe the lining of the intestines and prevent or reduce inflammation.

✔ Intake of anti-nutrient foods that may strip the body of important nutrients, for example over consumption of caffeine and tannins in tea and coffee can interfere with absorption of minerals such as magnesium and calcium.

✔ Toxins and chemicals ingested with foods such as pesticides on grains; heavy metals contained in fish oils; growth hormones, antibiotics, and other drugs given to commercially reared animals and fish.

✔ Weakened digestive systems due to intake of antibiotics and other medications that affect the balance of healthy bacteria in the gut.

✔ Improper digestive enzyme and stomach acid production due to irregular eating habits, not chewing food properly, eating too fast, chewing gum, and stress, leading to inadequate breakdown of foods in the stomach and malabsorption of nutrients.

✔ 'Leaky gut' syndrome whereby the gut becomes increasingly permeable due to inflammation and damage, and toxins and food waste products are passed back into the bloodstream.

✔ Food allergies and food intolerances (delayed onset food sensitivities), which mean that the body identifies 'safe' foods as 'invaders' and produces antibodies against them.

✔ Poor eating habits such as skipped meals (especially breakfast), bolting down food at a desk instead of taking lunch breaks, doing other activities (such as watching TV) while eating, eating late at night, and eating in-between meals.

✔ Bad cooking habits such as over-boiling food, cooking in lots of water, keeping food hot for long periods, and reheating food, which can lead to destruction and loss of nutrients in food.

✔ Lifestyle habits, such as stress, late nights, and overwork, that impair the body's physical functions including digestion.

✔ Exposure to environmental chemicals via pollution, paints, solvents, cleaning fluids, dental amalgam, and so on, which increase the toxic load in the body.

✔ Sedentary lifestyles and lack of regular exercise leading to loss of muscle tone and constipation, which contribute to a build up of waste products in the body.

✔ Less, and shorter duration of, breastfeeding of babies and too early, or inappropriate, weaning of infants onto solid foods, predisposing them to digestive problems as adults.

The aim of nutritional therapy is to identify and correct these sources of imbalance using dietary adjustment, nutritional supplements (if necessary), and lifestyle change.

TECHNICAL STUFF

What's the difference between nutritional therapists, nutritionists, and dieticians?

Since nutrition is not yet fully regulated as a profession, the differences between various professionals offering nutritional advice can be confusing and so it is a good idea to ask your practitioner about training, experience and membership of a professional body. At this point, anyone can call themselves a nutritional therapist or nutritionist, but the title dietician is protected.

Nutritional therapists are usually people who have taken some sort of nutritional therapy training that includes nutrition theory and clinical practice. In general, these courses are becoming increasingly comprehensive and many now have degree status. The new Nutritional Therapy Council (NTC) (www.nutritional therapycouncil.org.uk), which is spearheading self-regulation for nutritional therapists, recommends that anyone using this title should meet the National Occupational Standards for Nutritional Therapy and should complete a recognised training course with minimum requirements for training and practice. Nutritional therapists may be members of various bodies but are now being encouraged to register with the new NTC.

Some nutritional therapists prefer to call themselves *nutritional practitioners* or *consultants*. There is also a move to classify those who have done just short courses in nutrition as *nutritional advisors* rather than fully trained therapists/practitioners.

People using the title *nutritionist* are often those who have done a degree-level training in nutrition but who may have had no clinical experience in treating people with nutritional therapy and are unable to advise on the use of nutrition in the treatment of disease. Often such people work in public health, commercial, or educational settings, and give dietary advice based on the latest research and nutritional knowledge. Many of these degree-level nutritionists are members of the Nutrition Society (www.nutritionsociety.org), which operates a voluntary register for trained nutritionists and is seeking protection for this title. However, just to make this situation more confusing, some practitioners, using nutrition in clinical settings, like to call themselves nutritionists too, whether they have a degree-level training or not and even if they're not members of the Nutrition Society.

Dieticians are those who have taken a regulated degree-level training in dietetics and have had clinical training in the NHS. They can call themselves dieticians only if they have completed this training, and they must be registered with the Health Professions Council (HPC) in the UK to be allowed to work. Dieticians are trained to advise on special diets for people with different diseases, usually in hospital settings, and the professional body that represents them is the British Dietetic Association (BDA) (www.bda.uk.com).

Nutritional therapy today

With nutrition constantly in the media, from chef Jamie Oliver's focus on the poor state of school dinners; to the National Health Service's (NHS) focus on child obesity; to food scare stories and well-publicised government dietary guidelines, nutrition education, research and therapy are all becoming increasingly important.

As consumers become more aware of what they eat, highlighted by various popular television programmes on nutrition, increasing numbers of people are seeking out nutritional experts for help and advice.

Many different health professionals provide nutrition advice. These include nutritional therapists, practitioners or consultants, nutritionists, dieticians, doctors, nurses, and other complementary medicine practitioners such as naturopaths.

Exploring other types of nutritional therapy

Orthomolecular therapy, created by the double Nobel-prize-winning scientist, Dr Linus Pauling, in the 1990s, advocates the use of large doses of individual vitamins, minerals, or amino acids to treat different types of illnesses. Some support for this comes from research, which shows that high doses of Vitamin C may reduce the duration and severity of the common cold and may help clear blocked arteries, while high doses of magnesium may aid recovery after heart attacks and may help ease chronic fatigue syndrome. However, this approach remains controversial and research into it is ongoing.

Understanding How It Works

Nutritional therapy aims to strengthen your digestive system and rebalance nutrient status by means of the following:

- ✔ Providing you with a revised diet to improve your health. Often junk food items, refined foods, processed foods, and ready-meals are replaced with whole grains, and increased fresh fruit and vegetables, to give a more balanced intake of food components and nutrients.

- ✔ Dietary variety may be increased by introducing you to new foods, thus widening the range of foods eaten.

- ✔ Foods that trigger allergies or intolerances may be identified and removed from your diet or put on a rotation basis whereby you eat them only every other or every fourth day.

- ✔ Individual nutrient deficiencies may be identified and then corrected with either foods or nutritional supplements; for example, people low in iron may be encouraged to eat more iron-rich foods, such as prunes, or to take iron supplements.

✔ Excess nutrients, usually due to taking too much of a particular supplement, will also be corrected (usually by stopping or replacing the supplement). For example, some people take high levels of pure ascorbic acid (Vitamin C) and this can cause stomach irritation and diarrhoea. A 'buffered' type of non-acidic Vitamin C may be recommended in its place and the dose adjusted according to need.

✔ Individual foods or nutrients may be used to rebalance particular parts of the digestive system. For example, digestive enzymes from papaya, pineapple, or sprouted seeds, such as alfalfa, may be used to increase enzyme levels in the stomach to aid in the breakdown of foods. Or *probiotics* – beneficial bacteria – found in live and fermented foods such as live yoghurt or buttermilk, may be introduced to increase the levels of healthy bacteria in the intestines.

✔ Cleansing and detox diets may be used to cleanse the gut. For example, powdered psyllium husk and slippery elm compounds are sometimes used to facilitate the removal of waste products from the large intestine and to promote effective bowel movements.

The idea is that when the digestive system is working more efficiently, the diet is balanced, and correct nutritional status is established, better health ensues.

Discovering Whom and What Nutritional Therapy Is Good For

Nutritional therapy may be requested by those who just want general dietary advice, for example a young mother wanting advice on feeding her child, a teenager who wants to become vegetarian, or an athlete aiming for optimum sports nutrition. Increasingly, however, nutritional advice is being sought for specific conditions.

Conditions that nutritional therapists treat

Today's nutritional therapists commonly treat a wide range of disorders, including the following:

✔ Digestive problems including constipation, diarrhoea, indigestion, irritable bowel syndrome, Crohn's disease, and colitis

✔ Attention deficit and hyperactivity disorders

✔ Headaches and migraine

✔ Arthritis

    ✔ Circulation problems

    ✔ Respiratory problems such as asthma

    ✔ Menstrual and menopausal problems

    ✔ Eye, ear, nose, and throat problems

    ✔ Food intolerances and food allergies

Research evidence supports the use of nutritional therapy for a range of conditions but more good research is also needed.

Evidence that it works

A substantial body of research now exists linking certain foods and diets to particular health conditions such as high levels of fat intake with heart disease, high-sugar and refined carbohydrate diets with late onset diabetes, and diets low in fresh vegetables and fruits with certain cancers. The work of Professor Jane Plant has also suggested that intake of dairy products may be linked to breast and prostate cancers, and research by Dr Alan and Maryon Stewart has linked different types of diets with menstrual and menopausal imbalance.

Other research has shown that certain types of diet may lower risk and reduce symptoms. Examples of this type of research include evidence that high fibre diets can decrease the risk of colon cancer and that vegetarian diets can decrease the risk of conditions including gall bladder disease and the symptoms of some types of arthritis.

Increasing numbers of studies have also looked at the role of individual nutrients or foods in different diseases. Research at Bastyr University in the US has investigated the role of Vitamin C intake during pregnancy, the role of garlic in treating helicobacter pylori infection, and the role of chromium in balancing blood sugar levels, to name but a few examples. Other research has shown the role of B vitamins such as folic acid in reducing the risk of heart disease and preventing spina bifida in newborns (a condition where the spine and nerves don't form properly), the role of magnesium in treating chronic fatigue conditions, and the role of Vitamin B6 in treating premenstrual syndrome.

Sometimes nutrition research has been controversial, as in a large study using Vitamin E with patients with lung cancer, which had to be stopped because those taking the supplement were faring worse than those who were not. However, close investigation showed that *synthetic* Vitamin E, rather than natural form Vitamin E, was being used in the trial, which may have confounded results since synthetic Vitamin E is far less beneficial to the body and may even be harmful. This example illustrates how important it is to examine studies and their results carefully when drawing conclusions.

ANECDOTE

All in the mind? A case of food intolerance

I recently had a businessman as a patient who'd experienced digestive problems for 20 years. He suffered from abdominal pain, wind, bloating, indigestion, and vomiting, and was frequently unable to keep his food down. He had had every type of medical investigation possible and had seen a whole host of specialists, who could find nothing abnormal. On looking at his diet, I saw that certain foods were repeated over and over and decided to run a food intolerance test. His results came back showing a strong intolerance to some of these foods. I helped him to plan a new diet avoiding these foods and adding in lots of healthy alternatives. He kept to the new diet religiously, with the help of his family, although he was pretty sceptical about its likely effects. At the same time I recommended some digestive enzymes, essential fatty acids, and beneficial bacteria (probiotics) to rebalance his digestive system.

Within three weeks he was amazed to find his symptoms markedly improved, and within five weeks they had completely cleared. As a side effect, he was also feeling more energetic and clearer headed. He couldn't believe that 20 years of discomfort and pain could be resolved so simply, and he enthusiastically informed his doctor about his progress. The doctor completely rejected the idea of food intolerance, saying it was unproven, and suggested that his cure had been 'all in the mind' and resolved itself. So my patient did an experiment for himself. He reintroduced a few of the offending foods and within hours all his symptoms were back! He has therefore stuck to his new diet, gradually reintroducing some of the foods to which he was only mildly sensitive, and three years later he is still symptom-free.

For more on nutritional research, check out the Cochrane Library (www.cochrane.org/reviews/clibintro.htm), the NHS Complementary and Alternative Medicine Specialist Library (www.library.nhs.uk/cam), the Bastyr University site (www.bastyr.edu/research), and the PubMed database (www.nlm.nih.gov/nccam/camonpubmed.html).

When not to use nutritional therapy

Nutrition and diet play a useful role in most conditions but you must always consider medical treatment in the case of serious diseases such as cancer and diabetes. In such cases, keep your doctor informed about any dietary changes or nutritional supplementation.

Care also needs to be taken if you're on medication since some nutrients and drugs can interact. Always seek careful advice from an experienced and qualified nutritional therapist and your doctor in such cases.

Never take mega doses of nutrients unless a specific clinical reason exists and a trained professional is carefully monitoring their use. Nutritional supplements also need to be used with great care in the case of pregnant women, the elderly, and children.

Never use nutritional supplements as a substitute for proper, healthy eating.

What to Expect in a Typical Consultation

A consultation with a nutritional therapist generally starts with a discussion about your diet and health.

Questioning

The nutritional therapist will ask about your medical history and general health as well as your current symptoms. You'll be asked detailed questions about your diet and may be asked to complete a food diary for a week before attending. Also be prepared to be asked questions about your bowel movements, which give the practitioner valuable information about the functioning of your digestive system.

Diagnostic methods

The practitioner may examine your tongue, eyes, and skin and may palpate your abdomen to obtain information about digestive function. Tests may also be used to investigate your nutritional status. These tests can be any of the following:

- ✓ **Hair mineral analysis** to test for mineral levels and the presence of toxic heavy metals such as lead and mercury. This test is regarded as useful by many nutritional practitioners but considered unreliable by most medical practitioners.

- ✓ **Blood tests** to investigate your levels of different vitamins and/or minerals, essential fatty acids, and so on. These tests are generally considered to be reliable by both nutritional practitioners and medics.

- ✓ **Toxicity tests** that use urine analysis to investigate the levels of heavy metals and toxins stored in your tissues. These tests are used by doctors and naturopaths in the US and by nutritional therapists in the UK.

✔ **Bio-electrical tests** that use various types of electrical measuring devices to test for food sensitivities and allergies and 'energetic' imbalances. These devices are generally considered to be unreliable by doctors. Go to Chapter 22 on Energy Medicine for more details about these devices.

✔ **Kinesiology**, which is a form of muscle testing, is sometimes used to test for problem foods or nutritional deficiencies. Many regard this technique as unreliable. Read more about it in Chapter 16 on bodywork therapies.

✔ **Food allergy and food intolerance testing** using blood tests to determine immediate or delayed onset food allergies. See the nearby sidebar for more details.

Is the food you eat making you ill?

Food allergies and food intolerances are both sensitivity reactions to foods (or drinks, food additives, colourings, and so on) and can lead to a range of symptoms. Food allergies involve an immune system response and the production of specific antibodies called IgE antibodies. Common allergens are peanuts, shellfish, tree nuts, and eggs, and reactions can be swift and even life-threatening as the tissues swell and the airways become restricted.

In the case of food intolerances, also known as delayed onset food sensitivity, the reaction is less severe and may occur some time after the food has been eaten. In this case, the body is thought to produce different types of antibodies known as IgG antibodies, although this has not yet been conclusively demonstrated. Such sensitivities may also be linked to a lack of digestive enzymes for breaking down food effectively. Typical symptoms are bloating, wind, and an irritable bowel and may also include other conditions such as migraine, asthma, and eczema.

In the case of food allergies, any contact with the offending foods must be avoided completely, so sufferers need to read food labels carefully and take care in public places such as restaurants. Many food allergy sufferers carry emergency auto-injectors for the administration of a drug in case they inadvertently come into contact with an allergen and suffer a sudden extreme reaction, known as *anaphylactic shock.* In the case of delayed onset food intolerances, it may only be necessary to avoid the food for a period of time, after which it may be reintroduced on a rotation basis. Introducing a wider range of alternative foods, strengthening the digestive system and increasing digestive enzyme production may also help. In some cases where the food intolerance remains the food may need to be avoided on a more long-term basis. Common food intolerances are wheat, dairy, citrus fruit, tomatoes and potatoes.

The whole topic of food intolerance and food intolerance testing remains controversial in the eyes of many medics, and many people choose to do food intolerance testing privately. A recent study showed that more than 70 per cent of people using a home food intolerance test kit reported symptom relief after excluding the identified foods.

Types of treatment

Treatment involves recommendations on dietary adjustments, sometimes with food exclusion or food rotation, and often the introduction of new foods. Nutritional supplements may also be recommended.

Nutritional therapists may also recommend certain therapies alongside their nutritional advice. These may include the following:

- ✔ **Colonics:** A technique using water to flush the intestines and remove compacted waste matter. This is more thorough than an enema and involves special equipment and training. There is little research evidence to support its use however, and some critics believe that it can lead to weakening of the colon if done incorrectly or too often.

- ✔ **Chelation therapy:** This involves introducing certain nutritional compounds into the body intravenously to draw out heavy metals from the tissues. This treatment has been used for several decades but remains controversial as insufficient research evidence exists to support it.

Some nutritional therapists are also trained in other disciplines such as naturopathy, homeopathy, and herbal medicine and may incorporate approaches from these disciplines into your consultation.

Duration and frequency

The first nutritional therapy session is generally around 60 minutes, while follow-up visits may be 30 minutes. Follow-up sessions are usually after a few weeks, once you've had a chance to put the dietary advice into practice or to get started on taking nutritional supplements.

At the end of the first consultation, you may be asked

- ✔ To follow some sort of diet sheet outlining the dietary recommendations given to you. You'll need to rethink your food shopping, meal preparation, and eating habits to put these recommendations into practice.

- ✔ To take certain nutritional supplements. To make this easier you should be given details of when and how, and for how long, to take each one.

Follow the advice that you are given carefully and do not exceed the recommended doses for any supplements prescribed. More is not necessarily better and can be dangerous.

Munching your way through different diets

Your practitioner may recommend a specific type of diet for you. Here are some diets that are currently popular:

✔ **Atkins Diet:** A low-carbohydrate, high-protein diet devised in the 1970s, by American Dr Robert Atkins, this diet involves cutting out high-carbohydrate foods such as bread, pasta, and sugar while eating lots of high-protein food such as meat, cheese, and eggs. Critics have said that it can lead to heart and kidney problems and it is falling out of favour.

✔ **Blood Group Diet:** Formulated by American naturopath Peter D'Adamo, this plan involves basing your diet on your blood type. This diet has a celebrity following but many doctors and nutritionists don't believe that it has any scientific basis.

✔ **Detox Diet:** Many variations of this diet exist within the naturopathic tradition. It generally involves cutting out all refined and processed foods and following a vegetarian (no meat or fish) or vegan (no meat, fish, dairy, eggs, or any animal products) diet and drinking plenty of water.

✔ **Gerson Diet:** This controversial anti-cancer diet developed in the 1920s, by Dr Max Gerson is based on an hourly intake of juiced organic vegetables, an organic, low-salt vegan diet, and coffee enemas.

✔ **Hay Diet:** A system devised by Dr William Hay based on optimal food-combining. It involves avoiding combinations of proteins and carbohydrates at the same meal, and many people find it helpful. However, doctors generally reject it arguing that most plant foods contain both proteins and carbohydrates and that the digestive system is designed to deal with both mixed together.

✔ **Living Foods Diet:** Formulated by Dr Ann Wigmore from the 1950s onwards and based on raw, enzyme-rich live foods such as sprouted seeds, grains, and wheatgrass. Her work has also led to the popularity of many raw food diets today where no cooked food is consumed.

✔ **Life Choice Diet:** Formulated by American Dr Dean Ornish in the 1990s, this low-fat vegetarian diet emphasises vegetables, fruit, and beans and an intake of less than 10 per cent fat. Sugar and alcohol are also avoided.

✔ **Macrobiotic Diet:** Devised by George Osawa in Japan in the 1950s, this diet classifies foods according to their *yin* and *yang* properties (see Chapter 7) and excludes sugar and refined and processed foods.

✔ **Zone Diet:** Formulated by American biochemist Dr Barry Sears in 1990, this diet is based on keeping insulin levels on an even keel by having a balanced intake of proteins and carbohydrates and avoiding sudden high-carbohydrate/refined-sugar intake.

Users of these diets have claimed many health benefits from them; however, few are backed by conclusive research and many regard them as fad diets.

Inform your nutritional therapist of any medication that you're on and to inform your doctor of any supplements that you decide to take. Also inform your practitioner if you're pregnant or likely to become pregnant, because you'll need to avoid certain foods and supplements. A folic acid supplement is usually recommended to reduce the risk of the baby developing spina bifida (a condition where the spine and nerves don't form properly).

Knowing whether your nutritional therapy treatment is working

Sometimes people feel almost immediate benefits after making simple dietary changes, but others may find that reduction of symptoms can take time, as the body needs to readjust and heal. Nutritional supplements can also take time to become fully effective in the body.

Keeping a food diary and a symptom record to monitor changes can be helpful so that you can discuss your progress with your practitioner.

Finding a Good Nutritional Therapist or Nutritionist

The Nutritional Therapy Council (NTC; www.nutritionaltherapycouncil.org.uk) is leading the way with professional voluntary self-regulation of nutritional therapists and is establishing a register of practitioners and a process for accrediting nutrition training courses.

Other nutrition associations that currently maintain directories of nutritional therapists include:

- ✔ British Association for Nutritional Therapy (BANT; Tel/Fax: 0870 606 1284; www.bant.org.uk)
- ✔ The Register of Nutritional Therapists (RNT; www.nutritionalmed.co.uk)
- ✔ Wholistic Nutritional Medicine Society (WNMS; Tel: 0207 935 3533)

The Nutrition Society (www.nutritionsociety.org) also maintains a voluntary register for nutritionists.

In the US, many nutritional therapists are members of The American Association of Nutritional Consultants (AANC; Tel: 00 1 888 828 2262 or see www.aanc.net for an online directory). However, the credentials of some of its members have been questioned as some only have correspondence course training in nutrition.

The American Society for Nutrition (www.nutrition.org) is a learned society dedicated to nutrition research and education. Lots of nutrition information can be found in its journals; *The Journal of Nutrition* and *The American Journal of Clinical Nutrition*.

Because no formal registration currently exists for nutritional therapists, enquiring about the practitioner's level of experience and training is essential.

The following are some other suggestions for finding a nutritional therapist:

- ✔ Ask friends, family, and colleagues for personal recommendations of practitioners.
- ✔ Some sports and leisure clubs offer nutritional consultations.
- ✔ Consider visiting the teaching clinics at colleges with courses in nutrition. Students practise under close supervision from experienced practitioners and fees are low compared to private practice.

Counting the cost of nutritional therapy

Initial nutritional therapy consultations may cost between £35 and £100, while follow-up sessions are between £25 and £65. The cost of tests and supplements is usually extra.

Ensuring satisfaction

If you're dissatisfied with your treatment, first talk things over with your practitioner.

If you think that the practitioner has been negligent, unethical, or incompetent, contact their professional body and use the formal complaints procedure.

Helping Yourself with Nutritional Therapy

Here are ten dietary tips to help you achieve better health:

- ✔ **Eat more vegetables and fruit.** These foods are rich in nutrients, fibre, and health-giving antioxidants and including at least five a day in your diet is recommended.
- ✔ **Eat more healthy fats.** Decrease your intake of unhealthy, saturated or hydrogenated fats and increase intake of essential fats contained in seeds, nuts and plant oils and in oily fish (no more than three times a week for the latter, in case of contamination with heavy metals).

✔ **Eat more fibre.** Replace white bread, rice, and pasta with brown, whole grain versions.

✔ **Eat less sugar.** Cut out the sweets and sugary treats and satisfy your sweet tooth with fresh fruits and berries.

✔ **Go raw!** Try having a little raw food at the start of each meal, such as a side salad or a piece of fruit, to encourage digestive enzyme production.

✔ **Drink more water and less caffeine and alcohol.** Try swapping your latte for a healthy herbal tea or fresh juice and drink water throughout the day to stay hydrated.

✔ **Eat fresh organic and free-range produce.** Buy it whenever you can and support local producers to reduce your 'food miles'.

✔ **Cut down on table salt.** Flavour your food with a little seaweed or vegetable salt instead.

✔ **Maintain a healthy body weight.** And don't over- or under-eat.

✔ **Adopt healthy eating habits.** Always eat breakfast. Eat a wide variety of foods to meet all your nutrient needs. Eat little and often, if necessary, to maintain even blood sugar levels. Eat slowly in a calm environment to aid digestion. Chew your food well.

Chapter 13

Diving into Naturopathy

*N*aturopathy is a health philosophy and healthcare system based on the idea that the body has the power to heal itself. Unhealthy lifestyles are seen as the trigger for disease and various therapies and self-care regimens are used to help the body back to a natural state of health.

In this chapter you discover the thinking behind naturopathy and how it evolved over time from the Nature Cures of the 19th century to a popular form of healthcare today that has even influenced modern medicine.

You find out how naturopaths consider that the right food, water, air, light exposure, work/rest balance, and exercise are so important, and I introduce you to the range of therapies that are part of the modern day naturopath's healing repertoire.

On the way you also discover some tips on how to find a good naturopathic practitioner and what sort of questions you may want to ask, and I give you a naturopathic self-care technique that you may like to try out for yourself.

Finding Out about Naturopathy

The philosophy behind naturopathy dates back to Hippocrates, in ancient Greece, who stressed that proper diet, exercise, and rest could be used to maintain health and that cures should only be used to stimulate the body's natural healing ability. *Naturopathy*, or naturopathic medicine, therefore, seeks to help you make lifestyle changes that will support your health and uses natural therapies (that is, therapies that don't involve drugs or surgery) to support the self-healing process.

Naturopaths look for the underlying causes of disease, rather than focus on individual symptoms alone. They're interested in the whole person, rather than just the ailment, and seek to restore, maintain, and promote health as well as prevent future disease.

Naturopathic healing approaches utilise water (hydrotherapy), air and light, diet and nutrition, herbs, homeopathy, manipulation techniques, and acupuncture. Naturopaths also give you self-care recommendations to help transform your unhealthy habits into healthy ones.

Modern day naturopathy combines ancient knowledge of natural therapies with modern scientific knowledge about nutrition and health. Because it doesn't focus on individual disease or symptoms naturopathy can be used by anyone – even if you feel well! Naturopathy aims to help you attain your full health potential in terms of physical, mental, and emotional health.

A (very) brief history of naturopathy

Modern day naturopathy has its roots in the work of European and American Nature Cure practitioners in the 19th and early 20th centuries, such as Vincent Priessnitz, the founder of hydrotherapy (water cure) and Johannes Schroth, who was one of the first to show the importance of diet and nutrition. (For lots more about Nature Cure and its pioneers, check out Chapter 8.)

The term naturopathy, meaning 'natural treatment', was first coined in 1895 by John H. Scheel, a follower of the 19th-century Bavarian priest, Father Sebastian Kneipp, who became famous for his water and herbal cures. Another of Kneipp's students, Benedict Lust, who took Kneipp's ideas to America, bought the rights to this name in 1902 and established the first School of Naturopathy and a national organisation of naturopaths in the US.

Nature Cure and Natural Hygiene practices (both described in more detail in Chapter 8) had already been increasing in popularity in America and were being adopted by numerous medical doctors, chiropractors, and osteopaths, amongst others, disenchanted with the orthodox medical practices of the day. They were also becoming quite widely available through Nature Cure Sanitariums and private clinics.

Dr Henry Lindlahr, a medical doctor who became a celebrated naturopath, further established naturopathy by setting up several training institutions and writing best-selling books outlining naturopathic theory and practice.

Other individuals who made significant contributions to the development of this system of health and healing were: Bernarr Macfadden, who brought 'physical culture' to the fore and emphasised the importance of regular exercise, a whole-food diet, and fasting; Dr John H. Tilden, who promoted the idea of toxicity as the root cause of disease; Sylvester Graham, who promoted good nutrition through his wholemeal graham flour crackers and invented the dry breakfast cereal; and Dr John Harvey Kellogg, who established the famous Battle Creek Sanitarium and made several health inventions including the cornflake (you can read the story of the cornflake in Chapter 8 as well).

In the UK, the development of naturopathy as a profession was largely due to James Thompson, (a student of Henry Lindlahr) who set up the first naturopathic training college in Edinburgh in 1919, a healthcare home, and the Incorporated Society of Registered Naturopaths; and Stanley Lieff, who trained with Bernarr Macfadden and later established a Nature Cure Resort in the UK, founded the very popular *Health for All* magazine, and helped establish the British College of Naturopathy in London in 1949.

Other European practitioners also developed naturopathy as a field of practice and one of the most enduring has been the Swiss 'Nature Doctor', Alfred Vogel.

ANECDOTE

Dr Alfred Vogel and the Sioux medicine man

Alfred Vogel was born in a small town outside Basel in Switzerland in 1902. He learnt about plants and healing from his father and grandparents during his childhood and went on to establish a small health food shop, creating natural health remedies and reading, writing about, and practising natural therapeutics. The success of his publications, including the *Nature Doctor*, and his practice enabled him to travel widely during his lifetime to explore herbal therapy and natural cures in different parts of the world.

On one early trip to South Dakota in the US, he met Black Elk, a Native American Sioux elder experienced in plant remedies and healing.

Black Elk made Vogel a gift of a handful of seeds of the *Echinacea purpurea* plant, telling him that this was highly prized in his tribe for its medicinal properties.

Vogel carefully carried the seeds home to Switzerland and, with some difficulty, nurtured them into full grown echinacea plants. He was gradually able to cultivate and harvest the echinacea and is credited with having introduced this marvellous healing plant to millions of people worldwide. It is now cultivated widely and is an extremely popular over-the-counter cold and flu remedy. Modern research has confirmed echinacea's immune-boosting properties.

Mahatma Ghandi and Indian naturopathy

Mahatma Ghandi, a major spiritual and political leader in India in the early 1900s, was a strong supporter of Nature Cure and naturopathy since their methods were inexpensive and could easily be used by ordinary people. Indian naturopathy is closely linked to vegetarianism and yoga, which Ghandi also practised himself.

Nowadays Nature Cure and naturopathic clinics and hospitals exist all over India. Many Indian doctors train in both Western and naturopathic medicine and integrate the two in their practice.

I've studied and assisted in naturopathy clinics in India and have always been delighted to see the ready enthusiasm with which Indian people embrace naturopathic principles and practice.

I particularly remember the scene at one clinic where a group of us were out on the porch practising various yoga exercises, which were part of the clinic's health regime. Our actions attracted the attention of the town's street urchins who ran over and joined in by hilariously copying every move that we made with huge cheeky grins on their faces!

Naturopathy declined in popularity in the mid-1900s, as modern orthodox (allopathic) medicine and pharmaceuticals increased their influence, but more recently it has enjoyed something of a revival amongst people disenchanted with a pharmaceutical approach and interested in natural medicine.

Naturopathy today

Naturopathy is now widespread but its status and practice varies in different countries.

In the US and Canada, naturopaths are regulated and licensed in some, but not all, states, and they practise in a way similar to a general practitioner. In the UK, naturopaths are less numerous and not yet fully regulated and may have developed specialties in osteopathy, herbal medicine, homeopathy, or acupuncture as part of their training.

In Australia and New Zealand naturopathy is licensed and very popular and has been embraced by many doctors too. In Germany the naturopathic *heilpraktikers* (health practitioners) are well-established and some are also trained as medical doctors. In various other countries, including the Netherlands, Sweden, Switzerland and certain African countries, to name but a few, naturopaths are licensed and allowed to practise certain types of natural therapy but prohibited from the practice of particular aspects of medicine such as surgery.

Grasping the idea behind naturopathy

Naturopaths believe that the body is always trying to maintain a state of health balance, known as *homeostasis*. This delicate balance can be disrupted by poor diet, lack of fresh air or sunlight, inadequate exercise, stress, or mental or emotional upset. Naturopaths believe that as a result, the body's 'vital force', which determines health and healing, becomes weakened and leads to disease.

Other disease triggers are thought to be sluggish bowels and poor elimination of waste products, or accumulated toxins from chemicals, pollutants, and pesticides. These are thought to weaken the immune system, lowering resistance and making disease more likely.

Naturopathic practice is based on six principles that emphasise building health rather than fighting disease:

1. **The healing power of nature (*vis medicatrix naturae*)**

   Naturopaths believe that the body has an inherent ability to establish, maintain, and restore health. The aim of naturopathy is to support this ability.

2. **Identify and treat the cause (*tolle causam*)**

   Naturopaths aim to identify the underlying physical, mental-emotional, and spiritual causes of disease and to treat them rather than the symptoms, which are seen as signs of the body's attempt to heal itself.

3. **First do no harm (*primum no nocere*)**

   In naturopathy suppressing symptoms is considered harmful since they're seen as part of the process of healing. The naturopath's role is to support the body's natural healing power instead.

4. **Treat the whole person (*in perturbato animo sicut in corpore sanitas esse non potest*)**

   Naturopaths strive to treat the whole person, taking into account physical, mental, emotional, spiritual, genetic, environmental, and social factors, rather than just symptoms.

5. **The physician as teacher (*docere*)**

   Alongside accurate diagnosis and treatment, naturopaths seek to educate and encourage their patients to take responsibility for their own health.

6. **Prevention (*principiis obsta: sero medicina curator*)**

   The focus of naturopathy is on prevention, which is achieved by educating patients and promoting healthy lifestyle choices.

Iridology: It's all in the eyes

When the Hungarian Ignaz Von Peckzely was a child he caught an owl and accidentally broke one of its legs as it struggled to get free. He happened to notice that a black mark appeared in the iris (the coloured part) of the bird's eye as this happened and that it remained even after he nursed the bird back to full health. Later, having trained to be a physician, he noticed similar marks in the irises of people with broken bones. This aroused his interest in studying the links between eye signs and disease.

A similar experience happened to the Swedish clergyman Nils Liljequist, who noticed his eye colour darkening when he was given hefty doses of drugs to treat his malaria. He later trained as a homeopath and claimed to observe similar signs in patients who were on extensive medication.

Both von Peckzely and Liljequist formulated theories about eye diagnosis in the late 19th-century

that were later developed into *iridology*, the study of the iris to identify potential health problems. Pastor Felke, a German minister, took iridology further, by identifying different homeopathic remedies that he believed were indicated by different iris signs and the American chiropractor and Nature Cure practitioner, Bernard Jensen developed his own comprehensive method for iris analysis and taught it worldwide.

According to iridology different parts of the iris correspond with different parts of the body and specific signs and markings can indicate imbalance and malfunction.

Naturopaths may use iridology to identify health imbalance and early signs of disease. However no controlled trials have been done to validate iridology and orthodox medics remain sceptical about this practice.

Naturopaths also believe that health is more than just the absence of disease and so they're keen to promote and enhance general well-being.

Understanding how it works

By facilitating the body's natural healing mechanism, naturopaths believe that the body's 'vital force' can be strengthened and a homeostatic state of balance restored.

Naturopathic therapies such as hydrotherapy (water cure), massage, manipulation, and so on are also thought to help stimulate circulation and increase the oxygen and nutrient supply to the cells. In addition, detoxification and cleansing treatments are believed to promote more efficient function of the organs of elimination: The liver, kidneys, and intestines.

Exploring Naturopathic Diagnosis

Naturopathic practitioners diagnose using some or all the following:

- **Observation:** Looking at your tongue, face, skin, eyes (iridology), posture, and gait.

- **Questioning:** Asking about your general lifestyle and environment.

- **Physical examination:** The naturopath may palpate different parts of your body to check for muscle tone and tension, may test your body's reflexes, or may test joint mobility and check posture.

- **Clinical tests:** The naturopath may take your blood pressure or listen to your chest with a stethoscope (an instrument used to listen to the heart and lungs).

- **Laboratory testing:** Blood, saliva, urine, or stool tests, may be used to investigate different aspects of your health such as your nutrient status or the presence of parasites.

- **Live blood analysis:** Some naturopaths use a technique called Darkfield Microscopy whereby a drop of live blood is analysed using a special microscope enabling it to be illuminated against a dark background. Users claim that this technique yields valuable information about various aspects of health including vitamin and mineral status, parasitic infestation, and predisposition to degenerative diseases. However, the technique remains highly controversial and many feel it lacks scientific validity.

- **Subtle energy diagnostic methods:** Some naturopaths use subtle energy testing devices to measure 'vital force' (for more about these devices, take a look at Chapter 22).

Finding Out about Naturopathic Treatment

Naturopaths may use various self-care recommendations and/or therapies to support what they call the *Triad of Health*: The structure of the body (bones, muscles, and so on); the biochemistry of the body (cellular and organ function); and psychological health (mental and emotional well-being), as well as interactions between these three.

The self-care recommendations and therapies are designed to stimulate the body's self-healing capacity by increasing circulation, improving digestion, assimilation (the absorption of nutrients from food) and elimination (throwing off waste products via urine, stools, and sweating), boosting immunity, and building vigour and vitality.

The main therapies utilised by naturopaths are the following:

- ✔ **Nutritional medicine:** Dietary advice, and sometimes nutritional supplementation, is used to improve vitamin and mineral status and aid organ function.

- ✔ **Fasting and detoxification regimes:** Short or long, carefully supervised fasts, enemas, skin brushing, and colonics (irrigation of the large intestine with water under gentle pressure) may be used to cleanse and aid removal of accumulated waste matter and toxins, such as chemicals or other pollutants, in the body.

Fasting and restricted diets should only be carried out under supervision by an experienced practitioner. Fasting isn't suitable during pregnancy or while still breastfeeding, or for the very young or frail. It should never be used as a method for weight loss. Colonics should only be carried out by someone properly trained in their administration and strict hygiene procedures are essential for both colonics and enemas to prevent infection.

- ✔ **Hydrotherapy and Nature Cure:** Water, sunlight, air, and earth may be used therapeutically to cleanse and fortify the body. Practical applications include compresses, wraps, baths, and packs.

- ✔ **Herbal medicine:** Medicinal herbs may be used to stimulate healing, restore body balance, and help prevent disease.

- ✔ **Homeopathic medicine:** Based on the principle of 'like cures like', homeopathic medicines are used to promote healing on physical, mental, and spiritual levels. (For more about homeopathy, take a look at Chapter 10.)

- ✔ **Oriental medicine:** Acupuncture and its associated therapies such as acupressure (pressure-point healing) and moxibustion (heat treatment) may be used to clear physical or energetic blockages and promote healing. (Go to Chapter 9 on Acupuncture or Chapters 4 and 7 on Chinese and Japanese medicine for more.)

- ✔ **Manipulative therapy:** Gentle manipulative, soft-tissue and massage techniques drawn from osteopathy or chiropractic may be used to restore structural health and physical balance. (Take a peek at Chapters 14 and 15 if you want to know more about these therapies.)

Naturopaths offering osteopathic, chiropractic, homeopathic, acupuncture, or herbal treatment should have received specialist training in these therapies to enable them to use it safely and effectively. Not all naturopaths are trained in every therapy. Ask about their qualifications to determine their exact skills.

✔ **Therapeutic exercise:** Breathing exercises, yoga stretches, and physical exercises may all be recommended to improve flexibility and muscle tone and enhance relaxation. Water-based exercise may also be used.

✔ **Psychological therapy:** Counselling, affirmations, imagery, prayer, meditation, or some specific psychological therapy may be incorporated to help balance mind and emotions and to enhance spiritual development. (You can find out more about these in Chapters 18 and 21.)

✔ **Other treatments:** Some naturopaths also use other therapies such as flower remedies (Chapter 22), biochemical tissue salts (Chapter 8), electrotherapy (Chapter 8), and magnet therapy (mentioned in Chapter 22).

✔ **Minor surgery:** Some naturopathic practitioners (generally in the US) may be trained to perform simple minor surgical procedures such as superficial wound repairs or dealing with cysts.

Some of the above approaches are controversial and are not accepted by orthodox medical practitioners. Read more about the scientific evidence for each in the relevant chapters.

Since many naturopaths see their role as health educators, working in partnership with you, your treatment may also consist of giving you lots of health information and encouraging you to make lifestyle changes. These recommendations are based on naturopathic self-care ideas for a healthy diet, healthy exercise, and healthy work, rest, and play (and I don't mean Mars bars!).

Discovering Whom and What Naturopathy Is Good For

Naturopathy is suitable for anyone whether you feel well, and would like to optimise your health and prevent disease, or whether you have an ailment from which you'd like to obtain relief.

The conditions that are often treated by naturopaths include digestive problems, aches and pains, circulatory problems, menstrual problems, fertility problems, headaches, migraine, fatigue, and stress.

Most naturopaths see people of all ages and conditions and are used to dealing with both acute (recent and often pain-related) conditions and chronic (long-standing, degenerative) ones.

When not to use naturopathy

Naturopaths are trained to recognise serious medical conditions that require referral to a medical practitioner such as diabetes, tumours, other cancers, and so on. In such cases naturopathy may still be beneficial in a supporting role but diagnosis and treatment from an orthodox practitioner will be advised.

If you're taking Western medical drugs together with naturopathic remedies, always ensure that both your orthodox and naturopathic practitioner are fully informed so that they can be alert to any potentially harmful interactions.

Evidence that it works

Some naturopathic concepts, such as that of vital force, and some of the therapies used by naturopaths, such as homeopathy, have been dismissed by modern scientists and medics as having no real foundation. However, other aspects of naturopathy are gaining increasing support from modern day research. For example, many studies now support naturopathic dietary principles and the benefits of regular exercise and stress relief techniques, and some of these have even been incorporated into orthodox medical practice.

Extensive research at the Bastyr University in Seattle, in the US has also demonstrated the effectiveness of a naturopathic approach in treating a wide range of conditions including glue ear, sinus problems, digestive disorders, headaches, chronic fatigue, and auto-immune conditions including HIV-positive-related conditions. In one study of a group of 16 HIV-positive people who received naturopathic treatment for a year, none of them went on to develop full-blown AIDS and 12 reported feeling significantly better.

For details of research evidence for the different therapies used by naturopaths, see the relevant chapters on homeopathy, herbal medicine acupuncture, and osteopathy.

For more on naturopathic research, check out the Bastyr University Research database on www.bastyr.edu/research/default.asp. Other naturopathy research may be found via the Cochrane Library (www.cochrane.org/reviews/clibintro.htm), the NHS Complementary and Alternative Medicine Specialist Library (www.library.nhs.uk/cam), or the PubMed database (www.nlm.nih.gov/nccam/camonpubmed.html). You can find further information on US and Canadian trials at www.clinicaltrials.gov.

What to Expect in a Typical Consultation

First consultations with a naturopath normally last between 30 to 90 minutes. Your case history (details of your previous and current health and illness) will be taken and the naturopath will examine you using some or all the types of diagnosis described earlier in this chapter. You may be asked to go for further tests or to provide samples for them at home, such as urine or saliva tests.

The naturopath will discuss your health concerns and general well-being with you and will propose various lifestyle changes that you can implement to promote your health. These changes may cover diet, exercise, and other daily habits, and you may be asked to carry out a cleansing diet, or short fast, or to try some type of hydrotherapy (water therapy) at home. Certain types of therapy may also be suggested (this can be any from the list of therapies described in the 'Finding Out about Naturopathic Treatment' section earlier in this chapter).

Follow-up sessions are typically 30 minutes (depending on the type of therapy that is being provided). If you're being given osteopathy, or acupuncture, you may be advised to have two sessions in the first week and less frequent sessions thereafter depending on your health condition.

If you're feeling well and just want to optimise your health, you may only need to see your naturopath once or twice a year for check-ups and health advice. If, however, you have a specific health ailment that you're hoping to relieve, or decide to undergo a particular form of therapy with your naturopath, then you may need to make several repeat visits at regular intervals.

Knowing Whether Your Naturopathy Treatment Is Working

Remember that naturopathy is not really a form of treatment but more a way of life that may also involve having some therapy, depending on the orientation of your practitioner.

The key to getting benefit from naturopathic advice is really down to you – it depends on how committed you are to making the lifestyle changes recommended for restoring your health and maximising your health potential.

Making diet, exercise, and other lifestyle changes isn't always easy, so you may find it helpful to approach things one step at a time, with advise and encouragement from your practitioner.

If you're receiving some sort of naturopathic therapy such as hydrotherapy (water cure), herbal medicine, acupuncture, homeopathy, or osteopathy, then check out the chapters in this book about each of these for more tips on what to expect during treatment.

Be aware that many naturopathic therapies recognise the possibility of a healing crisis whereby symptoms may get slightly worse before they get better, due to the changes being initiated in the body. Such effects are usually short-lived but if you have any concerns about this, do discuss these with your practitioner.

Follow these pointers for safe treatment:

- ✔ If you're carrying out any kind of cleansing diet or short fast, follow the instructions you have been given *exactly* and contact your practitioner immediately if you have any concerns or unusual symptoms.

- ✔ If you experience a marked worsening of your symptoms, always contact your naturopath speedily for advice.

- ✔ Ask your naturopath what sort of health improvements you can realistically expect and over what sort of timescale.

- ✔ For best results carefully follow the exercise and lifestyle advice given to you by your naturopath.

- ✔ If you have no improvement after a course of treatment, then you may want to consider another form of therapy. Discuss doing so with your practitioner.

Common Questions about Naturopathy Treatment

Here are some questions that I'm often asked about naturopathy:

- ✔ **Can anybody fast?** Yes, just about everyone can benefit from a short fast such as a day on only organic vegetable and fruit juices or on a single food such as grapes. Such fasts can rest the digestive system and help to cleanse the body. However, fasts are not advised during pregnancy or while breastfeeding, or for infants, young children, or the very frail. Longer fasts require careful supervision and shouldn't be attempted by the inexperienced.

✔ **Are enemas and colonics uncomfortable or unsafe?** If performed correctly, with the gentle introduction of water at body temperature, then both enemas and colonics needn't be uncomfortable. Being relaxed and confident in your own ability to conduct the enema or your practitioner's ability to give the colonic also helps. Hygiene is crucial for the safety of these procedures and colonics should only be performed by properly trained practitioners using disposable equipment. Having probiotics (beneficial bacteria) reintroduced to the intestine (usually orally and anally) at the end of the enema or colonic, helps ensure that your intestines are populated with plenty of friendly bacteria vital for gut health.

✔ **Can I do hydrotherapy if I don't like cold water?** When your body is weak or you suffer from ill health, your resistance is often low and your ability to regulate body temperature is often impaired. As a result you can be quite sensitive to the cold and may find cold water immersion difficult. In such cases, starting with short exposure to tepid or slightly warm water and then gradually acclimatising your body to lower temperatures is best.

Never allow yourself to get chilled during cold water therapy, however. Simply get out of the water and warm yourself thoroughly. Remember cold water therapy isn't suitable for the very young, elderly, or frail, nor for those with heart or kidney problems.

✔ **What if I don't like whole-foods?** Changing your palate and dietary habits takes time. Your naturopath can advise you on how to make dietary changes slowly and how to experiment with a range of new foods to find healthy ones that you can enjoy.

✔ **How does the naturopath know what techniques to use?** Naturopaths are thoroughly trained in diagnosis, assessment, interpreting test results, and a range of therapies. Their training and clinical experience will enable them to determine which are the most appropriate lifestyle changes and/or therapies for you.

Finding a Naturopath

In countries where naturopaths are not yet regulated, such as the UK, anyone can call themselves a naturopath so check that your practitioner has had a thorough training at a recognised institution and is a member of a professional body.

In the UK, most naturopaths are registered with The General Council and Register of Naturopaths (GCRN; www.naturopathy.org.uk) and are members of its professional body, The British Naturopathic Association (BNA; www.naturopaths.org.uk) or Tel: 0870 745 6984. Both the GCRN and BNA Web sites have online directories of registered naturopaths.

The GCRN, set up in 1965, sets standards for naturopathy training, keeps a register of practitioners that meet its standards, and monitors members' professional conduct. GCRN-accredited naturopathy courses are currently three years of full-time study, including 500 to 560 hours of teaching and more than 400 hours of clinical training.

The British College of Osteopathic Medicine (formerly the British College of Naturopathy and Osteopathy) (Tel: 0207 435 6464; www.bcom.ac.uk) and Westminster University (Tel: 020 7911 5000 or 0207 911 5041; www.wmin.ac.uk) both run courses accredited by the GCRN and offer supervised student clinics where you can have low-cost naturopathy consultations.

The College of Naturopathic Medicine (CNM) (www.naturopathy-uk.com) also trains naturopaths in the UK. However, at the time of writing, their naturopathy course is not accredited with the GCRN. They maintain their own register of practitioners, The Association of Naturopathic Practitioners, on www.naturopathy-anp.com.

In the US and Canada, naturopaths can be located via The American Association of Naturopathic Physicians (AANP) (Tel: 00 1 206 298 0125; www.naturopathic.org) or the Canadian Association of Naturopathic Doctors (Tel: 00 1416 496 8633; www.naturopathicassoc.ca).

If you live in Australia, you can locate naturopaths via the Australian Naturopathic Practitioners Association (ANPA) (Tel: +613 9811 9990; www.anpa.asn.au) and in New Zealand via www.naturopath.org.nz.

India has no single body for naturopaths. Practitioners are recognised for their qualifications, which are generally either a Diploma in Naturopathy and Yogic Sciences (DNYS), awarded by the All India Naturopathy Council after a three-year course of study, or a Bachelor's Degree in Naturopathy and Yogic Science (BNYS) obtained after four or five years of university study. The following are some other suggestions for finding a naturopath:

- ✔ Ask friends, family, and colleagues for personal recommendations.
- ✔ Some sports and leisure clubs offer naturopathic treatment.
- ✔ Many integrated health centres and health spas offer naturopathy.

Questions to ask your naturopath

You may want to ask your naturopath about the following:

- ✔ **Qualifications:** Most practitioners are happy to give details of their training and qualifications. If you have any doubt as to the validity of these qualifications, check them with the respective professional body.

✔ **Insurance:** If your practitioner is a member of a professional register they will be required to have appropriate indemnity insurance.

✔ **Experience:** Ask your practitioner about their experience in educating about naturopathic principles and in treating your particular health condition.

✔ **Treatment:** If you've been recommended naturopathic therapy, ask about the likely frequency and duration of treatment and the costs.

Counting the cost of naturopathy

Initial naturopathy consultations may cost from £35 to £65 while follow-up sessions are usually £25 to £35.

Naturopathic treatment is rarely available on the NHS in the UK. Some private health insurances cover naturopathy treatment. Check with your provider for advice. Practitioners may offer concessions for retired persons or those on benefits. Ask for details.

Ensuring satisfaction

If you're dissatisfied with your treatment, first talk things over with your practitioner.

If you think that the practitioner has been negligent or unethical in any way, contact their professional association or registering body, which should have a formal complaints procedure.

Helping Yourself with Naturopathy

Skin brushing has been recommended by Nature Cure practitioners and naturopaths for more than 150 years as an excellent way of stimulating circulation and aiding skin cell renewal and body cleansing. Try the technique like this:

1. **Buy a natural bristle brush, preferably one with a long handle so that you can reach your back.**

2. **Strip naked in a warm and draught-free place.** On *dry* skin, move the brush in small sweeps, or small circular movements, starting at the feet and going upwards toward the heart. Brush towards the heart from the extremities inwards.

3. **Use gentle pressure.** The brushing should be vigorous and stimulating but not painful!

4. **Use very light strokes around the breasts and avoid the breast tissue and nipples.** Do not use on the face or near the eyes.

5. **Brush the whole body until your skin feels warm and tingling.**

6. **Take a warm shower and end with a cool rinse.** Also wash your brush and leave to dry out.

7. **Repeat this skin brushing every morning if you can, to thoroughly invigorate your body.** Don't use this technique at night because it may leave you too awake.

Part IV
Treating Your Body

The 5th Wave   By Rich Tennant

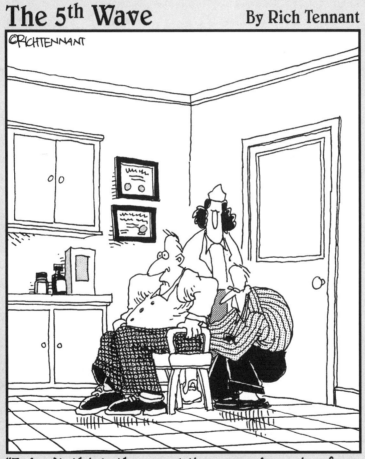

"I don't think the crackling sound coming from your lower back is as serious as you thought. Just relax and I'll have this Rice Krispie Square out of your back pocket in no time."

In this part . . .

This is the part that gets physical. Chiropractic, osteopathy, and massage are all very popular complementary therapies, and in the following chapters I tell you all about them and offer advice on how to find a good practitioner.

Delve into this part if you want to know your Alexander technique from your Bowen therapy, and explore body therapies from applied kinesiology to zero balancing.

Chapter 14

Opening Up with Osteopathy

*M*ention the word osteopathy and most people think of bone cracking and bad backs. Yet osteopathy is so much more than this image. Some even argue that osteopathy is a complete system of healthcare for restoring and maintaining equilibrium in the body.

I've called this chapter Opening Up with Osteopathy not only because it opens the Treating Your Body part but also because osteopathy really does seem to 'open' the body by releasing tension, facilitating movement, and creating a sense of 'space' in place of restriction.

In this chapter, I tell you a bit about the amazing life story of the founder of this therapy and describe the techniques that are in the modern day osteopath's repertoire. You'll get an idea of what it's like to have an osteopathic treatment and find out how even newborn babies are benefiting from it!

I also give you a checklist for the types of ailments osteopathy may be helpful for. You may be surprised by some of the things that are included in it.

Then I give you all the contact details that you need for tracking down fully qualified practitioners and tell you what those pesky letters after their names stand for.

Butter churns, blood-letting, and bones

Andrew Still, the founder of osteopathy, loved playing around with mechanical inventions all his life. He was born in a log cabin in Virginia in the US in 1828, the son of a preacher/physician, and the third of nine children. As a young boy he had to work hard helping his parents and was always looking for ways of improving the mechanical equipment that they used. He invented several labour-saving devices, including a more efficient churn for butter-making.

Still also applied his enthusiasm for mechanics to the physical body and became interested in finding ways of improving structural balance. He trained as a doctor by reading books and studying with his father and used his study of animal and human skeletons to begin to formulate his ideas about body mechanics.

Working as a doctor in the American Civil War, Still became disenchanted with the medical methods of the time – including blood-letting, crude surgery, and purging – which were not very effective in saving lives. This experience and the tragic loss of three of his children to meningitis, another to pneumonia, and his wife due to complications in childbirth, convinced him that a new form of medicine was needed.

Still went back to studying the body and came to believe that faulty body mechanics could affect organ function and the flow of blood and vital energy or 'nerve force'. He went on to develop methods for improving body balance and invented various devices to assist in treatment. These included a special brace designed to stop patients falling off the treatment table during vigorous manipulations!

Finding Out about Osteopathy

Osteopathy is a system of diagnosis and treatment that identifies and relieves structural and mechanical problems of the body. This therapy is concerned with the framework of the body, that is, the muscles, bone, tendons, ligaments, and cartilage – all the bony and sinewy bits – and the nervous system that co-ordinates their smooth functioning. This framework is sometimes referred to as the neuro-musculo-skeletal system – a bit of a mouthful but it manages to cover everything in one word! Osteopaths are interested in both the *structure* and the actual *functioning* of the components of this system.

A (very) brief history of osteopathy

Osteopathy was created by Dr Andrew Taylor Still, a rural physician in the US in the 1890s. He was not impressed by some of the more barbaric medical practices popular at the time and wanted to find a more natural way of treating the body. He thought up the name by combining two ancient Greek words, *osteon*, meaning 'bone', and *pathos*, meaning 'suffering' or 'disease'. Still believed that if you could create good neuro-musculo-skeletal balance, then the body would function better and self-healing could occur.

Still faced strong opposition from the medical establishment for his enthusiasm for natural medicine but he was an energetic and determined man who stuck to his principles. One of my favourite quotes of his, that seems to sum up his stance, is, 'I have no desire to be a cat, which walks so lightly that it never creates a disturbance'. He went on to establish the American School of Osteopathy in 1892 and trained thousands of osteopaths (including some of his own children and siblings) within his lifetime. He also admitted women and black people as students, which was highly unusual at the time, and was a vociferous opponent of the slave trade, which still existed. He continued to practise and teach osteopathy until his death in 1917 at the ripe old age of 89.

One of Still's graduates, a Scot, Dr John Martin Littlejohn, brought osteopathy to the UK and founded the British School of Osteopathy in 1917. This school still exists as a major osteopathic training institution. Gradually, other schools have been established.

Modern day osteopathy is still based on Still's work but has also developed to include new techniques and approaches. Psychological, social, and lifestyle factors are also considered important.

Osteopathy has been at the forefront of regulation in the field of complementary medicine and osteopathy practice is now governed by law in many countries. It is currently one of the most popular forms of complementary therapy in the West.

Grasping the idea behind osteopathy

According to Dr Still's osteopathic theory, all disease can be related to disorders involving the spine, muscles, joints, and nerves. He claimed that structural imbalance affected nerve and blood supply to the body's organs and termed these imbalances *osteopathic lesions*. Still devised methods of manipulation, stretching, and massage of the soft tissues to release blockages and areas of tension, increase mobility, and improve the flow of blood and lymph. In this way he aimed to restore normal function of the nerves and organs and enable the body's natural healing mechanisms to come to the fore.

Still maintained that osteopathy is a holistic system of medicine that takes into account not only the structural problem, or physical imbalance, itself but also underlying contributing factors in terms of lifestyle, diet, and emotional health.

The roots of imbalance

Imbalances in the neuro-musculo-skeletal system (the structural support of the body and its communication systems) can be caused by physical injuries, poor posture, bad work habits, repetitive strain, badly designed seating, and so on. Stress, emotions, and psychological factors can also play a part as they lead to tension, which in turn affects muscles, nerves, and blood supply.

The osteopath takes all these factors into account and each person is treated individually. So, for example, if a person has neck pain the osteopath may consider various possible contributing factors, including damage from past injuries or accidents, occupational factors such as long hours using computers or frequent carrying of heavy loads, poor bed or pillow support at night, stress and worry leading to muscular tension, pelvic imbalance leading to irregular gait, or child-bearing and pregnancy.

For example, John, 59, went to an osteopath complaining of a persistent stiff neck. He was surprised when the osteopath linked this problem to pelvic misalignment and his regular jogging. The osteopath eased stiffness in his ankles from an old sports injury, gave him exercises to strengthen weakened muscles, and fitted John with *orthotics* – specially made insoles for his running shoes – to balance his gait. To John's surprise, within just a few days of his treatment and wearing the orthotics his neck pain disappeared. He now wears the orthotics constantly in both his ordinary and running shoes, does the exercises regularly, and has occasional osteopathic check ups. The neck pain has not recurred.

Osteopaths therefore aim to identify underlying causes of imbalance and then to restore mobility, release restriction, ease tension, facilitate circulation, and enhance general well-being in order to affect improvements in body functions.

Osteopathy Today

The 1993 Osteopaths Act made osteopathy one of the first complementary therapies to be regulated and licensed in the UK. A register of osteopaths was set up in the UK in 1998 and the title 'osteopath' became protected by law in 2000. Since that time it is illegal for anyone to call themselves an osteopath unless they've completed a recognised training course and are registered with the General Osteopathic Council. Training is normally for a minimum of four years.

The General Osteopathic Council (GosC; www.osteopathy.org.uk) is an independent body set up following the Osteopaths Act in order to establish and maintain professional standards, accredit training courses, and maintain the register of osteopaths. The GosC also aims to make osteopathy a recognised medical specialty.

Seven approved osteopathic colleges exist in the UK and more than 5,000 practitioners. Some practitioners are medical doctors who have chosen to study osteopathy as a postgraduate course.

British trained osteopaths study for a minimum of four years and their training includes anatomy, physiology, differential diagnosis (accurate identification of disease from symptoms), clinical skills, and extensive clinical practice. Treatment is almost entirely based on manual therapy techniques, and students do not perform surgery or prescribe medicines. (However, they may be given these rights in the future since the British government has included osteopathy in their list of professions allied to medicine.)

In contrast, in the US, osteopaths undergo full medical training and are entitled to prescribe medicines and perform surgery. The US has had full licensing since 1972, and US osteopaths have been eligible for membership of the British Medical Association since 2005. However, these practitioners may have had quite limited training in manual manipulative therapy as compared to their British counterparts. For more information, consult the American Osteopathic Association at `www.do-online.osteotech.org/index.cfm`.

Within member states of the European Union, apart from the UK, France, and Switzerland, no standardised training in osteopathy is available. In Australia and New Zealand, osteopathy is a growing profession.

Exploring Different Types of Osteopathy

Once osteopaths have completed their general training, they may go on to do further specialist training. Popular forms of specialisation are cranial osteopathy, paediatric osteopathy, and visceral osteopathy. Other osteopaths may also specialise in sports medicine.

Cranial osteopathy

Cranial osteopathy was developed from the work of an American osteopath, Graham Sutherland, in the 1930s. Contrary to the orthodox medical view that the bones of the skull or cranium become fixed in adult life, Sutherland believed that they retain a degree of flexibility. He believed that the sheath, which encloses the cerebrospinal fluid (CSF) and attaches to these cranial bones and the spine – known as the *dural membrane* – can become less flexible due to birth trauma, injuries, and falls. He reasoned that this in turn would affect the flow of cerebrospinal fluid (CSF), circulation of blood and lymph in the body, and the drainage of sinus fluids in the head. Sutherland also believed this would affect normal bending and movement of the spine and cause joints to become restricted in their pattern of movement.

Sutherland claimed that the rhythmical pulsing of CSF, which should normally be around 6 to 18 times per minute, could be felt with the hands. Interestingly, this rhythm has been found to continue to pulse for a few minutes even after a person's heart and breathing stop in the process of dying.

He developed a range of gentle techniques to determine the quality and movement of this cranial rhythm, to release tension and restrictions and to restore balance.

Some people feel that nothing is going on at all during such treatment and simply feel pleasantly relaxed. However, the cranial osteopath has a highly developed sense of touch and is trained to detect real differences in cranial rhythm – although this ability is difficult to verify scientifically.

Because of the lack of scientific evidence, the theory and practice of cranial osteopathy remains controversial, even amongst osteopaths. However, it is practised by a growing number of osteopaths, particularly, but not exclusively, by those specialising in paediatric osteopathy, the treatment of babies and young children. Cranial osteopathy is also ideal for the elderly, weak, or frail, or for anyone who prefers a very gentle approach.

Cranial osteopathy has been used for premature babies; infant problems such as colic, teething, and sleeping or behavioural problems; ear and sinus problems; headaches and back, digestive, and respiratory problems, to name but a few.

Some osteopaths use cranial osteopathy as just one of the techniques at their disposal, while others specialise almost exclusively in cranial work. To find an osteopath who has completed a recognised postgraduate course in cranial osteopathy, contact the Sutherland Society (www.cranial.org.uk), which has more than 300 members both in the UK and overseas.

Paediatric osteopathy

Paediatric osteopaths use a range of gentle techniques, including cranial osteopathy, to treat newborns and young babies. This approach has been pioneered by British osteopath Stuart Korth, who founded the Osteopathic Centre for Children (OCC; www.occ.uk.com) and created diploma training in paediatric osteopathy for qualified osteopaths.

Which way did he come out?

My son first had cranial osteopathy from a very skilful osteopathic colleague and close friend of mine, Deidre Stubbs, the day after he was born. He had had a wonderfully easy, natural birth at home, without any sort of medication or difficulty, but Deirdre came over to see him and offered to check him over. I remember her gently laying her hands on either side of his head and telling me of some restrictions that she felt. To my amazement, simply from these sensations, she was able to correctly identify which way he'd come out of the birth canal (facing forwards, twisted slightly to my left-hand side, and with the umbilical cord around his neck!). She made some fine movements with her fingers to ease the restrictions that she felt and at the exact moment that she felt a release, my day-old son took a deep breath and then fell into a blissful sleep.

In the course of his early years my son was very fortunate to have further cranial osteopathy at times of need from the outstanding and renowned osteopaths, Professor Laurie Hartmann, a pioneer of minimal velocity (very gentle) manipulative techniques, and Stuart Korth, founder of the Osteopathic Centre for Children and developer of postgraduate training in paediatric osteopathy. Both recommend that treatment be given at major landmarks in children's development, such as when they first start to crawl, sit, stand, and walk, and after any major traumas such as falls or accidents. Being very active, fast growing, and accident prone, my son needed treatment quite a few times.

I sometimes wonder if one of the effects of these treatments was to give my son such good body balance that, as a teenager, he is now a competent and enthusiastic skateboarder and an outstanding climber.

The OCC has clinics in London and Manchester and treats children from birth to 18 years, as well as women during pregnancy. The OCC has become particularly renowned for its work with premature babies and children with cerebral palsy. However, as is the case for all paediatric osteopaths, it also offers treatment for a wide range of children's ailments, including ear infections, colic, teething, asthma, sleeplessness, growing pains, and epilepsy.

Various osteopathic colleges, such as the British School of Osteopathy (www.bso.ac.uk) and the European School of Osteopathy (www.eso.ac.uk) also offer specialist children's clinics. Contact the individual schools for further information.

Visceral osteopathy

Visceral osteopathy originally grew out of work done by two American osteopaths, H. V. Hoover and M. D. Young, in the 1940s, who attempted to synthesise the work of Dr Still, the founder of osteopathy, and John Upledger, the creator of cranio-sacral therapy.

The word *viscera* refers to the soft internal organs of the body – the lungs, heart, digestive organs, and reproductive organs. Jean-Pierre Barral, a graduate of the European School of Osteopathy in the UK, developed visceral osteopathy in the 1970s. He became interested in patterns of stress in the body tissues around these internal organs and how gentle osteopathic techniques could be used to release them.

Barral devised a system of soft manipulations of the internal organs and surrounding tissues to treat these abnormal stress patterns. He claims that this visceral osteopathic treatment can facilitate improved organ function, body system function, fluid circulation, mobility, and general wellness. He also developed a system of thermal diagnosis after discovering that areas of tension could be located by the increased heat that they give off.

In 1985, Barral established a training programme in visceral techniques at the Upledger Institute in the US, which has been taken by many osteopaths and other physical therapists.

Visceral osteopathy is considered to be particularly suitable for people after surgery, trauma, injury, or pregnancy but can also be used to rebalance the body after chronic illness such as repeated cystitis (bladder infection).

Cranio-sacral therapy

While cranial osteopathy is a postgraduate specialisation for registered osteopaths who have already had substantial training in anatomy and physiology and a minimum four years of study and clinical practice, another healing discipline also exists, cranio-sacral therapy, that may be learnt and practised by non-osteopaths with much shorter and limited training.

Cranio-sacral therapy was developed by another American osteopath, Dr John Upledger, in the late 1970s. He was a professor of biomechanics and clinical researcher at Michigan State University and became interested in the importance of the membranes that surround the central cord in the spine and the brain in the skull.

Building on the ideas of Dr Sutherland about the significance of the cranial rhythmic impulse

(CRI) and the ebb and flow of cerebrospinal fluid (CSF) in the spinal chord and the skull, Upledger came to believe that this could affect the function of every cell in the body.

He developed a system of using extremely light pressure on the cranium (skull), or sacrum (tailbone), or elsewhere on the body to ease these membranes and establish smooth, unrestricted flow of the CSF.

This work is even more controversial than cranial osteopathy in that no real research evidence exists to support its use. However, many people report finding cranio-sacral therapy deeply relaxing and beneficial. For more about this therapy, check out www.upledger.com.

However, little research evidence exists to support this practice and it remains controversial and not yet widely practised by osteopaths. No specific association has been established for visceral osteopaths. To find an osteopath who practises this approach, you have to simply ask around amongst osteopathic practitioners.

Understanding How It Works

The neuro-musculo-skeletal system provides the support structure for the body; the mechanics for movement in order to stand, sit, run, and carry out everyday activities; and the communications network for controlling this system. The neuro-musculo-skeletal system is made up of the following:

- ✔ **Bones:** The hard, solid bits that make up the human skeleton – more than 200 of them exist in the body

- ✔ **Joints:** The meeting point of two or more bones – usually to facilitate movement

- ✔ **Muscles:** Bundles of fibres that can contract in order to create movement of the bones

- ✔ **Ligaments:** The stringy bits that connect to your bones and keep your joints stable, stopping them from moving about all over the place

- ✔ **Tendons:** Strong, fibrous cords at the end of muscles that attach onto bones or other solid structures in the body

- ✔ **Soft tissue:** The collective name for all the tissues that connect, support, or surround the structures or organs of the body, including the ligaments, tendons, and muscles and also the tissues inbetween, fat, and nerves – basically all the soft and non-solid bits

- ✔ **Nerves:** Bundles of fibres that carry signals from one part of the body to another, such as the optic nerves that carry signals between the eyes and the brain

Damage to any of the above can cause pain and strain and have a knock-on effect on other body systems or internal organs.

Pain signals can build up, leading to increased inflammation and irritation and an accumulation of waste products produced by the body in response to the pain. These occurrences disrupt the normal flow of blood and fluids, which further exacerbate the pain and tension and may cause increased immobility. According to osteopathic theory, this disruption in normal fluid flow and body mechanics impairs the body's ability to regulate and heal itself.

Osteopathy is designed to break this cycle of pain, tension, and inflammation by relaxing the muscles, calming the nerves, easing restriction, and re-establishing normal circulation and function.

Discovering Whom and What Osteopathy Is Good For

Almost anyone is suitable for osteopathy. Most osteopaths treat men, women and children, the elderly, pregnant women, persons active in sports, and so on.

Conditions that osteopathy can treat

A typical osteopath's clientele may include manual workers, office workers, drivers, homemakers, musicians, dancers, athletes, and children. The most common complaints are bad backs, neck problems, and joint problems such as tennis elbow, frozen shoulder, and arthritis. Increasing numbers of doctors are incorporating osteopathy into their practices or referring to private osteopaths.

Acceptance of osteopathy is even filtering down to emergency medicine. I was involved in a road traffic accident recently and my passengers and I suffered severe whiplash. We were taken by ambulance to the A&E department of the local hospital and were surprised to be told by the examining doctor there to seek out an osteopath for treatment! We did this and it brought great relief.

However, osteopathy certainly isn't limited to joint pains and strains. An osteopathic colleague of mine recently did a clinical audit (a record of all the different conditions that patients have brought to him over the last year). It contained the following: Back pain; neck pain; joint problems (such as frozen shoulder, tennis elbow, arthritis); sports injuries; headaches or migraine; asthma or other respiratory problems; menstrual problems; sleep problems; digestive problems; ear infections and tinnitus (ringing in the ears); circulation problems; sinus problems; cystitis and bladder problems; repetitive strain injury; neurological problems such as head trauma and epilepsy; pregnancy related problems such as back pain, heartburn, and water retention; infant disorders including colic and teething; and developmental delays and learning difficulties. Quite a list!

Increasingly, osteopaths are finding that people are referring themselves for all kinds of problems and reporting benefits.

First visits to osteopaths are often made at times of crisis, such as when a person suddenly experiences acute back pain. However, more people are now using osteopathy preventively and going for regular or occasional mainte-nance treatments to maintain good ongoing structural balance.

Evidence that it works

Research trials investigating osteopathy for different ailments have yielded mixed results. Many early studies suffered from design flaws but increasingly good studies are being produced that do confirm the benefits of osteopathy for a range of problems, including back pain and middle ear infections in young children.

A lot of publicity was given recently to a review paper by researchers from the Peninsula Medical School at Exeter University, which claimed no evidence existed that osteopathic manipulation can effectively relieve any conditions including back pain! This claim has been vigorously refuted by the General Osteopathic Council, which argued that the review was very limited, did not take account of the multi-faceted nature of back pain, and excluded all good research carried out since 2000. For example, an excellent trial carried out in 2004, funded by the Medical Research Council, provided pretty good evi-dence that spinal manipulation plus exercise helped reduce low back pain.

For more about osteopathy research, check out the information and links of the National Council of Osteopathic Research (NCOR) at `www.brighton.ac.uk/ncor/about/index.htm`.

When not to use osteopathy

With care and experience, gentle osteopathic techniques can be used for any condition but vigorous manipulations should not be used in case of the following:

- ✔ Osteoporosis (brittle bones)
- ✔ Severe rheumatoid arthritis (bone inflammation)
- ✔ Osteoarthritis (bone degeneration)

Neck adjustments must be performed with great care in people with a history of stroke or high blood pressure.

Particular care must also be taken with the elderly and young children or infants. Gentle cranial techniques (check out the section on cranial osteopathy for more on this) are ideal for such people.

What to Expect in a Typical Consultation

A consultation with an osteopath will generally start with some questions and answers.

Questioning

An osteopathic consultation usually starts with detailed medical history taking and questions about your general health. You may have been asked to fill in a questionnaire beforehand to save time. The osteopath will also ask you details about your symptoms, how bad they are, how long they've gone on for, what makes them better/worse, and so on. Since the osteopath is interested in a holistic approach, you may also be asked questions about your diet and lifestyle.

Understanding diagnostic methods

The questions will be followed by a physical examination. For this examination you're usually asked to undress down to your underwear but sometimes certain garments can be retained; for example, if you have a neck problem you may only be asked to remove your upper outer garment(s). Some osteopaths provide a loose robe to be worn during examination and treatment.

Your osteopath diagnoses on the basis of:

- ✔ **Observation and movement:** The osteopath will observe your general posture, gait, and breathing pattern to learn about your structural balance. You may be asked to walk up and down as your gait is observed or to bend from side to side, or forwards and backwards, to assess the ease of movement of your spine. This observation may be followed by more detailed investigation of your range of movement for specific joints. For example, if you have a shoulder problem the osteopath may want to gauge how far you can raise or lower your arm.

- ✔ **Reflex testing:** The osteopath may test your reflexes – doing so can involve tapping at certain points on the body with a small rubber instrument, such as just below the knees. When the tap is made, your leg will involuntarily jerk as the nerve sends a message to the brain and this is then relayed to your muscle causing it to contract. (This jerk is the same mechanism as when you mistakenly place your hand on something hot and involuntarily draw it away.) The osteopath uses these techniques to check that all your reflexes are working properly.

✔ **Palpation:** The osteopath may also use hands and fingers to palpate the tissues surrounding your joints in order to assess the level of inflammation, muscle tension, and pain.

✔ **X-rays or scans:** Occasionally the osteopath may recommend that you have an x-ray or other medical test such as an MRI scan. If you've already had an x-ray taken of a joint or bone problem, take it with you to your consultation as all osteopaths are skilled in reading these.

Getting to grips with osteopathic techniques

Osteopaths have a range of specially designed techniques literally at their fingertips to help restore balance in the body, release muscular tension, ease pain and stiffness, increase mobility and range of movement, and improve circulation and general well-being.

Osteopaths have many techniques in common with other manual therapists, such as chiropractors, but tend to favour light manipulations, stretch and release techniques, and massage. In contrast, chiropractors often make more use of x-rays and more vigorous manipulations. Take a look at Chapter 15 to find out more about chiropractic therapy.

Here are some common techniques used by osteopaths:

✔ **Manipulations:** These are physical adjustments performed by the osteopath to joints, muscles, or their surrounding tissues. The aim is to release muscular tension or spasm and to ease restriction, thereby restoring better mobility and circulation.

A common type of manipulation is the 'high velocity low amplitude thrust'. This technique involves positioning the body carefully and then applying a rapid thrust to a joint, or the bones of the spine, in order to release restriction and tension. Sometimes an audible *crack* or *pop* is heard as the tissues are released. If this technique is done well, you can have an immediate increase in the range of movement afterwards.

This type of manipulation isn't suitable for those with weak or brittle bones.

More gentle forms of manipulation include positional release techniques, which are light adjustments used for areas of acute pain, inflammation, or injury, or on people who are weak or frail.

✔ **Joint mobilisation/articulation:** This involves the osteopath rhythmically moving a joint and applying gentle stretches to the surrounding tissue in order to release tension and ease restriction.

✔ **Myofascial release:** This technique employs slow stretching and easing out of muscles and surrounding tissues to release tension, increase range of movement, and facilitate healing.

✔ **Muscle energy techniques:** These are various techniques employing contraction and stretching of the muscles that are used, to release muscle tightness and restore range of movement.

✔ **Direct pressure:** The osteopath may apply direct pressure to certain trigger points in order to release tension and pain.

✔ **Massage:** Different types of massage may be used to ease muscle tension, stretch the tissues, and promote circulation.

These techniques are often accompanied by advice on posture, exercises, diet, and self-help techniques such as the use of heat treatments to enhance circulation or ice packs to ease swelling and inflammation.

The osteopath may also use other specialist techniques such as cranial osteopathy (very gentle techniques on the cranium (skull) and sacrum (tailbone)), or visceral (work on releasing tension in the soft tissues around the internal organs) techniques. For more about these techniques, check out the 'Exploring Different Types of Osteopathy' section earlier in this chapter.

Knowing what to expect at the end of treatment

After your osteopathic treatment has ended, your appointment is likely to conclude with the following:

✔ The osteopath may demonstrate or advise on certain exercises for you to practise between sessions.

✔ You may be advised that initially your symptoms may worsen – sometimes the tissues react to the treatment – and to take things easy. This effect normally subsides in a day or two and then real improvement can be felt.

✔ The need for further treatments and the time between them will also be discussed.

✔ You'll be advised to get up and get dressed slowly and to have a glass of water if you want. Ideally you need to rest, or at least avoid such activities as heavy lifting, manual labour, vigorous exercise, and long-distance driving immediately after treatment.

Anticipating treatment duration and frequency

Osteopathic treatments usually last half an hour but can be from 20 to 60 minutes. Treatments may be at weekly intervals initially and then become more spaced out once your condition improves. Sometimes just a single treatment may be all that is needed. More often a short series of two to six treatments may be necessary. For certain chronic conditions, regular maintenance treatments may be helpful.

Knowing Whether Your Osteopathic Treatment Is Working

The main reason you sought out osteopathy will probably have been because of pain, injury, and/or decreased mobility. So obviously if the treatment is working well you'll expect these to have improved.

However you need to bear in mind a few things:

✔ Don't expect immediate results. It may be a couple of days before things settle down and you feel the full benefit of your treatment. Allow your body to rest and heal after treatment.

If you experience a really marked increase in pain, or deterioration in your symptoms, contact your osteopath for advice.

✔ Discuss with your osteopath what improvements you can realistically expect over what sort of timescale. You may need a short course of treatments to obtain the full benefits.

✔ As treatments go on, you should feel more improvement in your symptoms and be able to have longer intervals between treatments.

✔ For best results, it is important to attend regularly and to follow the exercise and lifestyle advice given to you by your osteopath.

✔ If you have no improvement after a course of treatment then osteopathy may not be effective for your condition and you may need to consider another form of therapy. Discuss this situation with your practitioner.

Common Questions about Osteopathic Treatment

Here are some questions that I'm often asked about osteopathy:

✔ **Will it hurt?** Not usually, no. You may feel a slight click or hear a pop during manipulations but these are just signs that the manipulation has been successful. Gentle manipulation, stretching and massage techniques, and cranial techniques are usually very comfortable and relaxing.

✔ **Do I have to take my clothes off?** Not everything, no. You're usually asked to remove outer garments or wear a robe during treatment if you feel uncomfortable.

✔ **Will I be lying down or sitting up?** Some manipulations are performed when you're lying down on the treatment couch while some are done when you're in a sitting or standing position. Most treatment couches have a *nose hole* to enable you to get comfortable and breathe easily while lying on your front.

✔ **Will other equipment be used?** A rolled towel or pillow may be placed strategically against your body to cushion it during certain manipulations. Some osteopaths are trained in trigger-point acupuncture and may use acupuncture needles in selected sites to release tension and pain. Some also use lasers, magnet healing, or massage devices for the relief of pain.

✔ **How does the osteopath know what techniques to use?** The osteopath's long and rigorous training equips them well in deciding which is the most safe and effective treatment for your particular ailment.

✔ **What happens if I'm scared of vigorous manipulations?** Discuss your anxiety with your osteopath who can modify treatment to suit your needs.

Osteopathic treatment is most effective if you're relaxed and comfortable. Have confidence in your practitioner and ask for a blanket or towel for additional warmth if you feel cold during treatment.

If for any reason you feel faint or nauseous, or if you experience new pain during treatment, always let your osteopath know.

Finding a Good Osteopath

To find a qualified osteopath in your area contact the General Osteopathic Council (GOsC) at: 176 Tower Bridge Road, London SE1 3LU (Tel: 020 7357 6655; e-mail: info@osteopathy.org.uk; www.osteopathy.org.uk). Anyone using the name 'osteopath' must now be registered with this professional body.

Look for the letters after the person's name. All approved osteopathy colleges now offer courses to degree level. Therefore osteopaths who've completed courses since that date will have either BSc (Hons) Osteopathic Medicine, BSc (Hons) Osteopathy, B. Osteopathic Medicine or B. Osteopathy, after their name. British osteopaths trained before degree status became available on courses may use D.O. (Diploma in Osteopathy) after their name. Medical doctors who have done an accelerated course at the London College of Osteopathic Medicine (LCOM) have the letters MLCOM (Member of LCOM) after their name. American trained osteopaths have the letters DO (Doctor of Osteopathy) after their names.

Here are some other recommendations for finding an osteopath:

✔ Ask friends, family, and colleagues for personal recommendations.

✔ Some sports and leisure clubs provide osteopathy.

✔ Consider visiting the teaching clinics at the major schools of osteopathy. All students practise under close supervision from experienced practitioners and fees are often low, too. Contact the schools direct for details at:

- British School of Osteopathy, Tel: 020 7407 0222; www.bso.ac.uk
- College of Osteopaths, Tel: 020 8905 1937; www.collegeofosteopaths.ac.uk
- European School of Osteopathy, Tel: 01622 671 558; www.eso.ac.uk
- London College of Osteopathic Medicine (medical practitioners only), Tel: 020 7262 5250
- London School of Osteopathy, Tel: 020 7265 9333; www.lso.ac.uk
- Oxford Brookes University, Tel: 01865 484 848; www.brookes.ac.uk
- Surrey Institute Of Osteopathic Medicine (SIOM), Tel: 020 8394 1731; www.nescot.ac.uk

Questions to ask your osteopath

Consider asking your osteopath about the following issues:

- ✔ **Qualifications.** Normally practitioners are very happy to provide details of their training and qualifications. If you have any doubt as to their validity, check them.

- ✔ **Insurance.** To be a member of the Register of Osteopaths, your practitioner must be appropriately insured.

- ✔ **Experience.** Question your practitioner about their experience in treating your particular ailment and their usual degree of success!

- ✔ **Logistics.** Find out what fees you can expect and the likely frequency and duration of treatment that you may need.

Counting the cost of osteopathy

The majority of osteopaths work in private practice and their fees generally range from £25 to £55 per session. Practitioners in central locations or with extensive experience may charge more. Sessions are usually 20 to 30 minutes. Typically, two to six sessions may be required. Some osteopaths give discounts if a series of treatments are necessary.

Increasing numbers of osteopaths now work in GP practices and NHS clinics. Ask your doctor if you can be referred to an osteopath on the NHS. In such cases the treatment is usually free, although you may have a long wait.

Many private health insurances now cover osteopathy. You may need to be referred by your doctor in order to claim. Check this with your provider.

Some osteopaths offer concessions for retired persons or those on benefits. Ask your osteopath for details.

Ensuring satisfaction

If you're dissatisfied with your treatment, first talk things over with your practitioner.

If you think that the practitioner has been negligent or unethical in any way, including incompetent treatment and inappropriate touching, contact the

General Osteopathic Council. This independent organisation has a well-established complaints procedure for dealing with any concerns from members of the public.

Helping Yourself with Osteopathy

Osteopaths advise many self-help exercises to aid posture and breathing. Here's a great one that I find really helpful to ease a stiff neck when working at a computer.

1. **Sit with your back straight and imagine a string pulling you up from the top of your head, straightening your spine and lengthening your neck.**

2. **Tuck your chin in slightly so that your neck is in a straight line.**

3. **Put your hands behind your back and interlock your fingers with the palms facing upwards.**

4. **Pull down with your hands stretching your arms downwards and at the same time push your shoulders back and allow the shoulder blades to move towards each other.**

5. **Holding your arms in position, again check that your back is straight and chin tucked slightly in.** Imagine the string at the top of your head pulling you up a little farther.

6. **Hold for the count of ten, breathing evenly, and then release.**

This exercise gives an excellent stretch, improves posture, and releases tension in the neck and shoulders. If you're typing a lot, I suggest repeating it every hour.

I am indebted to the excellent medical osteopath, Dr Jovan Djurovic for teaching me this exercise. I've found it invaluable and hope you'll find it useful too!

Chapter 15

Getting to the Crunch with Chiropractic

*C*hiropractic is one of the most widely practised forms of complementary medicine in the West. In fact, even for many traditional doctors it is now one of the treatments of choice for bad backs and neck problems.

In this chapter, I tell you how chiropractic started as a therapy back in 19th-century America with its founder, Daniel D. Palmer, and how it developed into a popular and effective modern therapy today.

You find out about the types of assessments that chiropractors carry out to determine what's wrong with you. I also tell you about the moves chiropractors may make to put things right and the types of positions you may find yourself in during therapy!

Many chiropractors are also skilled in treating animals. So I let you know how even your dog, cat, racehorse, or bunny rabbit can have joint problems eased by chiropractic.

Finding Out about Chiropractic

Chiropractic diagnoses, treats, and prevents problems with the spine, joints, and muscles and is also concerned with their effects on the nervous system, internal organs, and general health. Chiropractors may use x-rays and other tests as part of their diagnosis.

The aim of treatment is to identify areas of restriction and muscle tightness or pain and to then free the restricted joints and relax the muscles. Treatment consists mainly of adjustments (also called manipulations) to restore normal movement to the joints, bring the body back into alignment and balance and to facilitate the body's own healing. These adjustments are usually performed with the hands but occasionally special hand-held devices are used.

ANECDOTE

Dr Diet, Dr Quiet, and Dr Merryman, and a case of deafness

Daniel David Palmer had already been a beekeeper and a grocer before he began to develop his interest in healing. He read widely on metaphysical ideas about healing that were popular at the time and probably read the works of Andrew Taylor Still, the founder of osteopathy. Whether the two ever met though isn't known.

The caretaker in Palmer's office, Harvey Lillard, had been nearly deaf for 17 years after hearing a 'pop' in his back one day after having been in a cramped position for a long time. Palmer claims to have manipulated Lillard's spine and that almost immediately Lillard could hear carriages in the street down below and regained his hearing. Palmer argued that there was nothing chance about this development but that it had been the careful application of his ideas in practice. Lillard's relatives dispute this story, saying that actually Palmer slapped Lillard heartily on the back one day, after he told a good joke, and then became interested in how his hearing miraculously returned!

Later, Palmer came to stress more strongly his belief in the religious and spiritual aspects of chiropractic and claimed that he'd been given the ideas of chiropractic from a deceased doctor during a séance and that he'd 'received chiropractic from the other world'. He later even likened himself to a spiritual leader who'd searched for and found the cause of all disease.

However, by this time chiropractors had organised themselves as a profession under the leadership of his son and successor, B. J. Palmer, and other prominent chiropractors, and Daniel Palmer became increasingly sidelined.

Palmer was fond of saying, 'The best physicians are Dr Diet, Dr Quiet, and Dr Merryman', but I don't know how merry he was himself. He was unhappy at being sidelined and in constant dispute with his son after selling him his chiropractic college. Palmer died controversially in 1913. The official cause of death was typhoid, but his widow later filed an unsuccessful lawsuit claiming his death was the result of injuries from being knocked down by a car driven at him by his son.

Chiropractic is most commonly used for back and neck problems but can also be used to treat headaches, sciatica (nerve pain from the lower back down into the legs), other types of joint pain, Repetitive Strain Injuries (RSIs), sports injuries, poor posture, and everyday wear and tear.

Chiropractors may also give advice on posture, exercise, lifestyle, and general nutrition.

A (very) brief history of chiropractic

Chiropractic's founder was Daniel D. Palmer, a Canadian, who moved to America with his family in 1865. He held several jobs and eventually worked as a *magnetic healer*. After using spinal manipulation to heal someone with deafness and another with heart problems, Palmer developed his theory of 'the science (knowledge) and art (adjusting) of chiropractic'. Together with a friend he came up with the term by combining the Greek words *cheir* meaning 'hand' and *praxis* meaning 'action', thus describing his manipulations done by hand.

In 1896, Palmer added a school of chiropractic to his magnetic healing practice and began to educate others. One of his first graduates, Solon Langworthy, later opened a second college and incorporated ideas from naturopathy and osteopathy in his practice. He also first coined the word *subluxation* to describe how malpositioned bones in the spine (vertebrae) can interfere with the surrounding nerves.

With the growth of the medical profession in the US, chiropractors became hounded and Palmer was thrown into jail twice for practising medicine without a licence. His son took over the development of chiropractic education and expanded it considerably. It was later successfully argued that chiropractic was a profession separate from medicine and the path to the development of modern, scientific chiropractic began.

Chiropractic was brought to the UK in the 1900s, and the British Chiropractic Association was formed in 1925. Several schools of chiropractic now operate in the UK, and since an Act of Parliament in 1994, all chiropractors must be registered with the General Chiropractic Council, which regulates training and standards.

Modern day chiropractic has long dropped the more metaphysical elements of Palmer's ideas and is now more firmly rooted in scientific theory and evidence-based medicine. However, research findings on chiropractic have been mixed (see 'Evidence that it works' later on in this chapter).

Grasping the idea behind chiropractic

Daniel Palmer believed that the body has an 'innate intelligence', enabling it to organise and heal itself if the right conditions are provided. He believed that the nervous system played an important part in this process and that interference with the nerve supply, due to spinal misalignment or other joint imbalance, was the basic cause of disease.

His theories developed over time. Originally he argued that displacements in the spine caused friction on the nerves leading to inflammation and disease. He later favoured the idea of nerve *impingement*, whereby pressure on the nerves caused by imbalance of spinal bones can affect internal organ function. He also adopted Langworthy's term, subluxation, and at one time argued that 'A subluxated vertebrae . . . is the cause of 95 per cent of all diseases. The other five per cent is caused by displaced joints other than those of the vertebral column.'

However, the concept of subluxation has remained very controversial in chiropractic, with it coming to have different meanings for different practitioners while others have opted to drop it altogether.

Palmer's idea was that if spinal and other joint imbalance can be corrected, and normal nerve function restored, then nerve irritation, inflammation, discomfort, and pain can be eased and related ailments relieved.

Resolving restriction and restoring normal function are still central to chiropractic today, but many of Palmer's original theories about how chiropractic works have been abandoned in favour of more scientific explanations based on an understanding of the physiological mechanisms of pain and pain relief.

Chiropractic today

Chiropractic was one of the first complementary therapies to be regulated and licensed in the UK, with the Chiropractor's Act of 1994.

As part of the Act, the General Chiropractic Council (GCC; www.gcc-uk.org) was established as an independent body to regulate the profession. The GCC sets standards for education and training in chiropractic and for professional practice.

Since 2001, it is illegal for anyone to call themselves a chiropractor unless they've completed a recognised training course and are registered with the GCC. Modern training is comprehensive and generally consists of a four- or five-year degree course incorporating clinical training.

Currently, the UK has three approved chiropractic colleges and more than 2,000 practitioners. In the US, where chiropractic is widespread, more than 50,000 chiropractors practise. Chiropractic is also established in Australia and New Zealand and elsewhere in Europe.

Modern treatment remains almost entirely based on manual therapy techniques. Chiropractors don't perform surgery or prescribe medicines (apart from some US chiropractors who are licensed to perform certain types of minor surgery).

Understanding How Chiropractic Works

The neuro-musculo-skeletal system is made up of the bones, joints, muscles, tendons, ligaments, soft-tissues, and nerves. It provides structural support for the body and the mechanics for our daily movements.

Accident, trauma, poor posture, stress, illness, or wear and tear can all cause damage to the neuro-musculo-skeletal system leading to loss of normal movement, misalignment and nerve inflammation. Nerve irritation can in turn lead to discomfort and pain, manifesting as back pain, neck pain, headache, or even organ dysfunction or it can contribute to *referred pain*, that is, pain in other areas of the body away from the site of injury or trauma.

Chiropractic adjustments open up the spaces between the spinal bones (vertebrae) and loosen up other joints, thereby increasing flexibility and range of motion. Adjustments also improve circulation through muscle tissue and help to reduce inflammation.

Chiropractic techniques also stimulate what are known as *joint movement receptors*, which can alter the messages sent to the brain about the joint's position and movement and can affect nervous system function.

As the nerve irritation is calmed and normal alignment and mobility are regained, then pain and discomfort may be relieved and normal function restored.

Discovering Whom and What Chiropractic Is Good For

Most people associate chiropractic with the treatment of bad backs and necks, and this certainly makes up a large proportion of the average chiropractor's daily practice. However, most chiropractors also treat a range of other conditions.

Conditions that chiropractic can treat

Today's chiropractors most commonly treat the following:

- Back, neck, and shoulder problems
- Joint and muscle problems and poor posture
- Nerve pain, including sciatica
- Headaches
- Whiplash injuries
- Sports injuries

Benefits have also been seen in the treatment of the following:

- Infant colic
- Digestive problems
- Respiratory problems such as asthma
- Repetitive strain injuries
- Menstrual pain
- Arthritis
- Migraines

A timely presentation

Many years ago I was invited to speak at a conference organised by the McTimoney Chiropractic Association. At that time I hadn't yet experienced chiropractic myself, although I had had osteopathy many times. As luck would have it I got stuck in a motorway traffic jam due to an accident and had spent almost six hours cramped in a car by the time I arrived at the conference. The cramped conditions, plus the stress of worrying that I might be late for my presentation (thankfully I wasn't), must have combined so that by the time I arrived I had a pretty bad backache. The organiser noticed that I was moving painfully and laughingly gestured towards the conference hall saying, 'Here are 200 people who can resolve the problem for you – you've come to the right place!' Right after my presentation one of the practitioners gave me some treatment. I was amazed at how gentle and effective it was. I felt better almost immediately and had a trouble-free and pain-free return home. Since that time I have worked regularly with chiropractors in my clinical practice and have found that the treatments have helped large numbers of my patients.

Evidence that it works

Studies in the UK, US, and Australia have shown benefits from chiropractic in the treatment of low back pain. In particular, a Medical Research Council clinical trial and its follow-up, reported in the *British Medical Journal* in 1990 and 1995, found that chiropractic treatment for back pain was more effective than hospital outpatient treatment.

Other trials have shown no specific benefits compared to orthodox or other treatments, and certain large scale review studies have concluded that overall the evidence is weak. However, some of these negative studies have been criticised because they don't take into account how multi-faceted back pain can be or because they analyse the effects of chiropractic manipulation alone, whereas in practice chiropractic often includes more than just manipulation.

Research on other conditions has also been inconclusive. Some have shown good results for infant colic and headaches whereas others for these conditions, and also asthma, carpal tunnel syndrome (nerve compression in the wrist), and painful menstruation, have not. However, many of these studies have had design flaws and more good research is needed.

For more information about chiropractic research, check out the Cochrane Library (www.cochrane.org/reviews/clibintro.htm), the NHS Complementary and Alternative Medicine Specialist Library (www.library.nhs.uk/cam), or the PubMed database, which can be accessed via www.nlm.nih.gov/nccam/camonpubmed.html. Further information on US and Canadian trials can be found at www.clinicaltrials.gov.

When not to use chiropractic

With care and experience, gentle chiropractic techniques can be used for most conditions, but don't use vigorous manipulations with the following conditions:

- ✔ Osteoporosis (brittle bones)
- ✔ Severe rheumatoid arthritis (bone inflammation)
- ✔ Unstable osteoarthritis (that is, serious bone degeneration as opposed to the mild osteoarthritic changes that are a normal part of ageing)
- ✔ Tumours

Neck adjustments should only be performed with great care in people with a history of stroke or high blood pressure. Particular care should also be taken with the elderly and young children or infants.

Chiropractic has a good safety record and the risk of serious complications from it is very low, although a very slight risk of complications with neck manipulations does exist.

What to Expect in a Typical Consultation

Chiropractic consultations usually begin with questions about your medical history and general health, as well as your current symptoms. You may also be asked questions about your diet and lifestyle.

Diagnostic methods

The questions are followed by a physical examination, for which you're given privacy to undress down to your underwear. Female patients are given a gown to wear, which is open at the back to allow the chiropractor to examine the spine.

The examination focuses on the spine, with the chiropractor checking which joints are moving freely and which may be restricted. Other joints and posture may also be checked. The chiropractor often manoeuvres you into different positions, while you are sitting or lying on the treatment couch, to check the range and ease of movement of your spine and joints and the functioning of your muscles.

You may be asked to bend forward or sideways to check your range of movement or to march on the spot to observe pelvic balance. Different muscle tests may be used to test for pain or immobility. Your skin may be palpated to assess levels of inflammation or muscle tension.

The chiropractor may also perform the following:

✔ Measure your blood pressure and pulse

✔ Test your reflexes

✔ Check your heart and lung functions by listening to your chest with a stethoscope, or by means of other tests

✔ Take x-rays if clinically necessary or recommend you for an x-ray or clinical scan elsewhere. If you already have recent x-rays of the affected joint or bone, take these with you to show your chiropractor.

McTimoney chiropractic

McTimoney chiropractic was developed by engineer John McTimoney, an Irish chiropractor, during the 1950s. After receiving successful chiropractic treatment himself, he studied with an American chiropractor, Dr Mary Ward, in England and went on to open his own school in 1972. He developed many of his own gentle techniques as well as specialised techniques for use with animals.

The key to McTimoney's techniques is using just the wrist to make the adjustment and then removing the hand immediately afterwards to allow the body to adjust itself appropriately, rather than having an adjustment imposed upon it. For more information, see www.mctimoney-chiropractic.org.

One of McTimoney's graduates, Hugh Corley also developed his own gentle *whole body* techniques and specialised treatments for animals, calling his method McTimoney-Corley chiropractic. For more information, see www.mctimoney-corley.com.

The chiropractor uses these methods to assess the nature of your symptoms and to identify or rule out any serious underlying disease. Treatment may be delayed until the second visit if diagnostic test results are required.

The chiropractor should explain to you the results of the examination and any test results, the proposed treatment plan, and outline any risks associated with your condition or the treatment.

Getting to grips with chiropractic techniques

Chiropractic treatment consists mainly of *adjustments*, carefully controlled movements, with the quick application of slight force, designed to increase the quality and range of movement in the area, or joint, being treated. The aim is to loosen and mobilise any areas that are locked or restricted.

Often the whole spine and other joints are treated, not just the affected part of the body, because each part is seen to have an effect on the other.

Chiropractors have many techniques in common with other manual therapists, such as osteopaths and physiotherapists but tend to focus on these adjustments.

Sometimes you hear a *crack* or *pop* when the joint is released. This may sound alarming, but is harmless and simply due to pressure changes causing the release of tiny gas bubbles around the joint. The treatment is usually painless. If the area is very inflamed or sore, treatment can be modified accordingly. Other techniques used may include the following:

- ✔ **Joint mobilisation:** Rhythmical moving of the joint and the application of gentle stretches to the surrounding tissue to release tension and ease restriction.

- ✔ **Direct pressure:** Direct pressure to certain *trigger-points* in order to release tension and pain.

- ✔ **Massage:** Different types of massage may be used to ease muscle tension, stretch the tissues, and promote circulation.

Most chiropractors also use other non-manual treatments. These may include the following:

- ✔ Heat and ice

- ✔ Ultrasound

- ✔ Electrical stimulation

- ✔ Exercise therapy

- ✔ Dry needle therapy (a type of trigger-point acupuncture used to relieve pain)

- ✔ Magnetic therapy

Chiropractors may also give nutritional, ergonomic and general lifestyle advice.

At the end of your treatment, you may receive the following additional tips and advice:

- ✔ You may be shown certain exercises for you to practise between sessions.

- ✔ You may be advised on the after-effects of your treatment. Some people experience mild aching, headache, or fatigue, but these are usually minor and ease after a day or so.

- ✔ You can discuss the need for further treatments and the time in between appointments.

- ✔ You'll be advised to avoid vigorous exercise, heavy lifting, and long-distance travel right after treatment to allow your tissues time to settle down.

Duration and frequency

The first chiropractic session generally lasts 30 to 60 minutes, while follow-up visits are typically 15 to 20 minutes (depending on the practitioner's choice of techniques). In the first week, you may be advised to have two or three sessions. Thereafter, sessions are usually once a week, according to need.

For recent conditions, three to six treatments are common, whereas more chronic conditions often require six to twelve treatments. Maintenance treatments at regular intervals to prevent recurrence are also often advised.

Exploring Chiropractic Approaches

Chiropractors use a variety of techniques and different chiropractors may go about your treatment in different ways. Their choice of technique depends on where they qualified, any special interests they have, and what type of additional courses they've attended.

ANECDOTE

An equine success story

Pronto was a horse used for dressage (a series of complex manoeuvres through which the horse is guided by slight movements of the rider's hands, legs, and weight to test the horse's physique and ability and the rider's skill). He'd won many competitions but had become over-bent after repeated practice with head carriage. As a result, the muscles of his neck and shoulders had become stiff and painful and movement of his forelimbs was becoming restricted. He was also becoming uncharacteristically temperamental and refusing to co-operate during practise sessions.

A chiropractor, specialised in dealing with horses, was recommended by the local vet and worked with Pronto, making adjustments to his neck and shoulders and massaging the muscles. She then showed Pronto's owner how to give him a series of stretches to loosen his muscles and joints, using a carrot as an incentive. (Nicknamed *carrot-practics*, examples of these exercises have been published in *Natural Horse Magazine,* and you can find them on www.todayshorse.com/Articles/HorseCarrotPractics.htm.)

After three treatments, a few days' rest, and daily *carrot-practics*, Pronto was performing better than ever, back to his usually happy disposition and soon in competition-winning form once more. His owner has maintained his exercise regime and occasional maintenance chiropractic treatments and the problem hasn't recurred.

Certain individual chiropractors have become known for particular styles of treatment that they have pioneered. The most well known of these is John McTimoney who developed what has become known as McTimoney chiropractic.

However, the common goal for all chiropractors is the same: To get your joints, muscles, and nervous system working properly, so that your body can recover and heal as quickly as possible.

Knowing whether your chiropractic treatment is working

Although you may experience immediate benefits from chiropractic treatment, symptoms do sometimes flare-up before they get better. You may feel a bit stiff or sore for a couple of days or feel more tired than usual. However, these effects normally pass after a day or so.

Here are some tips for successful chiropractic treatment:

- ✔ If you experience a marked increase in pain, or deterioration in your symptoms, contact your chiropractor for advice.

- ✔ Ask your chiropractor what improvements you can realistically expect over what sort of timescale.

- ✔ For best results, attend regularly and follow the exercise and lifestyle advice given to you by your chiropractor. Daily practise of the rehabilitation exercises can speed up healing.

- ✔ If you have no improvement after a course of treatment, then chiropractic may not be effective for your condition and you may need to consider another form of therapy. Discuss this situation with your practitioner.

Common questions about chiropractic treatment

Here are some questions that I'm often asked about chiropractic:

- ✔ **Will it hurt?** Not usually, no. You may feel a slight click or hear a pop during manipulations, but these are just signs that the manipulation has been successful.

✔ **Do I have to take my clothes off?** You're normally required to strip down to your underwear, but you may wear a robe during treatment if you feel uncomfortable.

✔ **Will I be lying down or sitting up?** Treatment may be given while you are sitting, standing, or lying down. Chiropractors use a specially designed treatment couch to maintain comfort during adjustments.

✔ **Will other equipment be used?** Some chiropractors use small devices to exert a measured thrust on a particular joint in place of their hands.

✔ **How does the chiropractor know what techniques to use?** Chiropractors are thoroughly trained in diagnosis, assessment, reading x-rays, and clinical practice to enable them to select the safest and most effective techniques for your particular ailment.

✔ **What happens if I'm scared of vigorous manipulations?** Discuss your anxiety with your chiropractor, who can modify your treatment if necessary.

Finding a Good Chiropractor

To find a qualified chiropractor in your area, contact the General Chiropractic Council (GCC) (Tel: 020 7713 5155; www.gcc-uk.org).

Anyone using the name chiropractor must now be registered with this professional body.

McTimoney chiropractors are also members of the McTimoney Chiropractic Association (MCA) (Tel: 01491 829211; www.mctimoney-chiropractic.org).

Look for the letters after the person's name. These will depend on when and where the person qualified but graduates of approved colleges currently have the following: Undergraduate MChiro (Anglo-European College of Chiropractic (AECC)); BSc(Hons) Chiropractic (McTimoney College of Chiropractic); and BSc(Hons) Chiropractic (University of Glamorgan).

American-trained chiropractors have the letters DC (Doctor of Chiropractic) after their names.

Here are some other recommendations for finding a chiropractor:

✔ Ask friends, family, and colleagues for personal recommendations.

✔ Some sports and leisure clubs offer chiropractic treatment.

✔ Many GPs have contact with their local chiropractor and may be happy to refer you.

✔ Consider visiting the teaching clinics at chiropractic colleges (listed below). All students practise under close supervision from experienced practitioners and fees are low compared to private practice.

- Anglo-European College of Chiropractic (Tel: 01202 436200; www.aecc.ac.uk).

- University of Glamorgan (Tel: 01443 482287; www.glam.ac.uk).

- McTimoney College of Chiropractic (Tel: 01235 523336; www.mctimoney-college.ac.uk).

Questions to ask your chiropractor

You may want to ask your chiropractor about the following:

✔ **Qualifications:** Most practitioners are happy to give details of their training and qualifications. If you have any doubt as to their validity, then check them with the General Chiropractic Council (www.gcc-uk.org).

✔ **Insurance:** To be a registered chiropractor, your practitioner must have appropriate indemnity insurance.

✔ **Experience:** Ask your practitioner about their experience in treating your particular ailment and their usual degree of success!

✔ **Treatment:** Ask about the likely frequency and duration of treatment that you may need and the cost involved.

Counting the cost of chiropractic

Initial chiropractic consultations usually cost around £40 to £65, while follow-up sessions are in the region of £25 to £35.

Some GP practices offer chiropractic treatment on the NHS. Ask your doctor for details. Some private health insurances cover chiropractic treatment. Check with your provider for advice.

Some chiropractors offer concessions for retired persons or those on benefits. Ask your chiropractor for details.

Finding chiropractors who treat animals

Chiropractors trained in animal manipulation, and able to treat animals with veterinary approval, hold a PGDip in Animal Manipulation from either the McTimoney College of Chiropractic (see the earlier sidebar about McTimoney chiropractic) or the Oxford College of Equine Physical Therapy (more information is available from www.mctimoney-corley.com or education@ocept.info). They may be located through either of these organisations or by logging on to www.natural-animal-health.co.uk/find-therapist.html.

Ensuring satisfaction

If you're dissatisfied with your treatment, first talk things over with your practitioner.

If you think that the practitioner has been negligent or unethical in any way, including incompetent treatment and inappropriate touching, you should contact the General Chiropractic Council, which has a formal complaints procedure.

Helping Yourself with Chiropractic

Chiropractors advise many self-help exercises to aid posture and strengthen muscles. Here's a good one for stretching the lower back and toning the muscles:

1. **Lie flat on the floor in a relaxed position with legs outstretched together.**

2. **Bend your right knee and bring it up towards your chest.**

3. **Place your hands around the knee and slowly and gently pull it down towards your chest.** Don't strain; simply pull down as far as is comfortable. Keep the left leg straight and flat on the floor while you do this.

4. **Hold this position for three to five seconds, breathing normally.** Release any tension and relax as you hold the position.

5. **Gently release and lower your leg.**

6. **Repeat the movement with the opposite leg.** Make sure that you keep the outstretched leg flat on the floor and straight out.

7. **If you want, you can develop the exercise by bringing both knees up to the chest together and holding as before.**

I use this exercise every day to help to prevent back problems that can be triggered by spending hours sitting at the computer writing books! It can be especially helpful to do this exercise first thing in the mornings.

If you have, or have had, any sort of lower back problem or injury, consult your chiropractor, doctor, or other manual therapist before performing this or any other back exercise.

Chapter 16

Moving with Bodywork Therapies

●●●

In This Chapter

▶ Finding out what bodywork therapies are all about

▶ Discovering what bodywork therapies can be good for

▶ Examining the evidence

▶ Knowing what to expect in a typical session

▶ Knowing where to find safe and effective practitioners

●●●

Complementary therapies offer so many ways to have your body moved, stretched, rocked, and restructured! Some of the therapies come from ancient medical traditions and have stood the test of time; some grew out of the pioneering development of osteopathy and chiropractic (check out Chapters 14 and 15 for more on these); others have been put together more recently.

The idea that all these therapies share is that misalignment and imbalance in your body can affect the function of your internal organs and body systems. Some also hold that your mental, emotional, and spiritual health can be affected too. The therapies are based on the belief that the body can be brought back into alignment or balance using physical manipulations, massage, stretches, or more subtle means. Some of the therapies mean working directly on your muscles, joints, and tissues – and you'll certainly feel what's being done to you! Others take a more subtle approach and focus on the so-called *energetic fields* around, or within, the body. In the case of these, you may not feel that much going on at all during actual therapy but transformations may start to occur afterwards.

Finding Out about Bodywork Therapies

In this section, I take you on a brief guided tour of popular bodywork therapies (in alphabetical order) and give you an idea what each involves, what evidence exists to support their use, and how you can find qualified practitioners so that you can try them out for yourself if you and your body are up for it!

Alexander Technique

The Alexander Technique was devised by an Australian actor, Frederick Matthias Alexander, in the late 19th-century after he suffered voice strain and voice loss and tried to devise ways to relieve his condition. Here's some info about the Alexander Technique:

- ✔ According to Alexander, years of poor posture, slouching, improper lifting, and muscular tension gradually have a negative effect on both the body and mind.

- ✔ The Alexander Technique teacher is trained to identify these patterns of misuse in the body.

- ✔ In a one-to-one or group session you're taught to increase your awareness of correct body posture and to re-educate your body towards correct posture and the release of muscle tension.

- ✔ Sessions generally last 30 to 45 minutes and are usually taken weekly, or sometimes twice weekly in the beginning, for at least 10 to 15 sessions.

- ✔ Research on the Alexander Technique has suggested beneficial effects for musicians, actors, and sportspeople as well as those suffering from certain types of pain.

- ✔ Costs vary from £35 to £100 per session.

- ✔ In the UK, you can find teachers via the Society of Teachers of the Alexander Technique (STAT; Tel: 0845 230 7828; www.stat.org.uk) whose members have all completed a three-year full-time training. You can also find teachers worldwide via www.alexandertechnique.com.

Applied kinesiology (AK)

Applied kinesiology (AK), derives from the term *kinesiology*, which is based on the Greek word *kinesis* meaning movement or motion, and was developed by American chiropractor, Dr George Goodheart, in the 1960s. He developed a way of muscle testing to determine the balance of structural, mental, and chemical (toxicity, allergies, and so on) health; three aspects that he called the *Triad of Health*. Here's the lowdown on AK:

✔ AK is used primarily for diagnosis and is based on the idea that every muscle is part of an *energy circuit* that can be disrupted by toxicity, blockage, or illness. The strength of the circuit can be tested by isolating individual muscles and challenging them (see below).

✔ Treatment consists of: (i) applying pressure to, or holding, certain energy points on the body to release blockages in the acupuncture meridian channels; (ii) gentle manipulation techniques to correct structural imbalances; and (iii) nutritional and lifestyle advice. Homeopathic, nutritional, or herbal supplements may also be recommended.

✔ In a typical session the AK practitioner places one of your arms or legs in a particular position and then challenges the muscle by pushing against it and asking you to resist. If the muscle is strong you can easily resist the challenge. If it is weak then you have difficulty resisting.

✔ AK challenges can be physical (directly pushing against the muscle), chemical (testing phials of allergens, bacteria and toxins, held against the body), or even mental (you, or the practitioner, holds a mental thought, such as of a nutrient or other remedy) while the muscle is tested.

✔ Medics and sceptics find it impossible to accept that such diagnosis can be accurate and argue that little scientific evidence exists to support the theories underlying AK.

✔ Research studies on AK (see the research section of www.icak.com for details), suggest that certain muscles testing weak may be linked to certain physiological changes in the body. However, the research to date has not been sufficient, or good enough, to change the mind of sceptics. Nevertheless, AK is utilised by large numbers of chiropractors, naturopaths, and other practitioners who say that they find this approach clinically useful.

✔ Sessions generally last 30 to 45 minutes and may be weekly at first and then spaced out according to the health problem being treated. At each follow-up session, the muscles may be re-tested for improvement.

✔ Costs vary from £40 to £70 per session and usually several sessions may be required.

✔ Various offshoots from AK have been developed, including Health Kinesiology, Nambudripad's Allergy Elimination Technique, BodyTalk, and more.

✔ You can find AK practitioners via the International College of Applied Kinesiology (UK) (Tel: 01403 734321; www.icak.com) whose members have all completed a 100-hour course.

Bates eye method

Bates eye method was devised by an American ophthalmologist, Dr William H. Bates, in the 20th century. He had really bad eyesight and his glasses broke one day while he was on holiday. He found that by the end of the holiday he could see better than before and determined to find out why. He concluded that misuse of his eyes and eyestrain had contributed to his poor eyesight and went on to devise a set of exercises to remedy these. Here's some more info about the Bates eye method:

- ✔ The Bates method consists of a series of eye exercises to *re-educate* visual habits.

- ✔ The exercises can be learnt from someone trained in the Bates eye method over six to ten weekly sessions or from self-help sources (such as books, videos, and online). The exercises require perseverance over a period of time and include splashing the eyes with alternating warm and cold water to increase circulation, blinking to cleanse the eyes and swaying while gazing on a fixed spot to relax the eye muscles, focusing on alternating near and far objects, and pressing warmed palms against the eyes to relax them.

- ✔ Although research by Bates and his colleagues and anecdotal evidence is supportive of this technique, recent scientific validation is lacking and modern ophthalmologists and opticians remain sceptical.

- ✔ Individual sessions are normally £40 to £50 per session but small group sessions may be as low as £8 per person.

- ✔ You can find teachers of the Bates method in the UK and elsewhere in the world via the Bates Association for Vision Education (www.seeing.org).

- ✔ The Bates method also forms part of the work by Meir Schneider for his method of self-healing, which combines massage, movement therapy, visualisation, and breathing exercises. For more information, check out www.self-healing.org or in the US call 00 (1415) 665 9574.

Bioenergetics

Bioenergetics was devised by American psychoanalyst Dr Alexander Lowen in the 1960s. Lowen had studied with the psychoanalyst Wilhelm Reich, a contemporary of psychiatrist, Sigmund Freud, and adapted their ideas to develop a body–mind therapy that he called *bioenergetics*. Here's the need-to-know stuff about bioenergetics:

✔ Bioenergetics is based on the idea that your body carries a physical memory of past traumas that are locked into the body in areas of muscle tension and rigidity.

✔ In a one-to-one or group session you're taken through various physical positions and situations and encouraged to express the feelings that these unlock. For example, you may be asked to lean against another person for support and then find out what emotions doing so brings up, or you may be asked to adopt an open or closed body position and then connect with the physical sensations inside your body.

✔ Sessions can be great fun and energising but can also be quite dramatic as emotions like anger, hurt, and fear get released. I took a bioenergetics course years ago and remember lots of tears and catharsis in the group!

✔ Bioenergetics may be used to relieve specific physical or emotional problems or as a tool for increasing awareness and for personal development.

✔ Sessions generally last about an hour and small groups generally meet on a weekly basis for six to ten weeks. Costs vary depending on whether you have individual or group therapy.

✔ Only limited research exists on bioenergetics. Most of it documents experiences that people have had with the therapy rather than clinical trials.

✔ Therapists using this method need to be well trained to deal appropriately with the raw emotions that can come up and the dynamics of the group.

✔ You can find certified bioenergetic therapists who have trained for four to six years via the International Institute for Bioenergetic Analysis at `www.bioenergetic-therapy.com`.

Bowen technique

The Bowen technique was devised by Australian Tom Bowen in the 1950s, and later taught extensively by his students, Oswald and Elaine Rentsch. Bowen had no previous training in any therapy or medical system. He simply wanted to alleviate suffering and always claimed that the technique was a 'gift from God'. Here's what you need to know about the Bowen technique:

✔ This therapy involves soft, rolling movements across different muscle groups through light clothing or on the skin, with the recipient lying on a treatment couch.

✔ Two-minute pauses occur between treatment of different muscle groups, during which the practitioner leaves the room in order to allow the body to *reset* itself by relaxing and readjusting itself.

✔ The technique is said to trigger electrical impulses in the nervous system that release muscle tension and increase the circulation of blood and lymph. It is held that this enables joints, tendons, muscles, and so on to recover normal function and movement.

✔ Sessions last 30 to 45 minutes and having three sessions at weekly intervals is normal, with follow-ups as necessary.

✔ The technique has been used to treat chronic fatigue syndrome, all kinds of muscular pain and injury, menstrual problems, and so on.

✔ As yet no rigorous research exists to support this therapy, although a frozen shoulder trial is currently underway at the Metropolitan University of Manchester.

✔ Costs vary from £35 to £45 or so per session depending on the practitioner.

✔ You can find practitioners of the Bowen technique in the UK and worldwide via the Bowen Association (Tel: 0700 269 8324; www.bowen-technique.co.uk), or the Bowen Therapists' European Register (Tel: 07986 008384; www.bowentherapists.com).

Feldenkrais technique

The Feldenkrais technique is a system of 're-education' for the body developed in the 1940s by Moshe Feldenkrais, who was born in the Ukraine and later settled in Israel. He applied his knowledge of engineering and his love of sports, especially judo – in which he was a second Dan black belt – to devise a technique that enabled maximum efficiency of the body with minimum effort. He was spurred on to create this therapy by the flare-up of an old knee injury that he wanted to be able to cure. Here's the lowdown on the Feldenkrais technique:

✔ This therapy's based on the idea that poor posture and inefficient movement of the body are linked to disturbances in the nervous system.

✔ Treatment consists of: (i) exercises that increase body 'awareness through movement'; and (ii) gentle manipulation and touch techniques, known as *functional integration* to help rebalance the nervous system and restore mobility.

✔ Feldenkrais technique may be learnt in groups or tailor-made in individual sessions, which usually last an hour and cost around £45.

✔ Feldenkrais has helped people with neck and back pain, stress, and tension, and is often used by dancers, actors, and sportspeople. Feldenkrais himself also pioneered its use with children and adults with severe disabilities due to, for example, cerebral palsy and stroke.

✔ Some studies have produced encouraging results for this technique but more research is needed.

✔ In the UK, you may find certified practitioners, who have trained for three to four years, via The Feldenkrais Guild UK (Tel: 07000 785 506; www.feldenkrais.co.uk). In the US, the Feldenkrais Educational Foundation of North America (FEFNA) lists qualified practitioners (Tel: 00 (1800) 775 2112 (toll free); www.feldenkrais.com).

Hellerwork

Hellerwork was devised by American engineer Joseph Heller in the 1970s. Heller was a prominent student of Ida Rolf (check out the section on Rolfing further on in this chapter), but later broke away to develop his own system with a greater emphasis on psychology and emotions. Here's what you need to know:

✔ This therapy's based on the same principles as Rolfing, namely that realigning the body and releasing tension in the muscle fibres can help alleviate pain and disease.

✔ It involves a series of eleven 90-minute sessions based on bodywork, movement, and dialogue. Costs are generally around £45 per session.

✔ The *bodywork* involves manipulation and deep pressure, similar to Rolfing; the *movement* involves re-educating the body to move in stress- and tension-free ways; and the *dialogue* is where emotions that surface with the release of tension are explored.

✔ Hellerwork is most commonly used to relieve pain, stiffness and injury, mental and emotional stress, poor posture, and sports injuries.

✔ Only very limited research into Hellerwork exists, so it currently remains unproven.

✔ In the UK, you can find Hellerwork practitioners via Hellerwork International (www.hellerwork.com).

Metamorphic technique

Practitioners of the metamorphic technique don't diagnose or treat particular symptoms or ailments. Rather, their aim is to facilitate the person's own natural metamorphosis by unblocking old *energetic patterns* in the body and enabling self-healing and personal development. Here's a snapshot of the metamorphic technique:

- ✔ The technique grew out of work by British naturopath and reflexologist Robert St John with autistic children in the 1970s. St John believed that certain physical, mental, and emotional patterns are established while in the womb and 'held' in the body. He found that by stimulating certain reflexology points on the feet that related to spinal reflexes (the reflexes connected to the spinal cord that send messages all around the body), these patterns could be released, and amazing, spontaneous changes would occur in the children's abilities and personalities.

- ✔ Gaston St Pierre, a student of St John, went on to develop this *metamorphosis* approach into the Metamorphic technique, emphasising a detached attitude on the part of the practitioner, allowing the person to be their own direct agent of change.

- ✔ The technique is based on the idea that the body develops energetic patterns based on life experiences and that light touch on the spinal reflex points of the feet, hands, and head can enable these patterns to be transformed without any other intervention by the practitioner.

- ✔ The technique is performed one-to-one over one or more sessions of about one hour. You remove your shoes and socks and sit or lie down while the practitioner works on your feet, and then hands, and finally head.

- ✔ The technique is safe and suitable for anyone from babies to the elderly.

- ✔ No research exists to substantiate the theory behind this technique or its usefulness, but those who have had it say that it is relaxing and enjoyable and that it can be a powerful facilitator for change.

- ✔ Costs vary from £35 to £60 per session.

- ✔ You can find practitioners worldwide via The Metamorphic Association (Tel: 01424 432 566; www.metamorphicassociation.org.uk).

Polarity therapy

This technique was devised by Dr Randolph Stone (formerly Bautsch), an Austrian who emigrated to the US. He qualified as an osteopath, chiropractor, and naturopath in the early 20th century, and made an extensive study of various Eastern spiritual disciplines, Oriental medicine, and the concept of Life Energy. The following is a summary of polarity therapy:

- ✔ This therapy's based on the idea that the body is surrounded by an electro-magnetic field. The head and right side of the body represent the positive electrical pole and the feet and left side of the body the negative electrical pole.

✔ The spine is the central axis for this energetic interchange and it has five energy centres corresponding to the elements of ether, air, fire, water, and earth, which relate to different areas of the body and body functions.

✔ For this therapy you lie on a treatment table in loose clothing or underwear and the practitioner uses light, medium, and deep pressure on certain points on the body to rebalance the energy fields while also engaging you in dialogue to increase self-awareness.

✔ Sessions last 60 to 90 minutes and are normally weekly over eight weeks or so, plus follow-ups as necessary. Dietary advice may also be given, based on a fresh food diet to clear toxins in the body. Polarity, yoga-type exercises, may also be recommended to aid this process.

✔ No research exists to prove the theory behind this approach or confirms its benefits, but it is rooted in such ancient traditions as Ayurveda and yoga, which have been practised for thousands of years.

✔ Costs vary from £35 to £60 per session.

✔ In the UK, you can find practitioners via the UK Polarity Therapy Association (UKPTA; Tel: 0700 7052748; `www.ukpta.org.uk`) and in the US via the American Polarity Therapy Association (`www.polaritytherapy.org`).

Rolfing

Also called *structural integration*, referring to the correction of mis-alignment and imbalance in the structure of the body, Rolfing was devised by US biochemist Ida Rolf in the 1950s. Rolf researched yoga, osteopathy, and physical therapy, and came to believe that body alignment is essential to well-being. Here's the lowdown on Rolfing:

✔ Rolf believed that poor posture, lack of fitness, emotional or physical stress, or injury can cause stiffness of the tissues, misalignment and later disease.

✔ She designed a system of ten, hour long treatments whereby the practitioner works through the body easing, stretching, and kneading the tissues to restore alignment.

✔ The practitioner uses fingers, knuckles, and elbows with firm pressure to achieve this 're-sculpting' of the body. When I had Rolfing I found this pressure a bit painful at times! As the sessions progressed it was certainly the most penetrating tissue work that I had ever experienced. Nowadays, however, increasingly light techniques are used for increased comfort and some people don't find it painful at all.

- ✔ The idea is to help your body to work with gravity rather than against it, and many people find this technique can ease pain and stiffness, relieve stress and tension, and more. Rolfing is often used by dancers, musicians, and sportspeople.

- ✔ A few research trials have confirmed that Rolfing can reduce stress, anxiety, and pain. Many medics and sceptics are prepared to accept Rolfing as a legitimate form of massage or therapeutic bodywork since the focus is specifically on realignment of the physical body.

- ✔ Rolfing is normally done over ten 60- to 90-minute sessions, with initial sessions on the superficial layers of the body, middle sessions at a deeper level, and final sessions on structural integration as a whole. Costs are about £75 to £95 per session.

- ✔ You can locate Rolfers worldwide via the Rolf Institute of Structural Integration (Tel: 00 (1303) 449 5978 or 00 (1800) 530 8875; www.rolf.org).

Tragerwork

Tragerwork was devised by an American physiotherapist and doctor, Milton Trager, who also studied transcendental meditation (see Chapter 18). He became interested in how the subconscious mind could be used to release mental *programming* concerning disease or disability. The following is a summary of Tragerwork:

- ✔ This therapy utilises rhythmical, rocking movements to stretch the body and release stress patterns.

- ✔ The practitioner enters a relaxed state known as *hook up* during which it is meant to be possible to sense areas of tension.

- ✔ When an area of tension is felt, then pressure is eased up, rather than increased, giving the recipient a sensation of lightness.

- ✔ The practitioner may also recommend special exercises known as *Mentastics* that are designed to reinforce positive subconscious programming for health.

- ✔ Sessions last 60 to 90 minutes and may be repeated weekly over several weeks. You wear loose, light clothing and lie on a padded treatment table for the therapy.

- ✔ Initial research suggests that Trager work can help ease pain and stiffness. More research is needed.

- ✔ Costs vary from £35 to £60 per session.

- ✔ In the UK, you can find practitioners via Trager UK (Tel: 01903 717987; www.trager.co.uk), and in the US via Trager USA (Tel: (001) 216 896 9383; www.trager.com).

The anaesthetic cure

One of the things that gave Trager the idea for his therapy was witnessing the remarkable transformation of someone under anaesthesia. He watched a patient who suffered from terrible stiffness and pain become limp and relaxed while under anaesthesia, but then observed how the patterns of rigidity returned as the anaesthetic started to wear off. This observation gave Trager the idea of tension existing as 'patterns' in the body that are reinforced by the subconscious mind. He then experimented with using touch to *repattern* the tension in the muscles and tissues while also using a meditative, relaxed state to change habitual subconscious thought patterns.

Yoga, qi gong, t'ai chi, kum nye, and do-in

Each of the ancient Oriental medical systems has a movement/bodywork therapy as an integral part of its healing tradition. The idea is that through your own therapeutic bodywork you can keep your body fit, flexible, strong, and healthy; ward off disease; and delay the ageing process.

The main bodywork approaches in these traditions are:

- ✔ **Yoga:** Part of the Ayurvedic tradition, and meaning 'union of body, mind, and spirit', yoga includes static and moving poses (*asanas*) and breathing exercises (*pranayama*) for physical health and as a preparation for spiritual development via meditation, service, devotion, and so on. For contact details of yoga organisations, see Chapter 18.

- ✔ **Qi gong:** Pronounced '*chee-kung*', and also written *Ch'i kung*, it means 'to work with'(or move) *qi*. This is an ancient system of static or moving exercises, originally based on observation of animal movements. Qi gong is a part of Traditional Chinese Medicine (TCM), involves breathing and meditation, and is sometimes used to direct healing energy to diseased parts of the body.

- ✔ **T'ai chi ch'uan:** Derived from Chinese characters meaning *great*, *ultimate*, and *fist*, and often translated as 'supreme ultimate power', this ancient Chinese system of therapeutic exercises and breathing techniques is said to have grown out of qi gong. Often described as a *soft* martial art, t'ai chi is usually performed as a set sequence of a small or large number of movements (called short and long forms). T'ai chi is designed to increase the flow of 'vital energy', or *qi*, in the body and to promote self-healing.

- ✔ **Kum nye:** Pronounced '*Koom nyay*', this oral tradition of meditative, self-awareness exercises and poses (static or moving) is part of the Tibetan medical tradition. In recent years, this tradition has been formalised and brought to the West by the Tibetan lama, Tarthang Tulku, and his students.

✔ **Do-in:** Pronounced '*Dough-in*', this system of exercises for personal and spiritual development is from the Japanese medical tradition and includes simple self-massage techniques and physical exercises.

These approaches are now practised worldwide by millions of people. They are quite different to the standard Western approach to exercise and body movement, which tends to focus on aerobics, exertion, and the 'no pain no gain' philosophy. In contrast, the Oriental bodywork systems are gentle and subtle, with a focus on breath and on moving 'subtle energy' in the body.

Yoga and qi gong have been the subject of increasing numbers of research studies that have shown both physical and psychological benefits but more research is needed to confirm how such benefits may be achieved.

Zero balancing

The Zero balancing technique was developed in the 1970s, by American doctor and osteopath Fritz Smith. He encountered acupuncture and became fascinated by the relationship between energy channels in the body and the structure of the body provided by the bones and muscles. Smith went on to train as an acupuncturist and gradually develop this approach, which got its name from a recipient who described the therapy as 'like being returned to zero'.

✔ This therapy's based on the idea that we have an invisible *energy body* as well as a physical one and that a relationship exists between the two. If the energy body becomes blocked the bones and muscles that make up the deep structure of the physical body will be affected and vice versa.

✔ Treatment aims to restore balance in the flow of this vital energy by working on the body and breathing, and by promoting self-healing.

✔ Special attention is paid to important 'shock absorber joints', such as those in the foot that support the body's weight, and also to your posture, breathing patterns, eye movements, and even the sounds of your stomach rumbling (all thought to give important clues as to the flow of this vital energy).

✔ In treatment sessions you lie fully clothed on a treatment table while the practitioner gently touches different points on the body and 'holds' stretches of the muscles. The stretches are held to a point of stillness, during which the body is thought to release tension and realign itself and the flow of *vital energy* is believed to be enhanced.

✔ Sessions usually last 20 to 45 minutes and three weekly sessions, with additional follow-up as necessary, are often recommended. Zero balancing is sometimes combined with other therapies, such as acupuncture.

✔ Little research exists to support the theory underlying zero balancing but those who have it report finding the therapy relaxing and enjoyable and some say that it helps reduce their pain and stress.

✔ Costs vary from £35 to £65 per session depending on the practitioner.

✔ In the UK, you can find teachers via The Zero Balancing Association UK (Tel: 01308 420 007; www.zerobalancinguk.org). For practitioners in the US or other countries, check out the Zero Balancing Health Association (Tel: 00 (1410) 381 8956; www.zerobalancing.com). All certified zero balancing practitioners have completed a series of training workshops including advanced training with Fritz Smith himself, who continues to develop the technique.

Helping Yourself with Bodywork Therapies

A really good way of relaxing, lengthening the spine, and easing tension, used as part of the Alexander Technique for re-educating the body, is the following:

✔ Grab yourself a couple of books of different thicknesses (content doesn't matter because you won't be reading them!).

✔ Lie on the floor (a hard surface is best but use a rug if the floor surface is cold) with your back flat and your knees bent up to allow the flat of your back to contact with the floor.

✔ Place two or three books under your head to allow your neck to feel relaxed and your spine straight.

✔ Adjust the position of your feet so that your knees and back feel at ease and comfortable. (If in doubt about your position, you can ask an Alexander Technique teacher to check it for you.)

✔ Place your hands comfortably folded on your abdomen.

✔ Breathe naturally.

✔ Focus your mind on your body and breathing and allow any tension to be released.

✔ Relax in this position for 5 to 15 minutes every day.

Chapter 17

Enjoying Massage Therapies

· ·

In This Chapter

▶ Finding out what massage therapy is all about

▶ Understanding how massage works

▶ Exploring different types of massage therapy

▶ Discovering what massage can be good for

▶ Knowing what to expect in a typical massage treatment

▶ Knowing how to find a safe and effective massage therapist

· ·

*M*assage is one of the oldest forms of therapy, having been practised since time immemorial. Touch is reassuring, relaxing, and healing, and even essential – in early life, babies and infants deprived of touch fail to thrive.

The touch of a mother's hand can soothe a crying infant or ease a child's pain; a neck and shoulder rub squeezed into a lunch hour can improve an office worker's performance and well-being; a massage from a sports thera-pist can ease an athlete's cramp; and self-massage of temples or belly can ease headache or abdominal pain. These are just some examples of how anyone can give and receive massage and benefit from it.

In this chapter I introduce you to a whole host of different types of profes-sional massage. You'll look at old and new massage therapies from both East and West and their benefits. You'll also explore just what it is about massage that makes you feel soooooo good!

I also tell you a bit about research that supports the use of massage and give you some tips on how to find a safe and effective massage therapist. At the end of the chapter I show you a quick massage that you can give yourself at any time, especially if you're short of time or money.

Finding Out about Massage

Massage is the use of different types of touch, pressure, and movement on the skin and underlying tissues to release tension, pain, and blockage and to help you feel good. The word *massage* is thought to have come from either the Greek word *masso*, which means 'to knead', or the Arabic *mas'h*, meaning 'to touch, feel, or handle'. The ancient Greeks, Egyptians, Romans, and other ancient civilisations are all known to have enjoyed massage.

Every culture and medical system has one or more different forms of massage, and massage techniques have also been incorporated into many different therapies used today, including osteopathy and chiropractic. Modern massage therapists may specialise in one type of massage or may have been trained in several and then use them individually or in combination.

Massage is believed to provide a range of benefits including increased circulation, improved immune function, relaxation of muscles, and relief from pain, inflammation, and fluid retention, as well as enhanced self-esteem and well-being.

Massage is a hugely popular therapy and is utilised in beauty salons, spas, health centres, hospitals, offices, schools, sports centres and gyms, homes for the elderly, and baby units, as well as, of course, in the home.

A (very) brief history of massage

Massage features in ancient Chinese scrolls that date back to 400 BC and in papyrus scrolls of the ancient Egyptians. The great ancient Greek physician Hippocrates recommended massage, and Julius Caesar and his Roman colleagues had it regularly, too.

Spared by the executioner!

Massage ability can even be life saving! The great French Renaissance doctor, Ambroise Paré, was a hearty barber-surgeon who became famous as an army doctor for devising humane and natural methods to save soldiers' lives. For example, he used eggs, oil of roses, and turpentine to treat amputation stumps and massage and physical therapy to rehabilitate injured soldiers. On one occasion he was captured by enemy soldiers and was just about to be executed when he was recognised. Because of his great healing skills he was spared and went on to write-up his healing techniques in a series of books and became personal physician to a succession of kings at the French royal court.

Massage continued to flourish down the centuries and in the 16th-century became popular in the French Court on the recommendation of the extraordinary royal physician, Ambroise Paré, who favoured natural healing methods. In the late-18th and early-19th centuries, massage came into its own as a stand-alone therapy due largely to the work of a Swede, Per Henrik Ling (1776–1839).

Ling was a gymnast and fencer who studied medicine and created a system of medical gymnastics that was later taught with government and medical approval at the Royal Gymnastic Central Institute in Stockholm.

The massage elements of Ling's system, based on a sound understanding of anatomy and physiology, were taken up by a Dutch practitioner, Johan Georg Mezger, who coined the French names for the different moves (see 'Exploring Different Types of Massage' later in this chapter to find out what these moves are). This system of massage, known as *therapeutic massage* or *Swedish massage* (except in Sweden!) is now practised around the world and has influenced many subsequent massage systems.

Massage continued to be popular in the 19th and 20th centuries with the development of physiotherapy, but fell out of favour as pharmacology and instrumentation (the use of mechanical devices for skin stimulation and therapy) came into vogue. Massage also gained a bad reputation by often being used as a misnomer for sexual services.

Nowadays, however, extensive research has helped to change people's perception of massage and it is now seen as a useful therapy as well as a form of relaxation and pleasure.

The range of massage therapies used today is very wide. They vary in terms of their origins (both East and West), their techniques (depth of pressure, type of massage movements), and their focus (physical effects, such as the release of muscular tension, or more subtle aspects, such as improving the flow of 'vital energy' in the body).

Grasping the idea behind massage

Massage has a direct effect on the skin, muscles, nerves, blood vessels, and lymph system (a network of vessels that transport a nearly colourless cellular fluid that plays a role in the immune system) and can also affect the functioning of the internal organs.

These effects are due to the mechanical action of massage and also the reflex action of the body. The *mechanical action* is the actual pressure and stretching movements of massage, which help to stimulate the release of built up acids and other toxins and to loosen up stiff joints. The *reflex action* is the body's response, which can trigger an effect in another part of the body.

Essentially, the massage stimulates skin receptors that relay messages to the brain via the nervous system. The brain in turn sends messages back to the area being massaged causing muscle relaxation, blood vessel dilation, and improved blood circulation.

Production of feel-good chemicals – the endorphins – is also triggered. These endorphins provide pain relief and also increase the sense of well-being – which is why people report feeling reassured, soothed, and relaxed after massage.

The benefits of massage

The effects of massage can be physical, psychological, emotional, and even spiritual. Physical benefits may include the following:

- Improved circulation
- Release of tension, stiffness, cramps, and pain
- Improved mobility and range of movement
- Breakdown of scar tissue
- Better muscle tone and flexibility
- Better sleep
- Increased energy and vitality
- Improved immune function
- Lowered blood pressure
- Improved removal of waste matter from the body
- Increased supply of oxygen and nutrients to the tissues
- Faster healing

Psycho/emotional benefits can include the following:

- Increased sense of well-being
- Greater self-confidence and self-esteem
- Improved concentration, memory, and creativity
- Less stress, anxiety, and irritability
- Greater sense of calm and relaxation

People also sometimes report feelings of bliss and 'oneness' or spiritual attunement during massage.

Massage today

Today, massage flourishes in most Western countries but none have a single governing body or formal regulatory system. This situation means that qualifications and standards can vary quite considerably.

In the UK, a new National Register for Massage Therapists was established in 2004 by the General Council for Massage Therapy (GCMT; www.gcmt.org. uk). Its members have all completed approved massage training courses, are bound by a code of conduct, and carry professional indemnity insurance. However, this council still only represents a small number of the many massage associations that currently exist.

Similar situations exist in other countries (see 'Finding a Massage Therapist' further on in this chapter).

Evidence that it works

Massage has been shown to be effective for a range of conditions including: back and other types of pain, fibromyalgia (chronic ache and pain), fatigue, stress, blood sugar control, insomnia, anxiety, and attention deficit and hyperactivity disorder (ADHD), to name but a few. This therapy has also been shown to improve your golf swing!

Additionally, massage has been shown to be effective in the treatment of premature babies, in the care of the elderly, and as an aid for recovery after surgery and during cancer treatment.

For examples of massage research take a look at the research pages of the General Council for Massage Therapy on www.gcmt.org.uk/research. asp.Other studies can be found on www.internethealthlibrary.com/ Therapies/MassageTherapy-Research.htm; the NHS Complementary and Alternative Medicine Specialist Library (www.library.nhs.uk/cam); the Bastyr University Research database on www.bastyr.edu/research; or the PubMed database on www.nlm.nih.gov/nccam/camonpubmed.html.

Exploring Different Types of Massage

Many different types of massage exist. These can be divided into Western forms (mainly Swedish, Danish, and Norwegian massage therapies), Japanese forms (Anma, Shiatsu, and Amatsu), Chinese forms (tui na and acupressure), and

Indian forms (Ayurvedic massage, Indian Head massage, Chavutti Thirumal, and so on). Thai, Tibetan, Mongolian, Indonesian, Hawaiian, and other forms of massage are also practised, as well as specialist types of massage including baby massage, hot stone massage, and sports massage.

Here's an A-to-Z of some of the most popular types of massage therapy:

- **Acupressure:** Originated in ancient China and uses finger pressure applied to acupuncture points on the skin to regulate the flow of *qi* (vital energy) in the acupuncture meridians. Acupressure techniques are a part of many other therapies, including Shiatsu, tui na, Shen Tao, and Jin Shin Do.

- **Amatsu:** Originated in Japan this is a modern day combination of anma massage, Seitai (bone adjustment), Shinden-jutsu (balancing of the ligaments and soft-tissue massage), and Kenkujutsu (Japanese cranial therapy). This therapy has recently been introduced to the West. For more, see www.amatsu.info.

- **Anma:** The oldest form of massage in Japan. Uses the thumbs, fingers, knuckles, elbows, knees, and feet to press, stroke, stretch, and percuss the skin. This massage is performed through clothing and no oils are used.

- **Aromatherapy:** Combines massage with the use of essential oils extracted from plants, which are inhaled as well as absorbed through the skin. For more about this therapy, see Chapter 19.

- **Ayurvedic massage:** Traditional Indian medicine, known as Ayurveda, employs several types of massage. Marma massage involves the application of pressure to a range of special *marma* points on the body, similar to the acupoints of acupuncture. Other types of massage are selected according to the person's *dosha* or 'vital energy' type and use different oils, pressure, friction techniques, and speeds. Specialist techniques include Chavutti Thirumal, a South Indian massage done with the feet and toes by a therapist suspended on ropes, and **Indian Head massage**, also known as *champissage*, which involves scalp, neck, face, ears, and shoulders massage. For more, see Chapter 5.

- **Baby massage:** Incorporates gentle massage strokes and stretches to stimulate the baby's immune system and aid digestion and relaxation.

- **Biodynamic massage:** Created by Norwegian physiotherapist and psychologist Gerda Boyesen, this massage therapy is designed to release physical and energetic blockages in the muscles and abdomen. For more, contact the Association of Holistic Biodynamic Massage Therapists (AHBMT) at www.ahbmt.org.

- **Chua Ka:** An ancient form of Mongolian massage using a stick, called a *ka*, and the hands to massage deep into the muscles and release tension and fear.

Re-drawing the meridian pathways

I had the great privilege to study shiatsu with Masunaga's successor, Suzuki Sensei, when I lived in Tokyo. He told us many stories about Masunaga and his amazing innovations. Masunaga read extremely widely but also let his hands and the bodies of his patients be his teachers. He spent countless hours trying out techniques and carefully palpating the body to observe and test its reactions.

The acupuncture meridian system had remained unchanged for thousands of years yet Masunaga redrew it! He followed the pathways of the arm meridians and extended them throughout the body. I was absolutely amazed by this extension of the pathways and found, on palpation and working with Masunaga's stretches, that they made perfect sense. I also found that his system of diagnosing and treating through the abdomen was extraordinarily effective as well as his system of self-help meridian stretches. Masunaga's marvellous techniques and exercises have been made available to all in the excellent book, *Meridian Exercises: Oriental Way to Health and Vitality* (Japan Publications, 1997) translated by Stephen Brown.

- ✔ **Deep-tissue massage:** Uses deep finger pressure and slow movements to break down scar tissue and compacted muscle fibres to release toxins, and ease tension and pain.

- ✔ **Do-In:** A traditional Japanese system for personal and spiritual development combining self-massage, acupressure, and shiatsu stretches with macrobiotic diet, breathing exercises, and meditation.

- ✔ **Hot stone massage:** Warm stones are placed on the body to increase circulation and relax muscles, or cool stones are used to reduce inflammation and swelling. For more information, see www.lastonetherapy.com.

- ✔ **Hydrotherm massage:** This massage is performed while you lie on a mattress filled with warm water.

- ✔ **Indonesian massage:** This deep massage uses the thumbs to penetrate deep into the muscles and soft tissue.

- ✔ **Jin Shin Do:** Meaning 'the way of the compassionate spirit', this is a modern day synthesis of acupressure, Qi gong exercises, and psychology, developed by Iona Teeguarden in the US. For more, see www.jinshindo.org.

- ✔ **Kahuna:** Sometimes called **Lomi Lomi**, this Hawaiian form of deep-tissue massage uses long, flowing strokes, rhythmical pressure and oils over the whole body.

✔ **Manual lymphatic drainage:** Danish physician Dr Emil Vodder developed this technique in the 1930s, using gentle touch and rhythmical movements to improve the flow of lymph (colourless fluid that surrounds the tissues and circulates via lymph vessels). J. R. Casley-Smith combined lymphatic drainage with skin care, compression bandaging, and special exercises to create complex physical therapy (CPT); while Australian Grace Halliday devised deep lymphatic therapy (DLT), by combining systematic lymphatic massage with hot foments (applied steam heat). For more information, see www.mlduk.org.uk.

✔ **Myofascial massage:** A technique used in Rolfing (see Chapter 16) and sports massage (see below) involving compression and skin rolling to stretch the fascia (tissues surrounding the bones and muscles), relieve pain and injury and increase mobility.

✔ **Neuromuscular therapy:** Also known as trigger-point therapy or myotherapy, this involves concentrated thumb/finger pressure to trigger points – tender points that have become sensitive due to lack of flow of blood and nutrients.

✔ **On-site massage therapy:** This is brief massage taken into the workplace using a special portable chair, which you sit on and lean forward in while massage is applied to the head, neck, shoulders, back, arms, and hands.

✔ **Pregnancy massage:** Gentle massage techniques to improve blood flow and reduce pregnancy discomfort.

✔ **Reflexology:** The application of fingertip and thumb pressure to points on the soles of the feet believed to be connected to different parts and organs of the body via the nerve reflex system.

✔ **Remedial massage:** A form of soft tissue massage used to treat muscle and joint pain and injuries.

✔ **Self-massage:** Simple pressure point and kneading techniques that you can do yourself to release tension and improve circulation. (For an example, see the end of this chapter.)

✔ **Shiatsu:** Meaning *finger pressure*, this Japanese therapy involves stretches and pressure from the thumbs, fingers, palms, elbows, knees, or feet while you lie on a padded mat, or *futon*, on the floor.

Various styles of shiatsu have been developed in Japan and spread to the West. **Namikoshi Shiatsu** (sometimes called shiatsu massage) was created by Tokujiro Namikoshi in Japan in the 1920s, and developed from instinctive pressure point massage that he gave his rheumatic mother as a child to ease her pain. In the 1950s, he took this therapy to America and his work is now continued by his son Toru, who has emphasised the role of Western anatomy, physiology, and pathology.

Shizuto Masunaga developed **Zen Shiatsu** by incorporating traditional Chinese medicine theory of *yin* and *yang* (called *in* and *yo* in Japanese – nip over to Chapters 4 and 7 for an explanation of these) and the concept of balancing deficiency (*kyo*) and excess (*jitsu*) in the meridian channels by means of shiatsu massage and stretches. He also devised a unique form of abdominal diagnosis and treatment called *hara* massage.

Another popular style is **Tsubo therapy** developed by Katsusuke Serizawa. This style focuses on stimulation of the *tsubo*, or acupoints, using massage, moxa (heat treatment), or electrical stimulation.

For more information on shiatsu and shiatsu practitioners, check out `www.shiatsu.org`.

✔ **Sports massage:** A combination of remedial, deep-tissue, and Swedish massage techniques used to relieve muscle stiffness and pain, improve athletes' performance and aid recovery from injury.

✔ **Thai massage:** Incorporates Ayurvedic and Chinese massage and uses pressure point therapy, muscle stretching, and firm compression techniques to release tension and relax the body.

✔ **Therapeutic massage (Swedish massage):** Developed by Per Henrik Ling in Sweden at the end of the 19th-century, and systematised by Dutchman Johan Georg Mezger, this influential type of massage employs five basic moves to stimulate the tissues and ease muscle tension:

- **Effleurage:** This massage is designed to stretch and relax the superficial muscles

- **Petrissage:** This technique involves kneading and squeezing the soft tissues (the tissues around the bones and organs of the body) and both the superficial and deep muscles of the body

- **Friction and compression:** These rubbing and holding techniques are designed to break down build-ups of scar tissue and to relax the muscles

- **Tapotement:** These are rhythmical, tapping movements, usually made with the edge of the hand or the heel of the palm, designed to increase blood circulation

- **Vibration:** These are rhythmical, vibrational movements designed to release tension and stimulate circulation

Swedish massage is usually performed without clothing and on a massage couch using oils and lotions. Most of the moves are directed towards the heart.

✔ **Tibetan massage:** This involves pressure to therapeutic points on the body as well as kneading, rubbing, and tapping techniques to relax the body and ease tension. Sesame, or other, oil may be used to warm the tissues and ease the massage moves (for more on Tibetan medicine, take a look at Chapter 6).

✔ **Tui na:** Meaning 'push and grasp', tui na is an ancient form of Chinese massage that uses fingers, hands, arms, elbows, and knees to vigorously rub, knead, and roll the skin and tissues. This massage is designed to release energetic blockage in the acupuncture meridians and to release muscular tension.

Thai massage and the golden Buddha

I once had a Thai massage in the Temple of Wat Pho in Bangkok, Thailand, which houses the longest reclining gold Buddha in the world. Instead of the privacy you might expect in the West, the massage room consisted (at that time) of an open hall with row upon row of simple beds on which the Thai masseurs worked on lots of people simultaneously.

Instead of being relaxing, the massage was incredibly invigorating! I remember being pulled into all sorts of positions and walked all over. At the end of the massage I felt as if I'd been beaten up but my level of energy was extraordinary. I felt as if I could run round that long, gold Buddha all night!

Understanding Massage Diagnosis

Massage therapists use their sense of touch, and palpation of the skin, to identify areas of pain, tension, inflammation, or water retention and to determine the condition of the skin tissues.

Shiatsu therapists also use the acupuncture meridian lines and acupoints to gauge information about the functioning of each of the internal organs (see Chapter 9 on Acupuncture for more about these), while reflexologists use reflex areas on the feet to identify possible problems with individual organs or body parts.

Massage therapists do not claim to make medical diagnoses. If you're concerned about a medical condition, consult your doctor.

Finding Out about Massage Treatment

Massage is best performed in a relaxed, peaceful environment by a practitioner, friend, or partner that you trust and feel completely comfortable with. Sometimes relaxing music, low lighting, or pleasant aromas from aromatherapy or incense burners may be used to add to the relaxing effect of the treatment.

Discovering whom and what massage is good for

Massage is suitable for anyone and may be used therapeutically to treat different ailments or used simply for pleasure and relaxation.

The types of conditions most often treated by massage therapists include back pain, headaches, arthritis, fatigue problems, Repetitive Strain Injuries (RSI), sports injuries, asthma, strains and sprains, digestive problems, insomnia, and stress.

When not to use massage

Don't use massage if you:

- ✔ Have an infectious skin condition (such as impetigo)
- ✔ Are suffering from flu or high fever
- ✔ Have sunburn
- ✔ Feel extremely unwell, or debilitated from some disease
- ✔ Are under the influence of alcohol or recreational drugs

Special care must also be taken in the case of small infants, pregnant women, and the elderly, and also for those suffering from high blood pressure, heart conditions, cancer, asthma, epilepsy, diabetes, or osteoporosis. Massage needs to be avoided at the site of scar tissue, varicose veins, sprains and fractures, cuts, verrucas, eczema, psoriasis, and so on.

If you're taking pharmaceutical drugs, such as for high blood pressure, epilepsy, diabetes, or asthma, make sure to inform your massage therapist.

What to Expect in a Typical Consultation

A massage treatment usually begins with some questions about general health and any problem areas of tension or pain in the body. You may then be asked to disrobe.

Many massage therapies are performed directly on the skin so you may be asked to undress to underwear and then be covered with towels. The room is usually kept warm to aid relaxation. Some massage therapies, such as shiatsu and Thai massage, may be performed through clothing. Wearing loose, cotton clothing for these types of treatment is advisable.

Massage may involve the use of oils, lotions, or talcum powder to ease friction on the skin (as in Swedish massage and Ayurvedic massage), or may be performed 'dry' such as in shiatsu massage.

You may be asked to lie on a treatment couch, sit on a massage stool, or lie on a mattress on the floor, depending on the type of massage you're going to receive.

The massage usually begins gently and then may become more vigorous depending on the style. Massage is usually very relaxing but some of the deep-tissue techniques, for example those used in Thai massage, may feel a bit tender or even mildly painful, depending on the area and type of tissues being worked on. If you feel discomfort, let your therapist know.

You may want to have your eyes open or closed during the massage and to talk or to be quiet. Some people feel so relaxed they even fall asleep during their massage!

Stretching exercises and dietary or lifestyle advice may also be part of the therapy.

To get the best results from your massage:

- ✔ Relax as much as possible.
- ✔ Drink plenty of water before and afterwards.
- ✔ Avoid stimulants such as coffee, tea, sugar, or cigarettes and also alcohol or recreational drugs for several hours beforehand.
- ✔ Avoid heavy meals prior to treatment.
- ✔ Get plenty of rest afterwards.

After the massage

After the massage is over you may feel tired or energetic, calm or emotional, as the massage can release deep-seated feelings. Some people experience mild muscle ache but this usually passes quickly. Finding that you need to go to the toilet (urination and/or stools) more often initially is normal because massage can stimulate the removal of waste products.

Duration and frequency

Massage treatments can last anything from 15 minutes (on-site massage) to 2 hours (Kahuna massage) but typically last around 60 to 90 minutes. Repeated massages, either daily or a few days or a week apart, may be advised in case of injury or illness and then spaced out. Therapeutic massages for relaxation and pleasure can be taken anytime.

Knowing Whether Your Massage Treatment Is Working

You may feel tired or slightly aching after massage but this passes quickly and you'll soon feel the benefits of increased relaxation, circulation, and vitality.

✔ If you experience a marked worsening of your symptoms, contact your massage therapist for advice.

✔ Ask your massage therapist what sort of health improvements you can realistically expect and over what sort of timescale.

✔ For best results, carefully follow the exercise and lifestyle advice given to you by your massage therapist.

✔ If you have no improvement after a course of treatment, you may want to consider another form of therapy. Discuss this situation with your practitioner.

Common Questions about Massage Treatment

Here are some questions that I'm often asked about massage:

✔ **Do I have to be naked?** No, not necessarily. Take a look at the different types of massage mentioned earlier on in this chapter and choose one that allows you to keep your clothes on if you feel self-conscious.

✔ **Will I feel embarrassed?** Normally, your massage therapist will help you feel comfortable by enabling you to disrobe in privacy and keeping you covered with towels when possible during the massage. As an experienced health professional, your therapist will be focused on giving you the greatest therapeutic benefit from your massage, rather than on what your body looks like.

✔ **What does massage feel like?** Pretty relaxing probably, blissful maybe, and tender perhaps, depending on the type of massage.

✔ **How do I choose which type to have?** Take a look at the main types of massage listed earlier in this chapter, see which tickles your fancy and give it a try! Things to consider include whether you're dressed/undressed; full body or specific body part; environment (quiet, individual room, or communal setting); technique (relaxing or invigorating).

Finding a Good Massage Therapist

Massage therapists are not fully regulated in the UK, US, Canada, Australia, or New Zealand, so anyone can call themselves a 'massage therapist'. Check that your practitioner is a member of a professional body and has had a thorough training at a reputable institution.

In the UK, many massage therapists are members of associations that are part of the General Council for Massage Therapy (GCMT), which maintains a practitioner register (www.gcmt.org.uk). Another register can be found on www.massagetherapy.co.uk.

In the US, numerous different massage associations exist, many of which represent a particular type of massage only. Many of them are listed at www.thebodyworker.com/associations_list.htm. One of the most well-established is the American Massage Therapy Association (www.amtamassage.org), which maintains a list of practitioners.

Following are some massage therapist associations in other countries:

✔ **Australia:** The Massage Association of Australia (www.maa.org.au) or the Association of Massage Therapists Ltd (www.amt-ltd.org.au)

✔ **Canada:** The Association of Massage Therapists and Wholistic Practitioners (www.amtwp.org) or the Canadian Massage Therapist Alliance (www.cmta.ca)

✔ **New Zealand**: The Therapeutic Massage Association (TMA) and the Massage Institute of New Zealand (MINZI) have joined forces and, from April 2007, will become a new unified body called Massage New Zealand (MNZ). More details on www.tmanz.org.nz

Finally, here are a few other ideas for finding a massage therapist:

✔ Ask friends, family, and colleagues for personal recommendations.

✔ Many sports and leisure clubs offer massage treatment.

✔ Check with local complementary medicine and alternative therapy clinics and magazines.

✔ Some beauty salons offer therapeutic massage, aromatherapy, and so on.

✔ Most health farms and spas offer massage.

✔ Massage schools may have teaching clinics with reduced fees or can refer you to graduates. One of the most established schools in the UK is the Clare Maxwell-Hudson School of Massage (www.cmhmassage.co.uk).

Questions to ask your massage therapist

You may want to ask your massage therapist about the following:

✔ **Qualifications:** Most practitioners are happy to give details of their training and qualifications and membership of a professional body. If you have any doubt as to their validity, check the qualifications with their respective professional body.

✔ **Insurance:** If your practitioner is a member of a professional register they'll normally be required to have appropriate indemnity insurance.

✔ **Experience:** Ask your practitioner about their experience and familiarity with your particular health condition.

✔ **Treatment:** Ask about the likely frequency and duration of treatment and the cost involved.

Counting the cost of massage

Massage costs from £15 to £90 depending on the duration and type of massage. Massage treatment is very rarely available on the NHS or covered by private health insurance.

Some practitioners offer concessions for retired persons or those on benefits. Ask your practitioner for details.

Ensuring satisfaction

If you're dissatisfied with your treatment, first talk things over with your practitioner.

If you think that the practitioner has been negligent or unethical in any way, contact their professional association or registering body, which should have a formal complaints procedure.

Helping Yourself with Massage

Self-massage can be a great way to relieve neck and shoulder tension.

1. **Support your right elbow with your left hand and place your right hand over your left shoulder.**

2. **Grasp the flesh close to your neck and squeeze it firmly.** Hold for a few seconds, then release.

3. **Repeat this squeeze-release movement three times.** Move the hand down slightly towards the shoulder and repeat the move again three times.

4. **Move your hand down over your shoulder itself and again repeat the squeeze-release movement three times.**

5. **Swap your hands over and repeat this on the opposite side of the body.**

Remember to breathe freely during the movements. At the end, your neck and shoulders feel tingling and relaxed.

This is a great technique to use when you've been typing for hours. I used it a lot during the writing of this book!

Part V
Healing Your Mind and Spirit

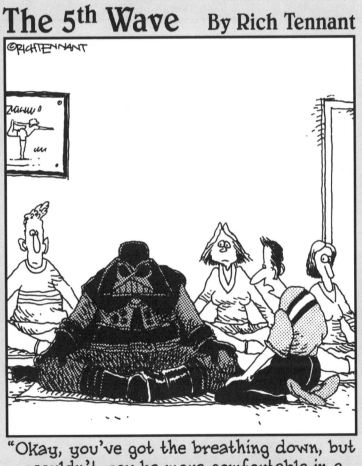

The 5th Wave   By Rich Tennant

"Okay, you've got the breathing down, but wouldn't you be more comfortable in a different workout suit?"

In this part . . .

Don't know your chakras from your auras? Always wondered what exactly reiki masters do for their money? Curious about crystals? Intrigued by aromatherapy? This is the part for you.

In this part, you can explore relaxation therapies, aromatherapy, healing, psychological therapies, energy medicine, and the creative therapies – all designed to soothe and stimulate your mind and spirit.

Chapter 18

Calming Down with Breathing, Meditation, and Relaxation Therapies

. . . .

In This Chapter

▶ Finding out what relaxation therapies are all about

▶ Exploring different ways to relax

▶ Discovering what relaxation therapies can be good for

▶ Examining the evidence

▶ Knowing what to expect in a typical session

▶ Knowing how to find safe and effective practitioners

. . . .

Do you suffer from stress? Then you're not alone. A moderate amount of stress can be a useful stimulant but too much wears you down and can contribute to a host of common ailments such as fatigue, lethargy, depression, insomnia, and headaches, as well as more serious conditions such as heart disease.

Relaxation of mind and body, healthy breathing, and meditation can all be powerful antidotes to stress as well as great health promoters. Many complementary therapies provide relaxation and stress relief as an indirect part of their healing approach but some therapies are also aimed specifically at promoting physical and mental relaxation. These therapies can be used in their own right or successfully combined with other forms of complementary medicine.

In this chapter, I outline some ancient and new ways of relaxing the mind and body. You'll find out about the importance of correct breathing and investigate techniques for releasing muscle tension and calming and expanding the mind. You'll also discover the evidence for the different therapies to determine what each may be helpful for.

At the end of the chapter, I pass on to you a simple self-help relaxation technique that you can use in your everyday life.

Finding Out about Relaxation Therapies

In ancient times people may not have been as stressed as we are now but they still valued relaxation and saw its health benefits! All the ancient healing traditions of China, Japan, India, Tibet, and so on (take a look at the chapters in Part II to find out more about these traditional healing systems) emphasise the importance of good breathing, of having a relaxed and healthy body, and of maintaining a calm, clear mind.

In the ancient medical systems of Asia and the Far East good health and relaxation almost always start with the breath.

In Traditional Chinese Medicine (TCM), for example, good breathing is said to facilitate the flow of *qi* (vital energy) in the *meridians* (vital energy channels), and to promote healthy internal organ function.

On a physical level, each of the great ancient medical traditions also employed techniques for relaxing the muscles and mobilising the joints. For example, Ayurvedic medicine involves yoga exercises and special *Panchakarma* hot oil massage techniques; TCM uses *qi gong* exercises and tui na massage; Japanese medicine utilises *Do-in* exercises, *anma* massage, and *shiatsu*; and Tibetan medicine involves *Kum Nye* exercises and various massage techniques (check out the chapters in Part II and Chapter 16 on body-work therapies for more about these).

These traditions also emphasised mental relaxation, so breathing and physical exercises were combined with training in stillness and meditation. Meditation techniques range from observing a flame or controlling the breath (Ayurveda and yoga), to visualisation of deities and reciting mantras (Tibet) and visualising the circulation of light, or observing the breath and practising 'mindful awareness' (Japan and China).

Some of these ancient therapies have become popular forms of relaxation today – such as yoga and yoga breathing techniques. Other techniques – such as Jacobson's progressive relaxation and Buteyko's breathing technique – have been developed more recently. In the next section, I take a look at these therapies in a bit more detail.

Looking at Popular Relaxation Therapies Today

First, I introduce you to some breathing therapies and then I tell you about some relaxation and meditation techniques. In this section, I cover the following:

- ✔ *Pranayama* (yoga breathing)
- ✔ Buteyko
- ✔ Yoga *asanas*
- ✔ Progressive relaxation
- ✔ Flotation
- ✔ Meditation

Breathing therapies

Breathing therapies have been an important part of healing systems across the ages. The underlying belief seems to be that abnormal breathing can contribute to disease and that by bringing it under conscious control and regulating it, health can be promoted and healing facilitated.

Not enough space exists within the scope of this book to go through the breathing techniques from each of the ancient traditions. So I concentrate here on one of those most commonly practised and researched types of breathing therapy – *pranayama*. Then I tell you about what could be the most important modern breathing therapy – the Buteyko breathing method.

Pranayama

The ancient Sanskrit word *pranayama* means bringing your *prana*, or life force, under control (*yama*). *Pranayama* breathing exercises were first described by the legendary Indian Yogi, Patanjali, said to have lived around the third century BC.

How does it work?

The exercises involve controlling your in- and out-breaths and holding your breath. Their role is to help cleanse the body, improve powers of concentration and to aid personal and spiritual self-development.

Practising pranayama

You can learn many different types of *pranayama*, from simple beginners' techniques through to quite advanced practices that should only be practised under the guidance of a qualified yoga teacher.

Introductory *pranayama* exercises include the following:

- **Diaphragmatic breathing:** Locating your *diaphragm* (the big bell-shaped muscle across your abdomen) and using it more effectively when breathing.

- **Full yogic breath:** Breathing in three stages, filling the lower part of the lungs, then the mid-section, and then the upper part, and then exhaling air from the lungs in the reverse order.

- **Anula viloma (alternate nostril breathing):** This technique involves using the thumb and forefinger to close each nostril alternately and enable in- and out-breaths through one nostril at a time. It may also be combined with breath retention. Take a look at the 'Helping Yourself with Relaxation Therapies' section at the end of this chapter for details on how to practise this technique.

- **Ujjayi pranayama (*victorious breath*):** This technique involves breathing in through the nose while tightening the throat to produce a throaty sound.

- **Kapalabhati pranayama (*skull cleansing* or *skull shining*):** This technique is a type of bellows breathing with a soft inhalation and then forceful exhalation achieved by contracting the abdominal muscles.

Whom or what is it good for?

Anyone can benefit from *pranayama*, but you need to practise the techniques properly and safely, ideally from an experienced yoga teacher. Only attempt the more advanced techniques under careful supervision, because an excess of deep breathing can cause dizziness and discomfort, and you need to avoid excessive strain on the lungs. Anyone with lung disease or a serious lung condition should not practise *pranayama* without medical supervision.

What's the evidence?

Research suggests that *pranayama* exercises can gradually increase lung capacity and improve the balance of oxygen and carbon dioxide in the body and may also slow brain waves, heart rate, and blood pressure.

The first-ever world survey of yoga, including a study of *pranayama*, is being carried out online in 2007. Visit www.yogainaustralia.com to find out more and register.

Where can I learn pranayama?

In the UK, the Yoga Biomedical Trust, founded by Robin Munro in the 1980s, has pioneered the therapeutic applications of yoga (Tel: 020 7689 3040; www.yogatherapy.org).

Worldwide, excellent *pranayama* training is offered by the Sivananda Yoga Vedanta Centres. (I did their yoga teacher training course myself in Grass Valley, California many years ago.) For details, see www.sivananda.org or, in the UK, contact London's Sivananda Yoga Vedanta Centre (Tel: 020 8780 0160).

Buteyko breathing training

Buteyko (pronounced *Bu-tay-ko*) is a method for re-training the way that you breathe devised by Russian medical researcher Konstantin Buteyko in the 1950s. Buteyko was assigned to monitor the breathing patterns of dying patients. He noticed that the sicker people became – especially shortly before death – the more they seemed to need larger volumes of air and took deeper breaths. He developed a theory that improper over-breathing (hyperventilation) contributed to disease and that the less you breathed the longer you'd live!

Buteyko then spent several decades devising a correct breathing technique and thoroughly researching its effects. Despite initial medical opposition his method was approved by the Russian authorities in 1981, for the treatment of asthma. Since then Buteyko breathing training has spread to Australia, New Zealand, Europe, and elsewhere.

How does it work?

Buteyko's method is based on the idea that incorrect over-breathing (hyperventilation) lowers carbon dioxide levels in the body – carbon dioxide is as necessary as oxygen for certain body processes and the two need to be in a correct ratio. He argued that over-breathing, and breathing through the mouth, means that the body cannot utilise oxygen efficiently and so people may become breathless, nervous, tired, or unwell.

His method emphasises breathing through the nose, using the diaphragm to breathe fully, and slowing down and holding the breath to correct this imbalance. The idea is that you train yourself to use a lesser volume of air more effectively.

Learning Buteyko

The Buteyko method is usually taught by a trained Buteyko teacher in a series of five 90-minute lectures and practical sessions taken over five days. However, some shorter training courses are also now available and follow-up, regular self-practice is essential. The aim is to reduce your number of breaths per minute from 12 or more down to 4. The exercises are easy to learn, and you can do them sitting in a chair. Simple stress-management and dietary advice may also be recommended alongside the breathing training.

Whom or what is it good for?

Children (from the age of four) and adults of any age can learn the Buteyko method. It has been reported to help relieve a range of respiratory problems including asthma, hyperventilation, panic attacks, sinusitis, bronchitis, hay fever, emphysema, and snoring, as well as arthritis, high blood pressure, and digestive problems.

What's the evidence?

A 1980 Russian trial by the Government's Committee for Science and Technology and many trials by Dr Buteyko himself, found significant improvements in people with respiratory and other symptoms after learning the Buteyko method. A 1994 Australian trial with asthma sufferers also showed that training in the technique led to a reduction of symptoms and inhaler use. However more controlled trials are needed and many Western medical doctors remain ignorant or sceptical about this technique.

How can I find a Buteyko teacher?

For lots more about Buteyko, see www.buteyko.com. In the UK, you can find a Buteyko teacher via The Buteyko Breathing Association (Tel: 01277 366 906; www.buteykobreathing.org).

Relaxation therapies

In this section, I introduce you to three relaxation therapies that are popular today: an ancient one – yoga, and two more modern ones; progressive relaxation and flotation therapy.

Yoga

The Sanskrit word *yoga* means 'union', and refers to union of the body, mind, and spirit. Yoga is believed to have originated several thousand years ago in India. Of the many different types of yoga, the type mainly used in the West for relaxation is known as *hatha yoga* and was first formalised in the 15th century by the Indian yogi Swatmarama.

Hatha yoga is based on a series of *asanas*, or 'body postures', that are primarily intended to improve physical health. However, their ultimate aim goes further and, combined with *pranayama* breathing exercises and meditation, the *asanas* are designed to help you on the path to mental peace, personal development, and spiritual upliftment.

Practising yoga asanas

The yoga *asanas* are a series of body poses, from simple ones to more advanced ones, either held statically or performed in a dynamic sequence. Different *asanas* are believed to stimulate different internal organs and body systems.

The *shavasana*, or 'corpse' pose, which is a resting pose performed lying down, is often used as the final pose of a yoga session and is especially useful for relaxation.

How do they work?

The *asanas* facilitate muscle stretching, toning and endurance, flexibility, relaxation, and correct breathing. On a more subtle level, the *asanas* are also believed to facilitate the flow of vital energy, or *prana*, in the energy channels known as the *nadis* – these are believed to correspond closely to the meridian system of acupuncture – and to promote healing.

Whom or what are yoga asanas good for?

Anyone, from young children to adults of any age, can practise the yoga *asanas*. Yoga has been found to be beneficial for many conditions, including back pain, digestive problems, and anxiety.

Only perform advanced poses under the guidance of an experienced yoga instructor. If you have neck problems or high blood pressure, don't perform the inverted poses (such as headstands).

What's the evidence?

Research suggests that practise of yoga *asanas* have a range of physiological effects including slowing brain waves, heart rate, and respiration rate; decreasing muscle tension and stress; and increasing the sense of well-being.

How can I learn yoga asanas?

Check out the resources listed earlier in this chapter in the section on *pranayama*, or, in the UK, contact The British Wheel of Yoga (Tel: 01529 306 851; www.bwy.org.uk) or, in the US, the Yoga Alliance (Tel: 00 1877-964-2255 (toll free) or 00 1301-868-4700; www.yogaalliance.org).

Progressive relaxation (PR)

Progressive muscle relaxation is a technique devised by an American doctor and researcher, Edmund Jacobson, in the 1930s. He noticed that anxiety was accompanied by muscle tension and reasoned that if you can relax the muscles you may be able to reduce anxiety. He also found that if you tense a muscle for a short period of time, when you release it, it will relax. He therefore devised a systematic sequence for going through each of the major muscle groups in the body and tensing and then relaxing them.

How does it work?

By isolating individual muscles and practising tensing and then relaxing them, you increase your awareness of muscular tension and become able to voluntarily release muscular tension.

Learning PR

To learn PR you need to sit or lie comfortably and then go through a sequence of tensing and relaxing each major muscle, or muscle group, from the hands, arms, and neck, down to the toes. Each muscle is contracted tightly and then held for about 10 seconds. At the end of the sequence you just rest for a while breathing normally. The whole sequence takes 15 to 20 minutes. You need to practise daily until you've mastered the technique.

Whom or what is it good for?

Anyone – from children to adults – can learn and use the PR technique.

What's the evidence?

Research has shown that PR is effective in reducing muscular tension and in promoting the relaxation response in the body.

How can I learn PR?

No association for PR teachers exists at present. You can train yourself in the technique from books or audio tapes.

Flotation therapy

Flotation therapy developed out of work in the 1950s, by American physiologist and psychoanalyst John C. Lilly on sensory deprivation, investigating the effects of being deprived of normal sensory experiences such as sight, hearing, and so on. He built *sensory deprivation chambers* that excluded light and reduced sounds, and contained several inches of a highly concentrated Epsom salt solution to make trial participants float and feel weightless. He found that when people were put in these chambers for short periods, they found the experience very relaxing.

In the 1970s, two other researchers, Peter Suedfeld and Roderick Borrie, coined the term 'restricted environmental stimulation technique', otherwise known as REST, to describe tanks that re-created these conditions for a specifically therapeutic purpose. Wet REST systems involve floating in a concentrated warm-water salt solution, while dry REST systems enable the person to lie on a piece of foam suspended on the water and stay dry.

Having flotation therapy

You float inside an enclosed tank, usually about 8 feet (2.5 metres) by 4 feet (1.25 metres) wide and with 10 inches (25 cm) or so of warm water that is highly salted so that you float easily. The tanks are often egg-shaped and have one whole side that lifts up or have a door by which you can enter. Once inside there may be a control panel to regulate light and sound. Earplugs can be worn to block out sound or some tanks have speakers and/or screens so that music or educational audios, or even videos, can be played. (It has been shown that learning is facilitated in this relaxed state!) Some tanks also have microphones so that you can communicate with a therapist or other person outside the tank. Sessions generally last for 60 to 90 minutes, but you lose all sense of time when floating and it feels like five minutes!

How does it work?

During flotation, the body and brain enter a deeply relaxed state. Your brain produces feel-good, relaxing chemicals known as *endorphins*, and your pulse rate, brain waves, and so on all slow down. Being freed from gravity appears to have a therapeutic effect that deepens the relaxation state, and the body's natural homeostatic mechanism for healing may be able to kick in as a result.

Whom or what is it good for?

Flotation is recommended for stress and pain relief, and for conditions such as arthritis, headaches, and fatigue. People also report that it helps their concentration and mental sharpness.

Flotation therapy isn't advisable for people who suffer from claustrophobia or serious mental disturbance.

What's the evidence?

Research shows decreases in blood pressure, muscle tension, and heart rate after flotation therapy, as well as a decrease in the production of stress hormones. Clinical studies have shown that flotation can be helpful in reducing pain and inflammation and may help ease a range of disorders, including high blood pressure, insomnia, premenstrual syndrome, and rheumatoid arthritis. More good studies are needed.

Where can I try flotation therapy?

You need a flotation tank! These tanks can be found in various complementary medicine clinics or you can buy your own for home use – but they're expensive.

In the UK and Eire, clinics and centres with flotation tanks can be located via www.floatationtankassociation.net and in the US via www.floatation.com (Tel: 00 1530 432 4502).

Meditation

Many different types of meditation exist and going into them all is beyond the scope of this book. I therefore concentrate on the therapeutic aspects of meditation, outline some of the main types for you, and then point you in the direction for further information.

What is it?

Meditation is a mental technique that, on a physical level, may be used to calm the mind and induce relaxation. It involves concentration on an object or image (such as a candle flame or religious picture), or a sound (such as the breath or chanting) in order to eliminate other external distractions or inner thoughts or feelings.

However, meditation also has a higher purpose. All the religions of the world involve meditation in one form or another, either in terms of prayer and contemplation, the recitation of mantras, or specific meditation techniques, and meditation is seen as a method of personal development and a way of transcending the material world in order to draw closer to the spiritual. Meditation may be devoid of religious trappings and used as a way of evolving consciousness and of entering a state of increased awareness and even bliss.

Types of meditation

Here are some of the main types of meditation (in alphabetical order):

- ✔ **Raja yoga meditation:** Taught free by the Brahma Kumaris World Spiritual University all over the world, this technique involves an exploration of universal values through meditation and positive thinking. For worldwide locations, see www.bkwsu.org.

- ✔ **Sufi meditation:** As part of the Sufi tradition (a mystic tradition derived from the Islamic faith), Sufi meditation uses chants, sacred dance, and philosophical lectures, taught in small groups under instruction from a master, to guide personal growth. For more details in the UK, see www.sufimeditation.org (Tel: 0794 44 89527), or for worldwide information, check out www.sufimovement.org.

- ✔ **Transcendental meditation:** Brought to the West by the Maharishi Mahesh Yogi, whose most famous students were the Beatles in the 1960s, this technique involves 20 minutes daily repetition of a simple mantra. For details of UK courses, check out www.t-m.org.uk (Tel: 08705 143 733), or contact the Association of Independent TM Teachers, who charge more affordable fees, at www.tm-meditation.co.uk (Tel: 01843 841 010 or 0191 213 2179). For worldwide and US information, see www.tm.org or, in the US, call 00 1 888 LEARN TM to find your nearest TM teacher.

- ✔ **Vipassana meditation:** *Vipassana* means 'to see things as they really are'. This form of mindfulness meditation is based on observing the breath. It was brought to the West by S. N. Goenka and is taught over ten days of silent practice with lectures and individual guidance from a trained teacher. The technique is derived from Buddhist teachings in India but can be practised by anyone regardless of religious background.

> The teaching is free and offered all over the world. For more information, see www.dhamma.org or, in the UK, call 01989 730 234.
>
> ✔ **Zen meditation:** This is also called the 'practice of no mind' and is based on emptying the mind of all thoughts and following the breathing. This technique is a Buddhist practice that travelled from India to the Orient and then to the West. It is practised sitting upright in either a cross-legged or kneeling position or seated in a chair. For a funny, visual, online introduction to Zen from the famous Kodaiji Temple in Kyoto, Japan, see www.do-not-zzz.com. Search online or in local phone directories for your local Zen centre.

How does it work?

During meditation you produce brain waves associated with relaxation and heart and respiration rate decrease.

Whom or what is it good for?

Anyone can benefit from meditation – both children and adults. It appears to be effective for stress relief and relaxation.

What's the evidence?

Meditation has been well researched for many decades, especially since the pioneering work of Professor Herbert Benson at Harvard University in the US from the 1970s onwards. Benson was the first to identify the 'relaxation response' showing the physical effects of meditation on the body. For more on this work, see the Mind/Body Medical Institute site at www.mbmi.org.

Helping Yourself with Relaxation Therapies

To relax yourself try the following alternate nostril breathing exercise from the yoga tradition:

✔ Sit in a comfortable position.

✔ Raise your right hand and place the thumb against the right nostril to close it.

✔ Inhale through your left nostril to the count of eight.

✔ Close your left nostril by pressing the ring finger against it.

✔ Release the thumb and exhale through the right nostril also to the count of eight.

✔ Repeat the process, this time inhaling through the open right nostril to a count of eight, then close this nostril with the thumb and release the ring finger, exhaling though your left nostril to a count of eight again.

✔ Repeat this sequence seven times slowly and gently.

This exercise helps to relieve stress and aid relaxation. In more advanced versions of this exercise, the sequence of counts varies and the breath may be held at the end of the out-breath.

Chapter 19

Scenting Out Aromatherapy

· ·

In This Chapter

▶ Finding out about aromatherapy

▶ Understanding how aromatherapy works

▶ Discovering what aromatherapy can be good for

▶ Knowing what to expect in a typical consultation

▶ Finding out about safe and effective use of aromatherapy

· ·

*A*romatherapy is the use of essential oils extracted from plants, flowers, trees, and seeds for therapeutic purposes. Scented oils have been used since ancient times for their healing properties, but more recently, scientists have investigated the psychological and physical effects of particular essential oils.

Nowadays, aromatherapy is one of the most popular forms of complementary therapy, and it is even used in schools, clinics, hospitals, maternity units, hospices, and work settings.

In this chapter, you'll explore the roots of aromatherapy and look at modern day practice from aromatherapy massage to medical aromatherapy (internal use of aromatherapy oils). You'll get the low-down on how aromatherapy may work, the evidence for its effectiveness, and key points for the safe use of aromatherapy oils.

Then I let you know what a typical aromatherapy consultation involves, and finally I give you some tips on how you can enjoy using aromatherapy oils at home.

Finding Out about Aromatherapy

Aromatherapy literally means 'treatment using scents' and involves the therapeutic use of fragrant essential oils extracted from plants and plant materials.
The oils may be massaged into the skin, inhaled, vaporised, or diffused
throughout the room. In France, under careful supervision from a medical
aromatherapist only, certain oils may also be taken internally.

Never take essential oils internally except under medical supervision
because they can be toxic!

The oils appear to work on the brain and nervous system via absorption
through the skin into the bloodstream and via the nose to act on the olfactory centres (the areas of the brain that respond to smells).

Aromatherapy may be used to relax or invigorate or to treat specific health
problems such as insomnia, nervous problems, circulatory or respiratory
problems, digestive disorders, and so on.

A (very) brief history of aromatherapy

The ancient Egyptians, Greeks, Chinese, Persians, Romans, Aztecs, Native
Americans, and Indians are all believed to have used aromatic plants and
scented oils, either in religious ceremonies, to perfume their clothes and
bodies or for massage.

Early aromatic oils were made by soaking herbs in olive or castor oil or by
expressing them, for example, by squeezing the oil out of citrus peel. Around
the start of the 11th century, however, the great Iranian philosopher, physician, and scientist Abu Ali Sina, also known as Avicenna, is credited with
inventing a new distillation process that used steam and a coiled pipe to
successfully extract volatile oils from rose and other plant materials.

The Crusaders brought this technique back to Europe, and traders over the
next few centuries brought an increasing array of novel herbs and oils from
different parts of the world.

In the 15th century, the alchemist Paracelsus is believed to have first coined
the term 'essence' and began using essential oils of plants medicinally. Soon
essential oils were being prepared and sold by apothecaries and perfumery
developed as an art and a science in its own right. Later, in the 19th and 20th
centuries, individual constituents of essential oils were isolated and research
on their aromatic and medicinal uses continued.

ANECDOTE

The father of modern aromatherapy

Story has it that in 1910, René-Maurice Gattefossé, a French chemist working in a perfumery, burned his hand in his laboratory one day and instinctively plunged it into the nearest liquid, which happened to be lavender oil. To his surprise his skin is said to have healed quickly and without scarring. This aroused his curiosity and he went on to investigate and then write about the protective effects of certain essential oils against infection. It is believed that he may have experimented by using them at military hospitals with injured First World War soldiers and that he discovered that lavender, thyme, clove, and lemon all had useful antiseptic properties. Gattefossé is credited with coining the term 'aromatherapie' and wrote a best-selling book under this title, which is still used today. He is widely regarded as the father of modern aromatherapy and influenced many French physicians to use his methods.

One of the physicians inspired by Gattefossé was French army doctor Jean Valnet, who successfully used essential oils to treat infections of soldiers during the Second World War and went on to pioneer their medical use for treating burns, diabetes, and even cancer. This work has remained a part of French medical practice to this day.

Modern aromatherapy grew out of the chance discovery in the early 1900s, by French chemist René-Maurice Gattefossé that lavender oil could heal burns.

The use of essential oils for therapeutic massage and beauty purposes was pioneered in the 1960s, by the biochemist, nurse, and beautician Marguerite Maury. She was born in Austria but moved to France, married a French physician, and spent decades studying and developing aromatherapy.

Modern pioneers who've promoted aromatherapy include Micheline Arcier, Shirley Price, Danièle Ryman, and Robert Tisserand.

Grasping the idea behind aromatherapy

Essential oils are concentrated volatile oils extracted from plants and plant materials by means of distillation, expression, or solvents.

- ✔ **Distillation:** Involves passing steam through a container holding plant materials, which causes the volatile oils to vaporise. As the vapour travels down a coiled glass tube, it is cooled and turns back into a liquid oil, which can then be collected. This method is used for the extraction of most essential oils such as eucalyptus, peppermint, or lavender. In this process, floral waters, also known as hydrosols or hydrolats, may also be produced as a by-product.

✔ **Expression:** In this method the plant material is collected and then pressed, usually using mechanical equipment, to extract the oil. Essences of lemon, lime, and orange are collected in this way by expressing the peel of the fruit.

✔ **Solvent extraction:** Some plants only contain minute quantities of volatile oils and so solvents may be used to draw them out of the plant material. An example of this process is the extraction of the essential oil Rose Absolute.

The term *essential* refers to the fact that the oil is the essence of the scent of the plant, or plant material, rather than that it is essential to the plant's survival.

The oils are extracted from the leaves, flowers, berries, peel, bark, seeds, roots, wood, and resins of plants and then used therapeutically for both psychological and physical ailments by means of inhalation or application to the body.

Aromatherapy today

In the UK, aromatherapy is currently going through a process of voluntary regulation under the auspices of the Aromatherapy Council (www.aromatherapy council.co.uk). In the US, no official form of accreditation or regulation exists at this time. In France, aromatherapy remains a part of orthodox medicine, cosmetology, and beauty therapy.

Aromatherapy is hugely popular as both a complementary therapy and a self-help therapy. It is widely used in Europe, North America, Australia, Japan, and elsewhere.

Finding Out How It Works

Aromatherapy is believed to work in two ways, via inhalation or absorption.

In the case of inhalation, as you breathe in the aroma of the essential oil, tiny receptors in the nose are stimulated and these in turn stimulate nerves, which are connected to the olfactory centres of the brain, that is, the areas stimulated by the sense of smell. These areas are linked to other parts of the brain connected to mood and so it is thought that somehow different scents can produce different moods such as feeling relaxed or happy.

Absorption of compounds in the oils takes place when the oil is massaged into the skin. These compounds pass into the bloodstream and from there affect the nervous system, which also can somehow affect mood and physical health. Exactly how this process works isn't yet known and the mechanism for specific effects of individual oils in the body is not yet fully understood.

Exploring Different Types of Aromatherapy

The main types of aromatherapy currently practised are:

- **Massage aromatherapy:** This therapy involves therapeutic massage (see Chapter 17 for more on massage techniques) using essential oils diluted in a carrier oil. Sometimes acupressure and other massage techniques are incorporated. This is the most common form of aromatherapy used in complementary medicine.

- **Cosmetic aromatherapy:** Here, essential oils are combined into various beauty products, such as skin or hair products, and used for beauty therapy treatments or home use. This is also practised by beauticians and beauty therapists.

- **Olfactory aromatherapy:** Essential oils are released into the atmosphere via vaporisers, burners, or sprays for inhalation. This type of aromatherapy is mainly for home use but is also used in some schools, hospitals, and work places.

- **Medical aromatherapy:** This therapy is sometimes called aromatology. It involves essential oils being taken internally. This is only practised by medically trained aromatherapists, mainly in France.

- **Culinary aromatherapy:** This uses essential oils in cooking, for example in the form of infused oils drizzled over vegetables or used to flavour rice or herb butters.

Discovering What Aromatherapy Is Good For

You can use aromatherapy to relax, rejuvenate, and energise, or to promote well-being and aid healing. It is often used for the following types of conditions:

- Stress, anxiety or insomnia
- Joint and muscular problems
- Chronic fatigue

✔ Hyperactivity

✔ Skin problems

✔ Sports injuries and pain relief

✔ Menstrual and menopausal imbalance

Aromatherapy is also used in cancer and hospice care and in burns and cardiac units in hospitals as well as sometimes in classrooms, to facilitate learning.

When not to use aromatherapy

Only use aromatherapy under careful supervision by an experienced aromatherapist with very young children or if you are:

✔ Pregnant

✔ Breastfeeding

✔ Suffering from asthma, high blood pressure, epilepsy, varicose veins, deep-vein thrombosis, or broken or infected skin

Always tell your aromatherapist if you are, or may be, pregnant; if you're trying to conceive; or if you suffer from any of the above mentioned disorders.

Possible side effects

Pregnant and breastfeeding women and young infants need to be careful because essential oils can be toxic. For this reason they should also never be taken internally except under medical supervision.

The oils are very concentrated and may cause irritation or allergic reactions if applied neat to the skin. For this reason always dilute them in a suitable vegetable carrier oil (exceptions are lavender oil for burns and tea tree oil for infections, which you can apply neat). Test a small amount of oil on the back of the earlobe to test for allergic reactions before full use. Avoid contact with the eyes.

Certain oils may interact with prescribed medicines so seek advice from your aromatherapist or GP if you're on medication. Some citrus oils also increase the skin's sensitivity to light, making it more prone to pigmentation.

Evidence that it works

Research on individual oils has confirmed their various properties. For example, tea tree has been shown to have potent antiseptic, anti-bacterial, and anti-fungal properties, while the sedative properties of neroli and lavender have also been confirmed.

In clinical studies, aromatherapy has been found to aid relaxation and help relieve anxiety and depression. Aromatherapy may also be helpful for other conditions such as dementia, premenstrual syndrome, and bronchitis, as well as in cancer care. However, many studies have only used small numbers of people and have had design flaws, so more research is needed.

For details of some published aromatherapy studies, check out the following:

✔ NHS Complementary and Alternative Medicine Specialist Library (www.library.nhs.uk/cam)

✔ The Cochrane Library (www.cochrane.org/reviews/clibintro.htm)

What to Expect in a Typical Treatment

Aromatherapy treatment generally starts with some questions about your health.

Questioning

Your aromatherapist may ask questions about your general physical and emotional health including current symptoms, medical history, stress levels, lifestyle and diet. You may also be asked whether you want the aromatherapy for general relaxation or to address a specific health concern.

Selecting the oils

The aromatherapist will use the information from your answers to questions to determine which essential oil, or combination of oils, may be the most therapeutic for you. You may also be asked to smell and choose between certain oils to determine your particular preferences.

Aromatherapists don't make any medical diagnosis, unless they're medically qualified, so if you're in any doubt about your condition consult your doctor first.

Good aromatherapists usually only use pure, and sometimes organic, essential oils rather than synthetic or diluted ones.

Aromatherapy treatment

For the treatment you're usually asked to undress down to underwear and then are covered with towels as you lie on a treatment couch in a warm room.

Most professional aromatherapists treat you with therapeutic massage (see Chapter 17 for more about massage techniques) using selected essential oils diluted in a vegetable carrier oil such as sweet almond, jojoba, sunflower, or grapeseed. Alternatively, the oils may be added to lotions or creams.

The massage may be for the whole body or just part of the body such as the neck and shoulders or a facial massage. Some aromatherapists also incorporate manual lymphatic drainage and/or acupressure techniques into the treatment (check out Chapter 9 on acupuncture and Chapter 17 on massage for more about these).

Other types of treatment

Sometimes you may be advised to use the oils at home as inhalants or added to bath water (see the 'Helping Yourself with Aromatherapy' section at the end of this chapter to find out how to do this). Your aromatherapist may also give you some general advice on diet and lifestyle.

At the end of treatment

You'll often be left alone for a short while to complete your relaxation, allow the oil residues to be fully absorbed into the skin, and to slowly bring yourself back to reality! You can then get dressed and it is a good idea to drink a glass of water or herbal tea to rehydrate after the massage.

Duration and frequency

Aromatherapy sessions usually last around 60 to 90 minutes for a full body massage or 30 minutes for a facial or neck and shoulder massage. Follow-ups can be as often as you like. Very tense people often choose to have aromatherapy at regular intervals – say weekly, fortnightly, or monthly – to ease tension and relieve stress.

Knowing whether your aromatherapy treatment is working

The success of aromatherapy depends on the quality of the essential oils used and the skill and experience of the practitioner. Pure, organic essential oils, carefully made and used within sell-by date, are the most effective. Essential oils adulterated with chemicals, pesticides, diluted, or left to go rancid are not likely to be effective and can even smell sickly or unpleasant. Reputable essential oil manufacturers provide information on the purity and quality of their oils. Well-trained aromatherapists are happy to confirm for you their level of training and experience. After the treatment you should feel relaxed and comfortable with an enhanced sense of well-being.

Common Questions about Aromatherapy Treatment

Here are some questions that I'm often asked about aromatherapy that are not covered in the chapter so far:

- ✔ **How are essential oils classified and combined into blends?** They can be classified according to their 'notes', that is their scent characteristics, as well as other characteristics. 'Top notes' are scents that give you a quick first impression and that are often fresh and uplifting. They include citrus essential oils such as lemon, lime, and orange as well as peppermint and eucalyptus. 'Middle notes' are rounder, softer scents such as lavender, rosemary, or chamomile. 'Base notes' are more solid, enduring scents such as sandalwood and cedarwood. Good blends often combine oils with top, middle, and base 'notes'.

- ✔ **What should the ratio of essential oil to carrier oil be?** Usually the ratio is between 0.5 and 3 per cent essential oil to carrier oil, depending on age, condition and body size.

- ✔ **What will I feel like afterwards?** You may feel very relaxed, tired, sleepy or thirsty at the end of the session. Allow yourself time to 'come round' before driving or operating machinery and, if possible, clear your schedule of demanding activities and avoid heavy meals and alcohol for a few hours after treatment.

Finding a Good Aromatherapist

The Aromatherapy Council (Tel: 0870-7743477; www.aromatherapycouncil.co.uk), is the new, voluntary self-regulatory body for aromatherapists in the UK and operates a directory of members who follow a code of professional practice and ethics.

In the US, where currently no national system regulates the practice of aromatherapy, and regulations for 'hands-on' therapy vary from state to state, the best way to find an aromatherapist is to look in local directories or contact local qualified massage therapists. You can find a lot of information about aromatherapy in the US online at www.aromaweb.com. However, always remember to ask about training, experience, licensing, insurance, and so on.

Counting the cost of aromatherapy

Aromatherapy sessions can cost from £30 to £90 depending on whether a full body massage or a partial massage, such as a facial, is carried out. Aromatherapy treatments on the NHS are usually free or subsidised. Private health insurance does not usually cover aromatherapy treatment.

Ensuring satisfaction

If you're dissatisfied with your treatment, first talk things over with your practitioner.

If you think that the practitioner has been negligent, incompetent, or unethical in any way, contact their professional association. The new Aromatherapy Council has a formal complaints procedure.

Helping Yourself with Aromatherapy

Here are some of the ways that you can enjoy using essential oils at home:

✔ **Baths**: Add five to ten drops of a relaxing essential oil such as lavender or geranium to warm bath water and stir vigorously before getting in. Soak for 10 minutes.

✔ **Inhalation:** Add two to three drops of essential oil to a bowl of steaming water, cover your head with a towel, lean over the bowl, and then breathe in the vapour. Oil of eucalyptus or lemon are good for clearing your head and easing colds or nasal blockage.

Make sure that the bowl is on a stable surface and won't tip and scald you. If you suffer from asthma get advice from a trained aromatherapist on the best and safest essential oils to use.

✔ **Diffusion:** Put five drops of essential oil in a vaporiser, aromatherapy burner, or light bulb ring (these can be purchased from health shops) and allow the room to fill with a wonderful aroma. Good oils for freshening rooms are geranium, lime, and ylang ylang, depending on your personal preference.

If using an aromatherapy burner with a dish for water and a lighted candle, take care that the water doesn't run dry and that the candle can't become a fire hazard. Keep safely out of reach of children and pets. Alternatively, use a plug-in electric vaporiser. With light bulb rings, make sure that no oil drops onto the light bulb itself as it may then overheat and blow.

✔ **Massage:** Mix five to ten drops of essential oil per 10ml of a carrier oil such as almond, jojoba, or good quality sunflower oil. Warm your hands and then massage the oil blend directly onto the skin.

Use towels to prevent staining clothes or bed linen. Ensure that the room is warm so that exposed skin doesn't get chilled.

✔ **Compresses:** Add three to five drops of essential oil to 300ml of warm/hot water and soak a clean flannel or soft cloth in this liquid. Wring out and apply to affected part of the body. Warm essential oil compresses can be used for menstrual pains, cystitis, and boils. For bruises, sprains, or headaches, first cool the compress in a bowl in the fridge for 20 minutes and then apply.

✔ **Gargles and mouthwashes:** Add one to three drops of lemon, tea tree, or thyme essential oil to a glass of water and mix well. Take a mouthful and rinse the mouth or gargle and then spit out – don't swallow.

Don't take essential oils internally unless under the supervision of a medical aromatherapist. Avoid bringing the oils into contact with the eyes. Halve dosages for children and get professional advice if you're pregnant, breastfeeding, or wanting to use aromatherapy with infants.

Chapter 20

Connecting with Healing Therapies

. . . .

In This Chapter

▶ Finding out what healing therapies are all about

▶ Exploring different types of healing

▶ Discovering what healing therapies can be good for

▶ Examining the evidence

▶ Knowing what to expect in a typical healing session

▶ Knowing how to find safe and effective healers

. . . .

*H*ealing therapies have existed in every culture from the dawn of time. At the most primitive they involve simple hand touch for comfort and support, but certain healing therapies claim to be able to radiate specific healing energy from the hands or to even 'channel' healing energy from an external source. Often healing has been linked to specific shamanic, religious, or spiritual traditions. Healing may focus on the physical body or on a more subtle level.

In this chapter, I explore some age-old healing traditions and some more modern ones. I look at their history and practice and find out what they're used for and what evidence supports their use. I also tell you how you can locate healers and give you some tips on self-healing.

A (Very) Brief History of Healing

All ancient cultures are known to have identified certain individuals as healers and to have called on their services at times of need. In early primitive societies, healers were often shamans, attributed with magical or healing powers, and the ability to enter trance-like states to get information on diseases and their cures. Some of these shamanic traditions still exist today.

In Medieval times in Europe, where Christianity held sway, healing was seen as a divine gift from God. Accordingly, healing came under the auspices of the Church and was achieved through prayer, laying on of hands in the name of God, penance, pilgrimage, and taking the waters at holy sites.

The Victorian era witnessed a great surge of interest in the occult, spiritualism, and the paranormal. During this time, mediums and spiritualists were often called on to give direct or absent healing at a distance.

More recently simple laying-on-of-hands, as a form of spiritual healing has become extremely popular with many thousands of lay people training in this kind of healing. Also, new forms of energetic healing have been developed whereby practitioners claim to be able to channel healing energy from a higher source.

Exploring Different Types of Healing

Several different types of healing are used in different healing therapies. The following list outlines the main types:

- **Absent healing:** This healing is done at a distance without the recipient being present. The healers usually close their eyes, visualise the recipient or connect with them via a lock of hair or other personal item, and then mentally direct healing to them.

- **Auric healing:** Auric healing is based on the concept of an energetic, electro-magnetic, or light body, also called an *aura* surrounding the actual physical body. Healers claim to be able to sense or see this aura and to remove blockages in it they believeare linked to diseases in the physical body.

- **Chakra healing:** This healing is directed towards rebalancing the seven main subtle energy vortices, known as *chakras*, according to the Indian yoga system. These *chakras* are not visible to the naked eye, but sensitive people claim to be able to perceive them and to be able to affect their functioning.

- **Faith healing:** This healing is where a so-called higher power or religious figure is invoked, such as Jesus, the Virgin Mary, the Buddha, Krishna, or a spiritual teacher, and the recipient needs to have faith in that higher power for the healing to be successful.

- **Laying on of hands:** In this type of healing, the healer's hands are laid on the body or held just off the body. Healing power is believed to radiate from the hands into the diseased or painful area in the recipient's body.

✔ **Psychic surgery:** In psychic surgery, the healer's hands are said to be guided by an unseen spirit or force enabling the healer to transfer 'healing energy' into the person or actually penetrate their body and remove the diseased tissue.

✔ **Spiritual healing:** Spiritual healing is similar to faith healing in that the healers believe that they are acting as channels for healing energy from a divine source but, in this case, no belief or faith is required on the part of the recipient.

✔ **Trance healing:** As the name suggests, this healing is performed while the healer is in a trance state and supposedly being guided by a healing entity rather than consciously directing their healing work.

A famous example of this type of healing was Edgar Cayce, an American who had little formal education, but was able to go into trance and then answer detailed medical questions and give extensive health and spiritual advice (for more about him, go to www.edgarcayce.org). Cayce did this work for decades yet appeared to have little knowledge of what had been said once he came out of his trance state.

Little evidence supports many of the claims for these different types of healing and many people remain sceptical, believing that any healing that occurs is merely a *placebo* effect; that is, a chance effect due to the person's personal belief in the healing.

Looking at Popular Healing Therapies Today

This section introduces you to the main healing therapies used today (in alphabetical order):

✔ Crystal healing

✔ Johrei

✔ Psychic healing and psychic surgery

✔ Reiki

✔ Shamanic healing

✔ Spiritual healing

✔ Therapeutic touch

✔ Other

Many healing therapies are given for free. Some practitioners, however, do charge or ask for donations. Charges vary according to the amount of time the therapy may take, the amount of training the person has undertaken, and what is involved in the healing.

If you're dissatisfied with your treatment, talk things over with your healer or therapist or make a complaint to their professional body.

Crystal healing

Crystals and gem stones have been valued and used in healing since ancient times and different types of crystals are attributed with different *healing* qualities. For example, rose quartz is said to be soothing and to facilitate heart and circulatory function, whereas amethyst is said to help calm the mind and aid throat function.

When you have crystal healing, the healer places crystals on or around your body, either individually or in patterns or grids. Alternatively, the crystal may be used in the form of a 'wand' to direct healing power, or crystals may be placed in the room or worn as jewellery.

Crystal healers claim to be able to use crystals for *aura cleansing* and *chakra purification,* which is essentially a form of spiritual purification of the person.

How does it work?

Crystals are believed to emanate vibrational frequencies that resonate with different organs of the body and the body's energetic centres, or *chakras.*

Who or what is it good for?

Anyone can utilise crystals and users claim they can help 'clear' the mind, relieve pain, and even ease common ailments.

What's the evidence?

No real scientific evidence supports the idea that crystals have specific healing powers, and many geologists and gem experts get quite hot under the collar about such therapeutic claims!

How can I find a crystal therapist?

There are no regulations in place or governing bodies for crystal healing. In the UK crystal healers may be located via the Affiliation of Crystal Healing Organisations (Tel: 07837 696 301; www.crystal-healing.org) or the International Association of Crystal Healing Therapists (Tel: 0161 702 8191; www.iacht.co.uk).

Currently, the US has no umbrella organisation for crystal healing, but two leaders in the field are the Association of Melody Crystal Healing Instructors (www.taomchi.com); and the Crystalis Institute (www.crystalisinstitute.com).

Johrei

Johrei (also written as *Jōrei*), meaning *purification of the spirit*, is a healing approach established by Mokichi Okada in Japan in 1934.

Okada believed that disease was linked to the intake of toxins, unnatural behaviour, and the separation of the soul and the body.

How does it work?

Universal energy or divine light is believed to be channelled through the palm of the giver towards the receiver a short distance away.

Who or what is it good for?

Anyone can learn Johrei and give it to anyone. Johrei is often used to treat stress or pain or as a form of absent healing. The aim is not to cure physical illness but to purify the spiritual body and increase happiness.

What's the evidence?

There is no firm scientific evidence to support this technique but some research is underway in the US. Check out www.johrei-institute.org for more details.

How can I receive Johrei?

For more on Johrei and its availability contact: the Johrei Association (UK) (Tel: 0207 281 1532; www.johreiassociation.co.uk), the Johrei Fellowship and Johrei Foundation via (www.johrei.com), the Izunome Association (USA) (www.izunome.org), and the Vancouver Johrei Centre (Tel: 00 1604 273 0212).

Psychic healing

As mentioned earlier in this chapter, psychic healing involves energy transfer or actual 'surgery' – cutting into the body without normal surgical tools or anaesthesia – by someone, often in a trance-like or meditative state.

How does it work?

The psychic surgeon is believed to channel a healing force or divine energy that enables healing to occur and/or the physical body to be penetrated.

Some psychic surgeons use their hands while others use instruments such as knives, to 'cut' the body open.

Interestingly, although these tools are unsterilised and the 'operations' are carried out in non-surgical conditions, no reported cases of infection exist.

Who or what is it good for?

Psychic surgeons are willing to attempt treatment for any type of ailment, even a serious or terminal one.

What's the evidence?

There is no conclusive evidence to support this type of healing and claims of miracle cures have not yet been substantiated to the satisfaction of sceptics.

ANECDOTE

Psychic surgery

I have both witnessed and experienced psychic surgery. Many years ago I travelled with a group to India. One member of the group was Stephen Turoff. He was a big bear of a man – tall and well-built but also softly spoken and affectionate and with a broad cockney accent. I had never heard of him but was told he was a healer. One day we were with a group of people and he was asked if he would do some healing. He agreed and underwent an extraordinary transformation. His whole demeanour and voice changed and he started to speak with a German accent! He then asked a woman to lie down, placed his hands on her eyeball and, moving it aside, quickly thrust a penknife a couple of inches into her eye socket, turned it quickly, and then pulled it out with some tissue-like material!

The whole thing happened very rapidly but everyone gasped as they saw the blade clearly disappear to some depth behind the woman's eyeball. Turoff then returned to his normal 'self' and said that the woman had had a tumour behind her eye that he had now removed. He said that she would have lost the sight of her eye if it had been removed surgically in the normal way. He claimed that during the surgery he was 'overshadowed' by a deceased German surgeon who enabled him to *operate*. To everyone's surprise the woman then said that she'd been having increasingly bad headaches and pain behind that eye for some weeks and been meaning to go to a doctor but had put it off. She had not mentioned these headaches to anyone previously but the next day reported that both the headaches and pain had completely gone.

Sometime later I took someone who was ill to see Stephen at his London clinic. I had expected simply to be an observer again but to my surprise he suddenly asked me to lie down and then rapidly cut into the side of my abdomen with a knife! I had the extraordinary sensation of his hands actually being *inside* my abdomen and then it was all over and he was out of the room without a word. I looked down at my abdomen and there was a thin, red line, just like a surgical scar, where I had been 'cut' open and which stayed for about three days. The whole area was also tender for that period of time and felt as I imagine it would feel if real surgery had been performed. I do not know what he was operating on but it was certainly a unique experience and a quite extraordinary sensation!

How can I find a psychic surgeon?

Many of the most famous psychic surgeons hail from the Philippines or Brazil, and several tour operators organise trips to visit them. Since some have been found to be fraudulent you need to be very wary before parting with your money or embarking on such a trip.

In the UK, one of the most well-documented psychic healers is Stephen Turoff, who practises at the Danbury Healing Clinic (Tel: 01245 348325; www.stephenturoff.org).

Reiki

Reiki (pronounced ray-key and meaning 'universal life energy') is a type of hand healing developed in Japan in the late 19th-century by Mikao Usui. He was an avid student of philosophy, medicine, and Buddhism who was inspired to make a form of healing readily available to the public. He developed a system of *attunement*, whereby you align yourself with universal healing energy, and then transfer it to the recipient by means of a series of hand positions and visualisation. One of Usui's students, Chujiro Hayashi, continued his work at a clinic in Tokyo and added more detailed hand positions, as well as a three-stage process of initiation. His work was then brought to Hawaii by one of his patients, Hawayo Takata, in the 1930s, and from there it has spread around the world.

The essence of Usui's original teaching is that Reiki be simple and accessible for all. Therefore, the complex series of initiations and levels, and the very high fees requested by certain teachers and practitioners is controversial. Other practitioners have developed their own techniques and made them freely available.

How does it work?

During Reiki healing the practitioner places hands in 12 different positions on or near your head, abdomen, and back holding each position for a few minutes. During this attunement the practitioner becomes aligned with universal energy and then uses the different hand positions and symbols to transfer this energy to different parts of your body to heal and rebalance it.

Who or what is it good for?

Anyone can receive Reiki. It is often used as a form of stress or pain relief but is also used for easing specific ailments and as a form of self-development. It can also be performed on yourself or used for absent healing.

What's the evidence?

No scientific studies exist to conclusively explain what goes on during Reiki or to prove that it is effective, but research is underway.

How can I find a Reiki practitioner?

Reiki practitioners in the UK have started a process of voluntary self-regulation and the newly formed Reiki Regulatory Working Group (www.reiki regulation.org.uk) lists various Reiki associations, which have directories of practitioners.

In the US, Reiki healers can be located via: the International Association of Reiki Professionals (IARP; Tel: 00 (1603) 881 8838; www.iarp.org); the International Center for Reiki Training (Tel: 00 (1800) 332 8112; www.reiki.org); and the Reiki Alliance (Tel: 00 (1208) 783 3535; www.reikialliance.com) that lists practitioners from the Takata lineage around the world.

Shamanic healing

Shamans use ritual, song, dance, trance, drumming, fasting, sweat lodges, visualisations, or the use of consciousness-altering plants, mushrooms, or other plant materials to heal or for self-development.

How does it work?

Shamans supposedly act as intermediaries and guides helping you to interpret dreams and symbols, interacting with 'spirits' and other entities on your behalf, and guiding you on the spiritual path. Some focus on visualisations, meditation, and dream work, enabling you to explore and change attitudes and beliefs and to open your eyes to new concepts and methods of understanding.

Other shamans have a good knowledge of plants, including hallucinogens, and may use these to enable you to enter altered states of perception.

Consciousness-altering plants can have very potent, and sometimes very disturbing, effects, and need to be used only under the careful supervision of someone experienced in their use.

Who or what is it good for?

Anyone can call on the services of a shaman. Some people use shamanic healing for specific ailments but many use it for self-development.

What's the evidence?

Many anthropological and sociological studies of shamans exist, as well as some scientific work on the effects of the hallucinogenic plants used by shamans, but there is no real evidence that specific shamanic rituals can heal.

How can I find a shaman?

You must be very careful when searching for a genuine and reputable shaman. Many Westerners now claim to have shamanic abilities but traditional shamans sometimes call these people *plastic shamans* – that is, people who have done little training and do not really understand what they're doing.

You can read more about shamanic healing via the Foundation for Shamanic Studies (Tel: 00(1415) 380 8282; www.shamanism.org); the Centre for Contemporary Shamanism (UK) (Tel: 01435 810233; www.shamanism.co.uk); and Living Magically (UK) (Tel: 015394 31943; www.livingmagically.co.uk).

Spiritual healing

Spiritual healing is the channelling of *universal healing energy* via a trained healer and is sometimes described as the simple transfer of 'love and light'.

How does it work?

The healer channels healing via hands held on, or just away from, the body. You do not need to have any particular faith or belief to receive this healing and it may also be used for absent healing.

As the body relaxes and tension is eased during healing, it is believed that this may stimulate internal self-healing.

Who or what is it good for?

Anyone may receive spiritual healing but it is often used to relieve stress, anxiety, and pain, and to ease discomfort in those with chronic or terminal illnesses.

What's the evidence?

Several studies have suggested that pain and anxiety may be eased with healing but more good studies are needed.

How can I find a spiritual healer?

The UK Healers Self-Regulatory Body is now very active in trying to get a consensus for regulations governing spiritual healing in the UK and lists all the

main UK healing organisations: (Tel: 0113 2741028; www.ukhealers.info).
Another useful resource is the Doctor Healer Network (Tel: 0208 800 3569;
www.doctorhealer.net).

You can locate healers in the US via the American Association of Healers
(www.americanassociationofhealers.com).

Therapeutic Touch

This type of laying-on-of-hands therapy was devised in the US in the 1960s,
by nursing professor Dolores Krieger and her healer colleague, Dora Kunz.
Krieger wanted to create a simple therapeutic healing system that she could
incorporate into nursing training. This technique is now widely practised by
nurses and other practitioners around the world.

How does it work?

The therapy has four main steps: attunement; checking the energy field by
placing the hands on or over different parts of the body; sweeping the body
to unblock any problem areas; transfer of healing energy.

Therapeutic touch is based on the idea that everybody has an energy field
that can be rebalanced through manual and visualisation techniques.

Who or what is it good for?

Anyone can receive therapeutic touch but it is especially widely used by
nurses in clinical settings such as hospitals or clinics to treat those with pain,
anxiety, diseases of ageing, and so on.

What's the evidence?

Quite a large number of studies have been done demonstrating lowered blood
pressure and decreased stress and anxiety after therapeutic touch. However,
some argue that these changes were due to placebo rather than any specific
healing effect and two review studies have found no real evidence of any therapeutic effect.

How can I find a therapeutic touch therapist?

In the UK, therapeutic touch practitioners may be members of the healing
organisations listed under UK Healers (Tel: 0113 2741028; www.ukhealers.
info) or the British Association of Therapeutic Touch (Redmire Farm,
Mungrisdale, Penrith, Cumbria CA11 0TB). You may also be able to locate
therapeutic touch practitioners through the Sacred Space Foundation (Tel:

017684 86868; www.sacredspace.org.uk). In the US, you can locate practitioners via the Nurse Healers-Professional Associates International (NH-PAI; Tel: 00 (1518) 325 1185 or Toll Free 00 (1877) 32 NHPAI; www.therapeutic-touch.org); and Therapeutic Touch at Pumpkin Hollow Farm (where the technique was originally devised and taught by Kreiger and Kunz) (Tel: 00 (1518) 325 3583; www.therapeutictouch.org).

Other healing therapies

Other healing therapies may focus specifically on healing the *energetic body* of the person, that is, the electro-magnetic field or aura, said to surround the physical body. One of the most well-known of these is the healing approach taught by Barbara Brennan's School of Light in the US, Germany, and Japan. Brennan, a former NASA physicist, has spent 30 years studying the human energy field and developed a system of healing that combines hand healing with psychological and spiritual approaches. For more information, contact the Barbara Brennan School of Healing (Tel: 00 (1800) 924 2564; www.barbarabrennan.com).

Helping Yourself with Healing Therapies

 You can do healing for yourself. The following is a simple technique that you may like to try.

1. **Sit in a relaxed and comfortable position, preferably in a quiet and warm environment.**

2. **Rub the palms of your hands together vigorously for a few seconds.**

3. **Place a warm palm, or both palms, on the area of the body that you want to heal.** You may alternate palms or place one hand over the other, depending on the area of the body being worked on.

4. **Leave the hands(s) in place for about 30 seconds, breathing deeply and relaxing your body.**

5. **Rub the hands together again and repeat the process.**

6. **If you want, you can also add visualisation while the palms are in place.** Imagine light streaming in through the top of your head and radiating out through your palms into the area that needs healing. Visualise the part of the body being healed.

7. **You can repeat this whole process several times during the day and also use it on other people as well as on animals.**

Chapter 21

Getting Your Head Around Psychological Therapies

*N*owadays the mind and body are generally accepted as interconnected. Your thoughts and emotions *can* have a bearing on ill health and may influence perceptions of pain, recovery time after surgery, and even the effectiveness of chemotherapy.

In this chapter, you explore some of the complementary therapies influenced by modern-day psychology that aim to help you have a healthy mind. You'll take a look at hypnotherapy, autogenic training, and re-birthing, and some quite recently developed therapies such as thought field therapy and the emotional freedom technique.

I let you know what you may be letting yourself in for with these therapies and how they may be beneficial. Then, at the end of the chapter, I give you a little tip on how to make positive thinking an everyday part of your life!

Finding Out about Psychological Therapies

Psychological therapies is a broad term that I use to refer to those therapies that specifically target your mind and emotions. However, this definition is really too narrow. The word *psychology* is nowadays taken to mean the 'study of the mind', but in its original meaning, it came from the Greek word *psykhe*, which means 'breath, spirit, soul' or 'animating spirit'; 'the invisible animating principle or entity, which occupies and directs the physical body'.

Thus, although these therapies target thoughts, emotions, and mental attitudes, the underlying aim is really to reach the soul, to create a sense of peace and happiness that can radiate throughout your life. Many practitioners also believe that such 'soul contentedness' can have a direct effect on the physical body. This effect is being increasingly backed up by modern-day research, which basically shows that happiness is good for you!

These therapies draw strongly on the work by famous psychologists and psychiatrists of the past such as psychoanalyst Sigmund Freud, behaviourists Ivan Pavlov and B.F.Skinner, psychiatrist Carl Jung, and psychologists Carl Rogers, Erik Erikson, and Erich Fromm, to name but a few.

The origins of psychology go back to the great Greek philosophers Socrates, Plato, and Aristotle, who wrestled with the concepts of the soul and the mind and what it means to be a human, thinking being. Over time, many more philosophers added to the mix and in the early 16th-century the term *psychology* first started to be used. (Marko Marulić, the Serbo-Croatian humanist and poet, is thought to have first coined the term.)

Psychology gradually developed into a study subject in its own right and over the last 200 years a whole host of theories and different types of therapies have been created.

More recently, individuals have taken inspiration from the fields of psychology, and sometimes combined elements from other complementary therapies to create new forms of therapy for balancing the mind.

Exploring Modern-day Complementary Therapies for the Mind

Defining psychological therapies as *complementary medicine* is difficult because some, such as hypnotherapy, are also used in orthodox settings by medical doctors. In this section I cover the main popular modern-day therapies that deal with the mind.

Autogenic therapy (AT)

Autogenic therapy (AT) was developed by a German neurologist, Johannes Schultz, in the 1920s, to ease stress, aid relaxation, and promote healing for a range of psychological and physical conditions. AT was later further developed by his Canadian colleague, Dr Wolfgang Luthe. *Autogenic* means 'generated from within' and gentle self-awareness is the focus of the exercises.

How does it work?

You are taught a series of six exercises over eight to ten weekly sessions, either one-to-one or in small groups. The exercises calm the mind and decrease the stress responses of the body. Studies have shown that during AT practice, the brain produces waves similar to those seen during meditation.

Who or what is it good for?

Anyone can learn and practise AT – from business people to children – and you can practise it anywhere that you can sit quietly or lie down. The therapy has been used to treat stress, migraine, asthma, and insomnia, among other ailments, and to facilitate pregnancy and birthing.

What's the evidence?

More than 3,000 studies have been conducted, and the studies suggest effectiveness for a wide range of physical and mental conditions.

How can I find a practitioner?

In the UK, health professionals who have taken a one-year part-time course to become a member of the British Autogenic Society are listed on `www.auto genic-therapy.org.uk`.

Biofeedback

Biofeedback is a method of therapy that measures 'autonomic responses' in the body – that is, physical responses that you normally cannot control voluntarily such as finger-tip temperature, heart rate, and brain waves – and then feeds back this information by means of a signal so that you can learn to control them. This work began in the US and the UK in the 1960s, as scientists became interested in trying to verify extraordinary feats by Indian yogis who appeared able to control their body's internal physical processes. Doctors Elmer and Alyce Green pioneered this work at the Menninger Foundation in the US.

How does it work?

Biofeedback devices measure a specific physical process and then feed back changes to the person being measured by means of numerical dials, beeps of varying sounds, or visual scales. The person then tries to control the process, such as lowering blood pressure or increasing finger-tip temperature, and the device tells them how successful they are. Over time, people develop the ability to control the process without the feedback being necessary.

What's it good for?

Biofeedback has been successfully used in the treatment of many conditions, including anxiety, insomnia, migraine, and bruxism (teeth grinding), and in helping to induce states of relaxation. *Neurofeedback*, which is biofeedback of brain waves, has been used to treat a range of conditions, including attention deficit hyperactivity disorder (ADHD), depression, epilepsy, and alcoholism.

What's the evidence?

Lots of studies since the 1960s, have now confirmed that biofeedback is effective.

How can I find a practitioner?

Practitioners vary hugely in their level of training and expertise. Some can be accessed via www.worldwidehealthcenter.net. In the US, a good source is the Biofeedback Certification Institute of America (BCIA; www.bcia.affiniscape.com).

Biorhythms

Biorhythms are supposed cycles of lows and highs related to emotional, physical, and mental (intellectual) function that are calculated mathematically (in the form of sine waves of fixed frequencies, for those who want to know!) from your day of birth. Biorhythms grew out of observations by Dr Wilhelm Fleiss (a great pal of Sigmund Freud and, incidentally, the one who tried to get him to give up the ten-cigar-a-day habit that gave him mouth and jaw cancer). Fleiss looked at medical records and noticed cycles for the occurrence of physical and emotional problems. Later, an Austrian mathematician, Alfred Teltscher, noticed what appeared to be intellectual cycles in the marks of his students. Subsequently, others have investigated, with varying results, cycles in accident rates of drivers, death rates following surgery in hospital, and so on.

How does it work?

You can purchase charts of biorhythms or access them via the Internet for free. You simply type in your date of birth and – hey presto! – a chart appears with cycles for physical, emotional, and mental function appearing in different colours.

What's it good for?

Biorhythms are good for fun, really. Some people claim that using biorhythm charts to foresee difficult times can help you weather the storm or even prevent accidents while planning activities on 'peak days'; for example, writing a book on days when you have an intellectual high can help to optimise performance. Certainly as a writer you have days that are easier and days that are harder but – for a bit of fun – I checked my biorhythm chart a few times during the long months it's taken to write this book and I really didn't find much correlation! Still, some people seem to find knowledge of biorhythms useful and I can't see the harm in it unless the charts are followed slavishly and start to take over your life. (I used to know someone who decided everything on the basis of the charts, which seemed to me to be taking things too far.)

What's the evidence?

Not much evidence exists – and is pretty erratic, to say the least. However, some interesting work in the field of chronobiology looks at rhythmical cycles of certain physiological processes such as hormone cycles or blood pressure. Some of these cycles appear to be linked to lunar cycles (the cycles of the moon) – for example, post-operative bleeding in patients during and after operations appears to be worse during full moons. This field of study can have huge implications for surgery and more work on this needs to be done.

How can I find a practitioner?

This therapy is do-it-yourself. However, some 'biorhythm experts' do offer to talk you through your chart – for a fee, of course!

Brief therapy

The term *brief therapy* was coined by American psychiatrist Milton H. Erickson to describe his way of addressing issues in therapy in just a few sessions. This idea was then picked up by American psychotherapist Steve de Shazer and his wife and colleagues in their solution-focused approach to family therapy. Basically, this approach is a talking therapy that focuses on solutions to problems in a few short sessions, rather than delving into the past.

How does it work?

The practitioner uses 'respectful curiosity' to help you identify your problem and then gives you a series of questions to help you identify solutions that can be tried out in practice. These include the 'miracle question', where you are asked how things would be different if a miracle happened and everything was sorted.

What's it good for?

Brief therapy's been used for all kinds of relationship problems, depression, anxiety, addictions, stress, and insomnia.

What's the evidence?

Research suggests that this approach can produce some lasting changes within quite a short time of therapy (usually no more than five sessions).

How can I find a practitioner?

In the UK, you can contact the Brief Therapy Practice (Tel: 0207 600 3366; www.brieftherapy.org.uk).

Emotional freedom techniques (EFT)

This therapy is a synthesis of a simplified version of Roger Callahan's thought field therapy (TFT) combined with neuro-linguistic programming (NLP) techniques – see the later sections about these. Created by American engineer and minister Gary Craig, this approach is now practised by more than 3,000 people around the world, and has been rapidly picked up as he offers the basics of the system free on his Internet site (www.emofree.com).

How does it work?

The tapping of acupuncture points is combined with affirmations such as, 'Even though I have this (*anxiety, depression, stiff neck, whatever*), I deeply and completely accept myself.' This therapy is said to aid release of stress, negative emotions, and so on, and to help balance the body's energies, based on the premise that negative emotions underlie all types of physical illness.

What's it good for?

EFT has been used for every kind of emotional and physical problem, including anxiety, depression, stress relief, phobias, and pain.

A mesmerising tale

Franz Anton Mesmer, an Austrian doctor in the 18th-century, was able to induce trance-like states in his patients. He claimed this trance was due to 'animal magnetism' (from the Latin *animus* meaning 'breath'), which, by the way, has nothing to do with animal behaviour. He used the term to refer to the 'life force' that he believed was in all living things and that was sensitive to influence. He claimed this force flowed in unseen channels of the body and that obstructions in this flow caused illness. This concept is very similar to that of acupuncture, described in Chapter 9.

In the beginning, he used magnets to influence this 'flow', but later believed that he could change it simply by staring deeply into the person's eyes and making a series of passes over their body with his hands. This approach came to be known as *mesmerism*, and he received some acclaim but was later (perhaps unfairly) denounced as a charlatan.

Around the same time an Indo-Portuguese priest, José Custódio de Faria, started to replicate Mesmer's work but insisted that the effects were all due to the openness to suggestion in the mind of the receiver rather than any special ability on his side. Mesmer's work was also picked up by a Scottish doctor, James Baird, who coined the term *hypnosis* and demonstrated how it could be used with suggestible people for surgery. French pharmacist Émile Coué, in the 1920s, went on to demonstrate the healing power of auto-suggestion (a type of self-hypnosis), and in the 1960s, modern-day psychotherapist Milton Erickson developed this approach into medical hypnosis.

What's the evidence?

A huge amount of anecdotal evidence exists but no published studies, which means that most of the medical profession dismisses this technique as unsubstantiated and mere placebo – that is, all in the mind (for more about the placebo effect, check out Chapter 10).

How can I find a practitioner?

Gary Craig's EFT Web site, www.emofree.com, lists practitioners all around the world and also offers a free download to learn the technique for yourself.

Hypnotherapy

Hypnotherapy involves the introduction of suggestions while the mind is in a receptive state and the body is deeply relaxed. Trance states and suggestion have been used since ancient times by shamans and healers. Modern-day hypnotherapy arose out of the work of a number of men, including Mesmer, Faria, Baird, Coué, and Erickson.

How does it work?

When the body is relaxed it is believed that the unconscious part of the mind can be accessed and is very open to suggestion. *Auto-suggestion*, or *self-hypnosis*, can be carried out when in a waking, fully conscious state, but some individuals are able to enter such a deep trance that they have no knowledge of what they have done or said when they come out of it. During this state it has been shown that brain waves change and various other biochemical changes also take place.

What's it good for?

Hypnosis has now become accepted and is practised by some doctors and dentists as well as specially trained hypnotherapists who use it to treat phobias, addictions, anxiety, insomnia, and so on.

What's the evidence?

Various studies have shown that hypnosis can affect relaxation and can have a beneficial effect on a range of conditions, including irritable bowel syndrome (IBS), asthma, headache, pain, and so on.

How can I find a practitioner?

In the UK, anyone can currently call themselves a hypnotherapist, and a very large number of different hypnotherapy associations and training bodies exist, all with varying requirements and standards. This situation also exists in other countries.

The UK Confederation of Hypnotherapy Organisations (Tel: 0800 952 0560; www.ukcho.co.uk) is an umbrella body for the hypnotherapy profession in the UK and lists a number of independent hypnotherapy associations, each of which has directories of members.

The General Hypnotherapy Register (Tel: 01590 683770; www.general-hypnotherapy-register.com) was set up by the General Hypnotherapy Standards Council in an attempt to create a single register of trained hypnotherapists.

Hypnotherapy associations in the United States include the following:

- American Association of Professional Hypnotherapists (AAPH; Tel: 00 (1650) 323 3224; www.aaph.org)
- American Hypnosis Association (AHA – set up by the Hypnosis Motivation Institute; Tel: 00 (1818) 758 2747 (also includes lay members); www.hypnosis.edu)

✔ National Guild of Hypnotists (NGH; Tel: 00 (1603) 429 9438; www.ngh.net)

✔ The American Board of Hypnotherapy (ABH; 00 (1808) 596 7765; www.hypnosis.com)

✔ American Psychotherapy and Medical Hypnosis Association (APMHA; Tel: 00 (1509) 662 5131; www.apmha.com)

✔ The American Society of Clinical Hypnosis (ASCH; Tel: 00 (1630) 980 4740; www.asch.net)

✔ The National Board for Certified Clinical Hypnotherapists (NBCCH; Tel: 00 (1800) 449 8144; www.natboard.com)

You can find some other hypnotherapy associations, including ones in Canada and Australia, on www.naturalbloom.com.

Please note: I am not endorsing any of the above associations, nor is this a comprehensive list.

Neuro-linguistic programming (NLP)

Developed around 1973 by Americans Richard Bandler, a psychology student, and John Grinder, a linguistics professor, with additional input from the social scientist Gregory Bateson, *neuro-linguistic programming* (NLP) refers to the study of neurology (the brain), linguistics (the use of language), and patterns of behaviour that you can observe (programmes). NLP as a therapy is a set of techniques for modifying language, behaviour, and experience.

How does it work?

Understanding how you have learnt to make sense of your experiences consciously and unconsciously via perception, thoughts, and feelings enables you to make changes in the way that you process information and communicate with others.

What's it good for?

NLP has been applied to everything from relationship problems and physical and mental conditions to the workplace and the training of salespeople!

What's the evidence?

NLP techniques are widely practised around the world and have been extensively researched. For lots of research papers, see www.nlp.de/research.

How can I find a practitioner?

You can find many organisations that represent NLP practitioners. Two good places to start looking are the following:

- ✔ UK Association of Neurolinguistic Programming (Tel: 0845 053 1162; www.anlp.org).

- ✔ Global Organisation of NLP (GONLP; Tel: 0845 141 2161; www.bbnlp.com). This site lists practitioners worldwide.

Psychosynthesis

A form of therapy that emphasises self-awareness and 'soul' knowledge, psychosynthesis was developed by Italian psychiatrist Roberto Assagioli in the early 20th-century. Assagioli had been a student of Freudian psychoanalysis but later rejected it to develop a more spiritual approach. The term *psychosynthesis* was used to represent the idea of synthesising different aspects of the self into a unified whole.

How does it work?

Painting, drawing, movement, meditation, creative visualisation, and other methods are used in one-to-one or group sessions to unify personality and develop potential.

What's it good for?

Psychosynthesis is suitable for anyone interested in personal development.

What's the evidence?

Psychosynthesis has been extensively researched and written about in psychological literature and journals.

How can I find a practitioner?

Look for a practitioner via the newly formed Psychosynthesis Professional Association (PPA; www.psychosynthesis.edu/ppa), or at the Institute of Psychosynthesis clinic (Tel: 0208 202 4525; www.psychosynthesis.org).

Rebirthing

Rebirthing is a therapy that uses breathing and other physical techniques to 're-enact' your birth so that you can resolve any traumas associated with it.

This therapy grew out of work by a small group of psychiatrists, psychotherapists, and psychologists, including Stanislav Grof and Elizabeth Fehr, interested in the influence of foetal and birth experiences on later mental health and personality. The therapy was utilised by Scottish psychiatrist R. D. Laing, who ran rebirthing workshops, and has been popularised by Americans Leonard Orr and Sondra Ray. Orr's rebirthing technique, which initially used water but later focused on special breathing techniques, has spread around the world.

How does it work?

Rebirthing is based on the idea that your mental life begins in the womb and that birth trauma can have a profound effect on the development of your personality, often leading to feelings of separation and anxiety.

What's it good for?

Rebirthing is supposed to reduce feelings of separation and resolve feelings of anxiety, depression, and so on, as well as help resolve relationship problems.

What's the evidence?

No solid research evidence supports this therapy although anecdotally many people report that they find it helpful.

ANECDOTE

Rebirthing with Ronnie

When I was a young psychology student, I became interested in the radical approaches to mental illness that were being proposed by innovative psychologists and psychiatrists such as Ronald David Laing. Ronnie, as he was known, was famous for establishing a therapeutic community where patients and therapists lived together. I went to live and work in one of these therapeutic communities for a while after I graduated and one day heard on the grapevine that Ronnie was going to lead a rebirthing workshop in an old church hall in London.

I went along, excited at the opportunity to meet the great man himself. He arrived about an hour late, rather tipsy but oozing charisma, and organised everyone into small groups. We had to make a human 'womb' over individual members of the group one at a time; the chosen one was to curl on the floor in a foetal position and then attempt to push their way out in order to be 'born'. As the 'birthings' got under way the hall became filled with the sound of grunts, groans, screams, and tears.

Many people seemed to find this experience an immense catharsis, with lots of group hugging and sharing of experiences. It was an unforgettable experience but it all seemed a bit crazy and haphazard to me so, when Ronnie slipped out, I gratefully took my 'reborn' self off home too!

ANECDOTE

A past-life therapy pioneer

Hazel Denning held two Master's degrees as well as doctorates in clinical psychology and metaphysical counselling. She spent more than 37 years working as a full-time past-life regression therapist and parapsychologist. I had the pleasure of meeting her in Japan one year when she came to visit Dr Hiroshi Motoyama's world-renowned Institute for Religion and Parapsychology, where I worked for some years. During her visit she presented a paper on past-life regression at the Institute's annual conference and did a live demonstration of regression in front of over 500 people. I knew the person that volunteered for this demonstration and was fascinated to see him go into a relaxed state and then suddenly apparently start to relive another life totally different from this one. From being a laid-back West Coast American journalist, he suddenly became a warrior from another age! Hazel was a wonderfully warm and sincere person with a sharp intelligence and participated in our research at the Institute for several days. She died peacefully in 2006 at the age of 98, saying she was looking forward to 'going dancing' with her husband on the other side (he had died over 20 years before!).

How can I find a practitioner?

You can find rebirthers in the UK via the British Rebirth Society (Tel: 0845 330 8214; www.rebirthingbreathwork.co.uk), whose practitioners use Leonard Orr's breathing techniques.

Leonard Orr's rebirthing Web site (www.rebirthingbreathwork.com) has a directory of US rebirthers.

Regression therapy

Regression therapy, also sometimes called past-life therapy or past-life regression therapy, involves deep relaxation and then being 'taken back' to specific times in your early life or even your past lives. This therapy was pioneered by, amongst others, the American clinical psychologist Hazel Denning.

How does it work?

In a deeply relaxed or hypnotic state, old memories may be accessed from the unconscious mind. Some claim that these relate not only to early childhood and forgotten experiences but also may even relate to time spent in the womb or to past lives, lived before the current one.

What's it good for?

Regression therapists claim to help treat phobias and other physical or mental conditions.

What's the evidence?

Most is anecdotal but some studies show that people's brain waves change in a novel way during regression therapy and that normal, healthy people are more likely to report past lives than mentally ill people. Some reported past-life experiences have been checked and supposedly verified, but not everyone is convinced by this 'evidence'.

How can I find a practitioner?

You can locate practitioners worldwide via the International Board for Regression Therapy (IBRT; www.ibrt.org).

Thought field therapy (TFT)

A technique devised in the 1980s, by American clinical psychologist Roger Callahan for treating stress and trauma, *thought field therapy* (TFT) links the mind and emotions with knowledge about the 'energetic body' taken from acupuncture and energy medicine (take a look at Chapters 9 and 22 for more about these treatments).

How does it work?

You are asked to visualise a relevant traumatic event or emotion while tapping different acupuncture *energy points* on the body in a specific sequence. Other techniques involve humming, counting, or moving your eyes in a particular direction while doing this tapping. These techniques are believed to re-programme the body and to balance your energy fields.

What's it good for?

TFT has been used to treat a range of psychological problems, including anxiety, insomnia, depression, addictions, phobia, and post-traumatic stress.

What's the evidence?

TFT practitioners claim high success rates, but this therapy remains controversial as no hard evidence exists to support its use. The American Psychological Association no longer recognises TFT as an acceptable form of study for continuing professional development (CPD) of psychologists.

How can 1 find a practitioner?

In the UK, you can find TFT practitioners via www.thoughtfieldtherapy.co.uk. In the US, look through the directory on Roger and Joanne Callahan's Web site at www.tftrx.com.

Visualisation

Visualisation, also called mental imagery, guided imagery, or creative visualisation, involves creating positive images in the imagination, while in a relaxed state, in order to change mental or physical problems or improve performance. This therapy has been used medically with cancer patients by Dr Carl Simonton in the US and has also been pioneered in the work of, amongst others, Shakti Gawain, Dr Larry Dossey, and Louise Hay.

How does it work?

You normally relax first with your eyes closed and then create a mental picture of how you would like things to be. Positive statements known as affirmations may also be used. Treatment may be done alone or with the help of a therapist. Studies have shown that during visualisation the right hemisphere of the brain is stimulated and changes in hormone production, and other aspects of the body's physiology, result.

What's it good for?

Visualisation has been used for many different things from relieving asthma, to overcoming interview nerves, to improving sports performance.

What's the evidence?

Some research has shown that visualisation can produce physical changes such as lowered blood pressure and increased production of breast milk in nursing mothers and also that it may help to reduce discomfort in sufferers of various ailments such as irritable bowel syndrome (IBS) and headache. Sports science research has also showed that having an 'inner game', for example visualising your golf ball going into the hole or your tennis ball going over the net, can improve performance results.

How can 1 find a practitioner?

Many different types of practitioners, such as psychologists, hypnotherapists, and counsellors, may employ visualisation and affirmation techniques. You can also teach yourself – see the 'Helping Yourself with Psychological Therapies' section at the end of this chapter.

Other therapies

Other psychological therapies include *dream therapy*, where your dreams are analysed for insight into current problems; and *laughter therapy*, where you are encouraged to laugh as a way of releasing tension, anger, and pain. Laughter has been shown to boost the immune system and promote various other healthy physiological changes.

Having Psychological Therapies

 Because so many different types of practitioners use psychological therapies with such varying levels and standards of training, satisfying yourself that your practitioner is properly trained and competent is essential. If you have any kind of history of mental illness, you must be particularly careful about selecting a therapy and practitioner. Some of these therapies may not be suitable for you and can aggravate your condition. Consult a trusted health professional if you are in doubt.

 Before embarking on therapy always enquire about training, membership of professional associations, experience in dealing with your particular condition, and so on.

The cost for any of the therapies discussed in this chapter may vary hugely – from £20 or so to £100 or more depending on the nature of the therapy, the duration of the treatment, and the experience of the practitioner.

If you're dissatisfied with your treatment, talk things over with your therapist or make a complaint to their professional body if they're a member of one.

Helping Yourself with Psychological Therapies

 Visualisation and affirmations are a great way to improve your daily life by making your experiences more positive! Here's a simple technique you can use every day:

  ✔ On waking, stay in bed for a few extra minutes and visualise your day ahead. See yourself doing everything well and easily and feeling happy and contented.

✔ Identify any parts of your day that you're worried about and then visualise things turning out well. For example, if you have an interview that you are nervous about, visualise yourself entering the room confidently, speaking well, and having a good rapport with the interviewers.

✔ If you want, add a verbal affirmation to support whatever you most need help with or are most concerned about. For example, with the interview situation, you can mentally say to yourself, 'I will be calm and relaxed in my interview and all will go well.'

✔ During the day, whenever you can, close your eyes for a few seconds and recall your positive image, or mentally or verbally repeat the affirmation to yourself.

You may not always get the outcome that you want – such as landing the job from the interview – but these visualisations can certainly make your day smoother and easier. Many people also say that these techniques help to boost their confidence and enable them to realise their potential.

Chapter 22

Feeling the Buzz of Energy Medicine

. . . .

In This Chapter

▶ Finding out what energy medicine is all about

▶ Discovering what energy medicine can be good for

▶ Examining the evidence

▶ Knowing what to expect in a typical consultation

▶ Finding a practitioner

. . . .

*E*nergy medicine is a broad term used to refer to the diagnosis, treatment, and/or enhancement of the subtle energy system in the body. It encompasses what is also sometimes termed *bio-energy medicine, functional medicine,* or *vibrational medicine.*

The concept of subtle energy is referred to in many forms of traditional medicine and was sometimes diagnosed by means of divining techniques and treated with magnetic stones, gemstones, and the like. Nowadays, a range of electrical and other devices have been designed that claim to be able to measure the flow of subtle energy in the body or to provide energy-based treatments intended to rebalance the body. A range of modern-day treatments are based on energy medicine including magnet therapy, gem therapy, and flower essences. Some medical doctors, acupuncturists, nutritionists, homeopaths, and others use these devices and therapies, but energy medicine remains highly controversial because little scientific evidence exists to support its use.

In this chapter, I give you some background to the roots and principles of energy medicine and then take you on a guided tour of the most common forms that you may encounter. I also let you know what can happen in an energy medicine consultation and the kind of results you may receive. At the same time, I let you know what (if any) scientific backing the different techniques have.

To some people, the whole world of energetic medicine is a step too far into the realms of the weird and wacky while for others it represents the medicine of the future. Delve into this chapter and decide for yourself.

Finding Out about Energy Medicine

Energy medicine is based on both ancient wisdom and modern scientific and technological advances. Each of the ancient medical traditions mentions a vital, subtle energy system in the body that is crucial to health. In Traditional Chinese Medicine (TCM), this subtle energy is called *qi*; in Japanese medicine, it is *ki*; in Tibetan medicine, it is *loong*, or 'wind', and in Ayurveda, it is *prana.* This subtle energy is said to flow through a network of invisible channels in the body known as the meridian system in acupuncture or the *nadi* system in yoga.

For decades researchers around the world have been interested in developing devices that may measure and treat the flow of this subtle energy, and the electro-magnetic field believed to surround the body. A range of these devices is now available and in use by complementary medicine practitioners. This chapter explores the most common ones, while also looking at some other forms of energy medicine, including radiesthesia and radionics (divining techniques using pendulums or electrical devices), magnet therapy, gem therapy, and flower essences.

A (very) brief history of energy medicine

Energy medicine in its oldest form consisted of divining techniques, often using a pendulum, rod, twig, or other instrument (known as *dowsing*), for detecting imbalances in the body and also for other purposes such as for locating water and evaluating the therapeutic properties of plants. The ancient Egyptians, Babylonians, Greeks, Romans, and Chinese are all believed to have used forms of dowsing and the technique is thought to have been fashionable in 18th-century France. Dowsing was resurrected by French Jesuit priests in the 1920s, who taught it to their missionaries as a way of determining the therapeutic properties of plants in areas where no medicine was available.

The French priest Abbé (Father) Alex Bouly coined the term *radiesthésie*, from the Latin *radius* meaning a ray or beam, and the Greek *aisthesis* meaning a feeling or perception. This term has been translated as *radiesthesia* and is used to mean literally 'perception of the radiation or vibration of a person or thing'.

Dowsing with a pendulum

Pendulums are usually made of metal, such as brass, or wood, generally have a point at the end, and are suspended by a thread or chain. To begin using a pendulum, you first determine what its line of movement will be to indicate 'yes' or 'no'. Users suggest that you hold the pendulum suspended directly below your fingers without moving it and then ask it to give you a 'yes'. After a short time, the pendulum may gather momentum and move in a clockwise or anti-clockwise fashion or move forward and back or side to side. You then repeat this exercise asking the pendulum to give you a 'no'. For many people, a clockwise movement is 'yes' and an anti-clockwise movement is a 'no'.

Next, you suspend the pendulum in the air, or over the body part, plant, or object that you're investigating and then mentally ask questions about it. The way that the pendulum swings determines the answer. For example, you may ask questions about the therapeutic value of a particular plant. Dowsers believe that the pendulum amplifies the unconscious mind and tunes into the vibrational frequency of the matter being investigated. This idea may sound far-fetched, and no real scientific evidence supports this technique, but in fact dowsing is used by the military, local authorities, and mineral companies to detect water and mineral deposits, and it has even been used by the police in criminal investigations.

Abbé Bouly and two other Jesuit priests, Abbé Alexis Mermet and Abbé Jean Jurion, pioneered the medical use of dowsing. They surmised that if dowsing could be used successfully for divining water, it could also be used to determine the circulation of blood and the condition of the tissues in the body.

At the turn of the 20th-century in another part of the world, American doctor Albert Abrams formulated the idea that disease was caused by an imbalance of electrons (tiny sub-atomic particles) in affected tissue rather than imbalance in the cells. He believed that these electrical particles radiated a charge that could be detected outside of the body and that different electronic reactions were linked with different diseases. He developed devices for measuring these changes and called his system *radionics*.

Although a recognised medical expert at Stanford University in California, Abrams was ridiculed for his ideas, as was Dr Ruth Drown, a chiropractor who took up his work and developed ways of diagnosing and treating at a distance using samples of hair or blood. However, in the UK, Abram's work found more acceptance after a medical committee tested his findings and replicated them and an American living in the UK, David Tansley, popularised his work in the 1960s. Dr Cyril W. Smith, a retired UK lecturer in engineering, has also done pioneering work on the body's electro-magnetic field, summarised in his fascinating book, *Electromagnetic Man*.

In Germany, a modern-day pioneer of energy medicine was Reinhold Voll, a doctor who studied acupuncture in the 1950s, and then, together with a group of colleagues, became interested in the electrical properties of acupuncture points.

Voll developed a simple electrical device to measure these points and used them to map the acupuncture meridians, verifying the known ones and adding some of his own along the way. He also converted some of the traditional Chinese medical terminology into Western physiological terms, which made his system, that he called EAV (ElectroAcupuncture according to Voll), more widely acceptable amongst medics.

Voll used the application of tiny micro-electric currents to abnormal points to bring their measurements back into the normal range and held that this procedure could help relieve illness and imbalance. He also claimed that incorporating homeopathic remedies, nutritional supplements, or medicines into the circuit could alter abnormal measures and could be effective in treating a range of conditions including inflammation and allergies.

Voll's method was simplified by some other German doctors who developed *Bioelectronic Functions Diagnosis and Therapy (BFD)*, which reduced the number of points being measured to around 60 and also limited the number of medications tested.

A German pioneer

The innovative Dr Helmut Schimmel was always interested in bridging the gap between orthodox and natural medicine and between science and religion. He studied dentistry, medicine, naturopathy and homeopathy and was constantly striving to make a synthesis between orthodox and alternative disciplines. He felt he had a lifelong calling to work in 'bio-energy (functional) medicine' and believed that this really was the medicine of the future. Schimmel summed up this belief by saying:

'I personally believe that functional medicine will prove to be the medicine of the 21st-century. Orthodox medicine has no answers and no means of coping with the problems of chronic and degenerative diseases. I regret having to say this, but something dreadful will probably have to happen before functional medicine can free itself of its isolation. This means that chronic diseases will have to increase drastically, that the health insurance companies will probably become bankrupt due to the immense costs, and that the normal patient will finally understand that orthodox medicine has to be complemented by functional medicine. The public will demand changes in our public health system. Traditional medicine will be forced to do something, just because of the pressure of public opinion. I'm afraid that these changes will be fundamental and drastic. But these are the forces that move the world. When such idealistic thoughts coincide with these materialistic events, the result will be a break-through.'

The BFD system is still in use today but has been overtaken in popularity by the VegaTest method developed by Dr Helmut Schimmel in the 1970s. His system was a further refinement because it involved measuring trays of ampoules of test substances rather than different points on the body. The VegaTest method, or VRT (vegetative reflex test), has been constantly updated and is now used in many countries including the UK, Germany, Australia, the US.

Researchers in other countries, such as Dr Hiroshi Motoyama in Japan and others in Russia, Hungary, the US, and elsewhere, have also done pioneering work investigating different ways of measuring the body's subtle energy flows and electro-magnetic fields. With the advances in information technology, energy medicine devices for assessment and treatment are now increasingly available both in clinical settings and for home use. However, many practitioners remain sceptical about them because little evidence supports their claims for effectiveness.

Understanding how energy medicine works

Energy medicine approaches such as radionics, magnet therapy, and flower essences are based on the idea that every living thing has an electro-magnetic 'field' or 'vibration', which is different in health and disease and which may be affected by different remedies, types of healing, or devices.

Many energy medicine devices are types of *electro-dermal screening (EDS)* devices – that is they measure changes in the ability of the skin to conduct electricity, known as the *electrodermal response (EDR)* or *galvanic skin response (GSR)*. This ability changes according to physical and emotional states and environmental influences such as dryness or humidity. High speed computerised versions have also been developed, known as *computerised electro-dermal screening (CEDS)*.

Other devices use different forms of measurement, such as skin tissue sampling (the AMI device) or infra-red pulses (the MERID).

Treatment devices then add a substance into the electrical circuit with your body and it is believed that this can then directly influence your own body's electro-magnetic field and indirectly help to rebalance internal organ function and restore health.

However, little scientific evidence supports these theories or assessment and treatment approaches.

What's the evidence?

Not much evidence currently exists to verify the principles underlying energy medicine or the effectiveness of energy medicine treatments. Some studies confirm the link between EAV (Voll) assessment and allergies, and other studies have suggested a link between skin polarisation values (as measured by the Motoyama AMI – see below) and different types of health conditions. However, many of these studies have used only very small samples, have had design flaws or have not been replicated.

More damaging are investigations that have shown that people can get different results when measured by the same machine in different places, as shown for example with Vega food intolerance testing in high street chemists. Critics argue that people who get better after being tested on the Vega device do so because of cutting out obvious foods that may be causing problems, such as dairy and wheat, rather than the accuracy of Vega diagnosis.

However, in the hands of well-trained practitioners, large numbers of patients do claim to have benefited from following advice and treatment regimes based on VEGA test results.

Currently, insufficient evidence exists to support the methods of assessment and treatment used in energy medicine, but the numerous testimonies of benefits by both practitioners and their patients suggest that further consideration and investigation may be worthwhile.

The healing power of magnets

Stones with magnetic properties (lodestones) have been used for healing since ancient times. More recently extensive research into magnet healing has been carried out in Russia, Eastern Europe, Austria, Germany, the US, and the UK.

Fixed therapeutic magnets are usually encased in plastic or ceramic material and then placed against the skin by means of a plaster or wrap. They may also be embedded in items such as mattress covers and shoe insoles. Pulsed electro-magnetic devices are usually hand-held and moved over the affected area.

Magnets vary in strength, size, and thickness, and magnet products vary in terms of how many magnets are used and their placement. To be effective therapeutically, the magnets must be strong enough to penetrate the skin tissues and the product must contain enough magnets.

Magnet strengths of 800 to 1,000 gauss are needed and thicknesses of ¼ to ⅜ inch are helpful. Generally, the stronger, thicker, closer, and more numerous the magnets are, the greater the therapeutic effects are likely to be. Horseshoe, bar, and fridge magnets are not suitable for healing as they aren't strong enough!

Magnet therapy is used by vets, podiatrists, acupuncturists, osteopaths, physiotherapists, and sports coaches to heal injuries and ease conditions such as arthritis, headaches, foot pain, and more.

Magnetic devices shouldn't be used by people with pacemakers, defibrillators, insulin pumps, or other electro-insulin devices, as the magnets may interfere with their activity, nor by pregnant women, as the effect on the foetus or on babies is unknown.

Energy medicine today

Energy medicine isn't regulated in the UK. Some of the energy medicine devices used have now obtained a CE mark in Europe, which means that they satisfy European Community directives, or have FDA (Food and Drug Administration) approval in the US. However, these approvals relate mainly to issues of safety and don't necessarily verify what the devices claim to be measuring or the effectiveness of their treatment.

Countries such as the UK, Germany, and the US have attempted to establish training standards for the use of particular devices, but the range of devices and the many different types of practitioners who use them have made establishing any universal standards or unifying association or training body difficult.

Radionics, magnet therapy and flower and gem essence therapy also remain unregulated at this time.

Introducing Different Types of Energy Medicine

Energy medicine devices currently in use that assess and/or treat the body include the following:

- ✔ The **AMI** (new version is called **AMICS**), devised by Dr Hiroshi Motoyama in Japan, measures polarisation values at acupuncture *source* points on the fingers and toes to determine meridian balance and, it is claimed, the health of corresponding internal organs.

- ✔ The **ASYRA**, a device approved by the US Food and Drug Administration (FDA), was developed by Mark Galloway and uses fewer point readings than the BEST system, incorporating software that scans a vast range of remedies, including all the single and nosode homeopathic remedies, Scheussler tissue salts, Dr Reckweg formulations (see Chapter 10 for more about each of these), flower remedies, and so on.

- ✔ The **BICOM** (BIO-ogical COM-puter) takes electro-magnetic readings from the body and compares them across 400 preset therapeutic programs.

- ✔ The **LISTEN** system, which developed into the **BEST** (MSAS, or meridian stress assessment system) BioMeridian system, also uses devices that measure electrical changes over acupuncture points and tests for food intolerances, vitamin and mineral deficiencies, environmental sensitivities, and so on.

✔ The **MERID**, a device developed in Holland by Derk Buiskool Leeuwma, uses pulses of infra-red light, at gradually increasing levels of intensity, to measure responses at 24 points on the hands and feet and provide information on the energetic state of meridian channels.

✔ The **MORA**, devised by German physician Dr Franz Morrell and electronics engineer Mr Eric Rasche in the 1970s, was named by combining the first letters of their names. The various MORA devices now available measure 'ultra-fine electro-magnetic oscillations' by taking electrical measurements at acupuncture points on the body and also using pre-set programs to assess toxicity and imbalance.

✔ The **NES** (Nutri-Energetic Systems) device, developed by Peter Fraser and Harry Massey, involves the client placing a hand on an input device, which then relays information to a computer that analyses disturbances in the human body field.

✔ The **OBERON** is a device developed by a team of Russian scientists that scans the body with a range of different frequencies of magnetic field and identifies areas of diseased tissue in the body.

✔ The **QXCI (Quantum Xxroid Consciousness Interface) and SCIO (Scientific Consciousness Interface Operations System)**, developed by American William Nelson, is a computerised biofeedback system that collects data from measurements via wrist, ankle, and head electrodes and then assesses them across sophisticated software for a wide range of remedies and conditions.

✔ The **SCENAR** (Self-Controlled Energo Neuro Adaptive Regulation) is a hand-held biofeedback device with an electrical contact that is passed over areas of inflammation, injury, or infection on the body to stimulate healing.

✔ The **VEGA** electro-dermal screening (EDS) devices measure electrical changes at an acupuncture point and are used to test for food intolerances, vitamin and mineral deficiencies, and environmental sensitivities.

✔ **Kirlian photography** is a controversial technique used in energy medicine involving *energetic photography*. Developed by Russian engineer Semyon Kirlian and his wife Valentina in 1939, it measures electromagnetic fields around the hands and body and reproduces these on photographic paper. Luminous, regular patterns are claimed to be signs of health, whereas broken outlines are believed to indicate disease. Kirlian photography produces beautiful images but as a method of diagnosis it has not yet been proven to be very reliable or accurate.

Other forms of energy medicine include dowsing and radionics, mentioned at the beginning of this chapter and also the following:

✔ **Magnet Therapy:** Magnets are placed directly on the skin or electromagnetic devices are used to pulse a magnetic field around the affected body part. Some research suggests that the magnets may stimulate cellular activity and tissue repair and reduce inflammation.

The flower essences of Dr Edward Bach

Dr Edward Bach (pronounced *batch*) a Harley Street doctor and homeopath in the 1930s, came to believe that mental attitude and emotional health played a vital role in illness and recovery. He identified 38 primary negative states of mind and, over years of careful research, created a flower or plant remedy to treat each one. These came to be known as the Bach Remedies and are used individually or in combination and taken as drops on a daily basis. One combination of five remedies created by Dr Bach is known as *rescue remedy* and he recommended its use during emergencies or traumas.

More recently people all over the world have started to develop flower, tree, mineral, gem, rock, desert plant, and even dolphin remedies based on Bach's principles. Some of the most well-known ones in use today include the Bailey Essences, created by Dr Arthur Bailey in 1967, the Australian Bush Flower Remedies, created by Ian White, The Findhorn Flower Essences, The Alaskan Essences, and the Perelandra Essences.

✔ **Gem Therapy:** Gemstones or crystals, such as rose quartz, amethyst, jade, and lapis lazuli are placed on different parts of the body, or worn as pendants. The gemstones are believed to emit certain frequencies that trigger healing of physical, emotional, and even spiritual problems. This type of therapy has been practised since ancient times but little scientific evidence exists to support its use.

✔ **Flower and vibrational essences:** Flowers, or other plant materials such as bark, are soaked in spring water in the sun or boiled to extract their essence. Alcohol is added to this *mother tincture* as a preservative. You take a few drops of the essence daily to treat emotional states such as anxiety, grief, and disillusionment. These flower and other remedies are now made and sold worldwide and it is believed that the vibrational energy contained in the essences can alter mental, emotional, physical and spiritual states. However, no scientific evidence supports this.

Discovering Whom and What Energy Medicine Is Good For

In clinical ecology, also known as environmental or functional medicine, *electrodermal devices* (electrical devices used to measure points on the skin) such as the ones mentioned earlier on in the chapter may be used to determine whether your body is reacting to the following:

✔ Irritants inhaled through the air, such as pollens

✔ Components of certain foods, such as lactose in dairy products

> ✔ Chemicals ingested with your food or otherwise swallowed or inhaled, such as chemicals from the linings of tins of food or mercury from tooth fillings
>
> ✔ Stored toxins, such as from previous chemical or pesticide exposure

See Chapter 12 for more details about this and other ways of testing for food intolerance and food allergy.

Flower and gem remedies are widely used to treat emotional states; magnet therapy is often used to treat pain and inflammation; and radionics and dowsing may be used for any condition.

Little scientific evidence exists to support these therapies and approaches as yet.

What can energy medicine treat?

The devices mentioned earlier in this chapter are used to treat allergies and other sensitivities (such as to chemicals), asthma, joint problems, digestive problems, and a whole host of chronic diseases. Often people who go to energy medicine practitioners have tried everything else, which makes the oft-reported dramatic improvements all the more interesting. Radionics practitioners treat any condition, even at a distance, by claiming to be able to *broadcast* remedies far afield using devices or simply mental intention. Flower remedies are believed to be especially helpful for emotional states.

To sceptics such treating at a distance, or the healing of emotional problems using water with trace amounts of plant material seems impossible. Yet perhaps, once we understand more about subtle energy fields, we may get closer to an explanation.

When not to use energy medicine

Energy medicine is generally believed to be entirely safe because no direct physical intervention is involved. The only exception is magnet therapy, which isn't suitable for pregnant women or for those with pacemakers. However, people with serious diseases or chronic conditions need to ensure that they seek medical advice rather than relying entirely on the assessments and treatments as mentioned in this chapter.

What to Expect in a Typical Consultation

Energy medicine is unusual amongst complementary therapies in that you may not need to answer questions, give a medical history, complete a questionnaire, or even be physically present! In the case of radionics, diagnosis and treatment given at a distance sometimes all that is required is a lock of your hair or just your name on a piece of paper! In the case of the energy medicine devices, however, you do need to be present and you'll be in some way connected to the device either by means of electrodes or by holding an electrode and then being tested with a probe touched to a point, or points, on the skin.

Diagnosis

Diagnosis is made on the basis of the swing of the pendulum, the measurements of the radionics device, or the manual or computerised measurements of the electro-dermal measuring devices. In the case of flower and gem remedies, diagnosis is made either online after answering questions about mood and emotions; by yourself with the help of books or dowsing; or in consultation with a trained therapist.

Treatment

In the case of radionics, treatment may be 'broadcast' by means of a pendulum or radionics device. The 'matter' being broadcast may be a homeopathic remedy, a nutrient, a herb, or even a word or loving thought.

In the case of the devices, treatment is more sophisticated and may be a homeopathic or other remedy that is 'put into the circuit' and transferred into drops or pills or onto a magnetic strip on a card and worn on the body.

For magnet therapy the magnets are worn on the body or received from a pulsed magnetic field device. For flower and gem essences you take the remedy as drops in water several times a day.

What to expect once you start treatment

Treatment is very subtle, so you may notice nothing very much at first. However, people often report having effects similar to those created by homeopathic remedies (see Chapter 10 for more about these) – for example, they may initially get a flare-up of symptoms and then a decrease. Many people report improvements in how they feel within a relatively short period of time.

Your first consultation with a practitioner may last from 30 to 60 minutes. Subsequent visits may be shorter, usually 30 minutes or so. You may need to return for one or two follow-ups or until your health problem has cleared up.

If you're given a remedy in the form of drops, pills, or magnetic strip card, you need to continue to take or wear them as directed by your practitioner. In the case of magnet therapy, the magnets are usually worn until you feel better and may be used continually for health maintenance and prevention (as in the case of magnet mattress pads or insoles).

Knowing Whether Your Energy Medicine Treatment Is Working

You may experience immediate benefits from your energy medicine treatment or remedy, or you may find that you get an initial worsening followed by an improvement. Some people feel more tired than usual afterwards. This effect should pass quickly. Here are some more pointers about using energy medicine:

- ✔ If you experience a significant deterioration in your symptoms, contact your practitioner for advice.

- ✔ Ask your practitioner what improvements you can realistically expect over what sort of timescale.

- ✔ For best results, carefully follow the directions for taking the remedy, using the magnet, as well as any diet and lifestyle advice given by your practitioner.

- ✔ If you have no improvement after a course of treatment, it may be that energy medicine isn't effective for your condition. Discuss this situation with your practitioner.

Common Questions about Energy Medicine Treatment

Here are some questions that I get asked about energy medicine:

- ✔ **Does this type of measurement hurt?** No. The most you may feel is a tiny tingle from the application of the tiny electrical micro current.

✔ **How do I know which device to go for?** Each device has its strengths and limitations. Read up about them and ask the practitioner lots of questions before committing yourself. Also, check that your practitioner is thoroughly trained in using the device and knows how it works!

✔ **Does it matter if the magnets get wet?** Usually the magnets are encased in plastic or ceramic and are fairly waterproof, but try to keep them dry or they lose their power. I washed some of mine in with the laundry once by mistake and they were too weak to pick up a single key afterwards, whereas before they could pick up a whole bunch!

✔ **Can radionics be used for someone at a distance without their consent?** Not usually, no, because an individual needs to be involved in their own healing, and ready to play an active part in it.

Finding a Good Practitioner

No formal national registers of energy medicine practitioners exist. In the UK, two of the foremost centres for energy medicine are the Centre for Complementary and Integrated Medicine in London, run by Professor George Lewith and his colleagues, and the Dove Clinic, run by Dr Julian Kenyon:

✔ Centre for Complementary and Integrated Medicine (Tel: 020 7935 7848; `www.complemed.co.uk`).

✔ Dove Clinic for Integrated Medicine (Tel: 01962 718000; `www.doveclinic.com`). The Dove Clinic also has a London practice (Tel: 020 7580 8886).

You can find flower and Vibrational Essence practitioners in the UK via the British Flower and Vibrational Essences Association (`www.bfvea.com`).

Alternatively, ask friends, family, and colleagues for personal recommendations, or try accessing names of practitioners via online directories such as The Institute for Complementary Medicine `www.i-c-m.org.uk` (for the UK) or `www.EnergyMedicineDirectory.com` (mainly for students of Donna Eden in the US and around the world).

Questions to ask your practitioner

You may want to ask your practitioner about the following:

✔ **Qualifications and training:** Most practitioners are happy to give these details. If you have any doubts as to their validity, check them with the organisations themselves.

✔ **Insurance:** Check that they're a member of a professional association and have appropriate indemnity insurance.

🖊 **Device:** If your practitioner is using an energy medicine device, ask what exactly it is measuring, how it works, what the research is behind it, and what the evidence is of its usefulness in therapy.

🖊 **Experience:** Ask your practitioner about their experience in treating your particular ailment and their usual degree of success!

🖊 **Treatment:** Ask about the likely frequency of consultations that you may need and the costs involved.

Counting the cost of energy medicine

Initial energy medicine consultations may cost from £35 (for high street chemist VegaTest consultations for food intolerances) to £100 or so for more sophisticated forms of measurement. The cost of remedies may be separate. Magnet therapy prices range from £15 for a disc magnet to around £90 for a pulsed magnetic field device. Pendulums can be obtained from £5 to £15 upwards. Gemstones vary from a few pounds to hundreds of pounds depending on the size and quality of the stone. Flower and other vibrational essences range from £5 upwards.

Ensuring satisfaction

Because no formal registration of energy medicine practitioners exists, your only recourse if you're not satisfied with your therapy is to talk things over with your practitioner or contact their professional body if they belong to one.

Helping Yourself with Energy Medicine

You can have fun using a pendulum, as described earlier in this chapter, to dowse anything from lost objects to remedies for your health. However, if in any doubt about a remedy, always contact a specialist practitioner for advice, and if in doubt about a medical problem, always consult a qualified health professional.

Chapter 23

Having a Go with Creative Therapies

Creative therapies utilise art, music, sound, light, movement, colour, and the placement of objects as forms of self-expression and for their therapeutic effects. These therapies have a long history as treatments for both mental and physical health problems and some are also used in conventional medical settings, such as hospitals and clinics.

In this chapter, I take you on a creative journey from clay modelling to psychodrama and demonstrate who and what these therapies may be good for and the evidence to support their use.

I let you know what each of the therapies involve and give you some tips on how to decide which might be good for you and how to find an appropriate therapist to guide you on your creative journey. At the end of the chapter I give you some creative tips, based on the art of Feng shui, that you can try out for yourself!

Finding Out about Creative Therapies

Creative traditions have existed since the birth of culture – even cave men and women drew in their caves, and all ancient tribes and civilisations have had music, dance, and other creative past-times as part of their lives.

Creative therapies refer to creative expression via different mediums that is used for a therapeutic purpose. Take painting, for example, apart from painting for pleasure painting may be used to express difficult emotions or memories that are hard to talk about or to explore unconscious feelings.

An art therapist may help you consider why you selected particular materials, shapes, images, or colours in your work and to find out what insights your selections can give into your current situation. Sometimes, the creative act is healing in its own right as it can enable you to leave your troubles behind and immerse yourself in a playful and enjoyable activity that gets the creative juices – and the 'life force' – flowing.

Creative activities can also help you to re-connect with your *inner child*. Sometimes with the pressures of study, work, family life, and so on you may forget how to play, and may lose sight of the joy that was experienced as a young child when you could just dabble in finger painting, build models out of egg boxes, or whatever! Creative therapies can enable you to step outside of your busy, stress-ridden life and remember the simple joy of letting time, and the world, slip by as you enjoy being part of a unique, creative process.

Completing creative works can give you a sense of achievement and can help boost your self-esteem and confidence. No judgement or competition is involved; the focus is on the *doing* of the activity, whatever the end result.

Exploring Modern-day Creative Therapies

The formal use of creative traditions in a therapeutic way has developed in the last 100 years or so to the point where creative therapists, such as music, art, or drama therapists, are now well-established.

Each tradition has its own special features, which I tell you about one by one, going in alphabetical order.

- ✔ Art therapy
- ✔ Bibliotherapy
- ✔ Colour therapy (including aura-soma)

- Dance therapy
- Dramatherapy (psychodrama)
- Feng shui and geomancy
- Light therapy
- Music therapy
- Play therapy
- Sound therapy

Art therapy

The use of art (painting, drawing, collage making, sculpture, clay modelling, and so on) to promote physical, mental, and emotional well-being developed partly from the work of Rudolf Steiner (see the nearby sidebar 'Anthroposophical medicine') and of European psychoanalysts and psychotherapists such as Sigmund Freud, Carl Jung, and Melanie Klein (see Chapter 21 for more on psychological therapies) and also from the work of the American educator/therapist sisters, Margaret Naumburg and Florence Cane. The term *art therapy* is credited to the UK artist Adrian Hill, who used art to aid the healing of himself and his fellow inmates while in a sanatorium with tuberculosis in the 1940s.

How does it work?

Producing artwork is said to enable difficult or suppressed emotions to be safely expressed. Art therapists are trained in psychology, imagery, symbolism, and non-verbal communication to facilitate exploration of difficult issues and an increase in self-awareness.

What's it good for?

Art therapy is found in schools, clinics, hospitals, prisons, rehabilitation centres, and so on and has been used to aid a wide range of mental, emotional, and physical imbalances and also as a form of stress relief or a self-development tool. The good news is that you don't have to have any specific artistic talent to benefit from this therapy!

What's the evidence?

Art therapy is now an accepted profession in several countries, including the UK and US. It has been studied extensively and appears to be helpful in various contexts, such as helping children with behavioural or emotional problems, assisting adults with relationship issues, and aiding people with addictions and mental health problems.

How can I find an art therapist?

British and American art therapy associations have been in operation since the 1960s, and offer a wealth of information:

- ✔ British Association of Art Therapists (BAAT): www.baat.org
- ✔ American Art Therapy Association (AATA): www.arttherapy.org

In the UK, art therapy has been registered as a 'Profession Supplementary to Medicine' in the NHS since 1997. A recognised training and membership of the BAAT are a requirement for employment.

Within NHS settings, art therapy is free but some art therapists also work privately. Art therapy is also offered as part of anthroposophical medicine.

Bibliotherapy

The roots of bibliotherapy are unknown but it seems to have grown out of psychotherapist Anna Freud's work on play therapy (discussed later in this chapter). Bibliotherapy involves the use of literature (normally books, but nowadays also writing, film, theatre, and so on) in a therapeutic way to help resolve trauma or emotional problems.

JARGON ALERT

Anthroposophical medicine

Rudolf Steiner, a highly innovative philosopher and educator, whose work spanned the fields of medicine, education, agriculture, culture and spiritual thought in the 20th-century, coined the term *anthroposophy*, to describe a new form of 'spiritual science'.

Steiner believed that medicine should treat not only the physical body but also the subtle 'bodies' described by esotericists of his time, namely the *etheric*, or energetic body; the *astral*, or unconscious body; and the *ego*, or consciousness body. He believed that these aspects of the self could be reached through creative therapies such as art and movement and could be treated via homeopathic and herbal remedies. He also believed in the power of wholesome food and a healthy lifestyle, and he advocated *biodynamic gardening*, that is, planting and harvesting according to the cycles of the moon. In fact, he believed that cosmic cycles had a profound effect on all life forms, influencing not only plant growth and potency but also human thought and feeling. Steiner's anthroposophical clinics, schools, and medicines are popular even today although critics argue that there is no scientific validation for his approach.

Intensive journaling

Ira Progoff, a 20th-century American psycho-therapist who studied with Jung in Switzerland in the 1950s, devised a novel creative therapy in the form of intensive journal writing. More than just noting down your thoughts in a diary, this method involves a series of writing execises designed to stimulate self-awareness and promote creativity. The exercises explore, amongst other things, relationships, career, health, dreams, and the meaning of life! The technique involves creating a loose-leaf journal with sections for dialogue, remembrances, meditations, and so on. Today, Progoff's method is used in clinics and prisons and by individuals such as writers, dramatists, and artists to stimulate their creativity. For more info, check out www.intensive journal.org.

Bibliotherapy may involve using a story of a real-life trauma situation to help people work through their own feelings on the issue. For example, children suffering from the death of a parent, or separation from a parent due to marital breakdown, may find it helpful to read or be read a story about a child in a similar situation. Reading of the story may also be combined with play, art or drama therapy as ways of bringing the child's own story to life. Alternatively, bibliotherapy may be combined with writing therapy, where the self can be expressed through the story's characters, or journaling, where feelings can be expressed privately and then reflected on with the therapist later.

How does it work?

The idea is that children (or adults) can identify with the characters in the story and use them to explore their own current experience. The characters can also be used as models to introduce new or alternative ways of dealing with a current issue.

What's it good for?

Both children and adults can benefit from bibliotherapy, and it is thought to be especially helpful for dealing with personal, family, or relationship problems, as well as trauma and emotional issues.

What's the evidence?

Not a lot of research exists on bibliotherapy, so the evidence is mainly reports from individuals who've found it helpful.

How can I find a practitioner of bibliotherapy?

Among those who practise bibliotherapy are psychologists, creative therapists, and educationalists. Though no specific training or member organisation exists, you can find more information about bibliotherapy via The Bibliotherapy Education Project (www.bibliotherapy.library.oregonstate.edu/index.php).

Colour therapy (including aura-soma)

Colour has been used since ancient times for health and healing. The ancient Egyptians and Greeks both used colour in the form of garments, ornaments, wall hangings, drapes, oils, and ointments to treat physical and mental conditions. The ancient Chinese also associated colours with each of the seasons and internal organs and felt that different coloured foods had different effects on the body.

Ayurvedic medicine (see Chapter 5) and yoga have long regarded colour as a form of divine energy that is filtered through the body's energy centres called the *chakras*.

The great Persian physician Avicenna first devised a system linking different colours to different diseases and using them as a type of treatment. At the turn of the 20th-century, American Edwin Babitt, who had studied Hinduism and Ayurveda, compiled this knowledge into a huge text, *The Principles of Color*, and made this information available to Westerners. He also devised *chromatology*, whereby water is radiated with sunlight via different coloured filters and the 'potentised' coloured water is used for healing.

In the 20th-century, Rudolf Steiner also taught that different colours could influence mood, development, and learning.

Another great colour pioneer was the Swiss psychologist and psychotherapist Max Lüscher, who devised a colour test that is now used all over the world. In the test, you order your preference for eight colours and your selection is used to analyse your personality and state of mind. Lüscher believed that colour could be used for diagnosis and healing and this work has been further developed in the UK by Theo Gimbel.

How does it work?

Every colour has its own wavelength and frequency, and colour therapists think that each of these can affect the body in different ways. Colour therapists variously argue that colours can affect the glandular system, the functioning of the chakras, or the aura that surrounds a person.

Aura-soma

Aura-soma is a type of colour therapy that uses an array of bottles that each contain two coloured liquids. The idea is that you choose four bottles, with each one representing a different aspect of yourself. The first bottle represents your life's mission, the second your difficulties and obstacles, the third your progress on the path, and the fourth your future possibilities. A therapist then helps you interpret your choices. The therapy was developed by Vicky Hall in 1984. She was a chiropodist, herbalist, and pharmacist, then 66 years old, who had been clairvoyant since birth but whose extra-sensory abilities were said to have increased after she started to lose her normal sight. In a series of visions, she claims that she was 'told' to create this system from essential oils, herbal extracts, and spring water as a form of 'soul therapy'. For more details, see www.auro-soma.net or to find a practitioner contact the Aura-soma International Academy of Colour Therapeutics on www.asiact.org.

In a colour therapy session, you may be wrapped in coloured cloths, sat in front of a device that emits coloured light into a darkened room, or have coloured light applied to different parts of the body via a special torch.

What's it good for?

Colour therapy is believed to help alleviate both physical and mental ills and may help relieve depression, anxiety, and high blood pressure. However, little scientific evidence supports this.

What's the evidence?

A lot of work has been done on the effects of individual colour by Max Lüscher and his associates in Switzerland and at universities around the world. These studies have shown that, for example, certain colours are exciting while others are calming, and this information is widely used in advertising and in commerce. However, the therapeutic and spiritual aspects of colour therapy have not yet been widely researched.

How can I find a practitioner of colour therapy?

Various types of therapist use colour therapy, and no one association regulates it. The Lüscher institute (www.luscher-color.com) offers training in Max Lüscher's methods while the International Academy of Colour Therapeutics lists aura-soma practitioners (see the nearby 'Aura-soma' side-bar).

To find out more about colour in general, log onto the colourful, fun, and informative Colour Museum site at www.colour-experience.org.

Dance therapy

Dance therapy employs movement and dance, either one-to-one or in groups, to promote mental and physical well-being. Dance has always been part of many different cultures as a way of expressing emotion, storytelling, exercising, promoting co-ordination, and enjoying oneself!

Dance as a method for expression featured in the work of psychoanalyst Carl Jung and Rudolf Steiner. Modern dance pioneers such as Martha Graham also showed how free movement could be a vehicle for expressing moods and feelings. The Austro-Hungarian dancer, choreographer, and social activist Rudolf Laban pioneered dance therapy in the 1950s, in his work with industrial workers and sick people.

Various professional dancers have devised ways of using dance in therapeutic settings, notably Marion Chace in the US and the wonderful Audrey Wethered in the UK, under whom I long ago had the privilege of training in drama and movement therapy. Audrey was a private pupil of Laban, as well as a graduate of the Royal Academy of Music, and she used his work to develop movement therapy with psychiatric patients, people with learning disabilities, patients undergoing psychotherapy, and maladjusted children.

How does it work?

Being able to move freely, alone or in groups and with or without music, can be an extraordinarily liberating experience that seems to free up the physical body and may also help release mental and emotional blockages.

What's it good for?

Dance therapy has been used therapeutically in facilities such as hospitals, clinics, and schools with people with various mental, emotional, and physical difficulties, as well as a form of self-expression. You don't need to be a good dancer or even have a sense of rhythm as freedom of expression is the key!

What's the evidence?

A great deal of work exists that describes the beneficial effects of dance therapy, and scientific studies are now emerging. For more details on dance therapy research, see the research page on the American Dance Therapy Association Web site (www.adta.org).

How can I find a dance therapist?

To experience dance movement therapy, check out the Association for Dance Movement Therapy in the UK (www.admt.org.uk) or join expressive dance classes at the Laban School (www.laban.org). In the US, you can obtain further information from the American Dance Therapy Association (www.adta.org).

Dramatherapy and psychodrama

Dramatherapy uses theatrical techniques to promote mental and physical well-being and self-awareness. Drama has been used since ancient Greek times as a form of expression and catharsis (emotional cleansing).

Dramatherapy developed out of work by the Russian psychiatrist Vladimir Iljine, who developed *therapeutic theatre*, involving performance and reflection, and Russian playwright and producer Nikolai Evreinov, who used theatre and role play as a way of exploring human behaviour.

In the 1920s, Romanian psychiatrist Jakob Moreno, developed *psychodrama* using dramatic techniques in group therapy. Another dramatherapy pioneer was Peter Slade in the UK, who spent decades demonstrating how the therapy could be used as an important tool for expression and self-development, as well as to combat delinquency!

From the 1950s, onwards, occupational therapists working in psychiatric hospitals started to incorporate dramatherapy techniques in their work, as did some psychotherapists. Remedial drama, using drama in clinical settings, was established in the UK by Sue Jennings and Gordon Wiseman and also Audrey Wethered (mentioned in the section on dance therapy earlier in this chapter) in the 1960s.

Dramatherapy has been state registered in the UK since 1997.

How does it work?

Dramatherapy exercises enable you to explore thoughts, feelings, relationships, and behaviours in a novel way that combines role-playing with both language and movement. Techniques used include improvisation, role-playing, puppetry, mask work, theatrical production, mime, pantomime, and psychodrama.

Dramatherapy can give you a safe way of exploring new communication, social, or behavioural skills. It can also help build self-confidence and can be great fun to do, too.

What's it good for?

Dramatherapy has been used with both children and adults to help deal with emotional, relationship, social, and mental health problems.

What's the evidence?

Dramatherapy research is developing and studies have suggested benefits for autistic children, those with special needs, and adults suffering from mental health problems such as dementia, schizophrenia, and thought disorder but more research is needed. You can find examples of studies on the research page of the British Association of Dramatherapists (www.badth.org.uk).

How can I find a drama therapist?

In the UK all registered drama therapists are members of the British Association of Dramatherapists (Tel: 01242 235 515; www.badth.org.uk).

In the US, contact the National Association for Drama Therapy (NADT) (Tel: (585) 381-5618; www.nadt.org).

Feng shui and geomancy

Feng shui (pronounced *fong shway*) is an ancient art that has been practised in China, Japan, Tibet, India, and elsewhere from long ago to the present day. The word *feng* means 'wind' while *shui* means 'water', and *Feng shui* relates to the balancing of energy flows in order to create a harmonious living environment and increase the chances of health, happiness, and prosperity.

In recent years, *Feng shui* has become increasingly popular in the West where it is often associated with simply moving furniture around, clearing clutter, and placing wind chimes, gold coins, dragon symbols, or models of toads in strategic places in the home or office.

However, this rather trivialises the art of *Feng shui* as traditionally it was seen in a much wider context and intended as a way of understanding and building a harmonious relationship between humankind, the natural world, and the heavens. *Feng shui* was used to understand subtle energy flows as a way of working with the natural landscape to arrange the best sites for buildings, burial places, and more, and of creating harmonious work, home, and public environments. Even today, many buildings in the Far East are designed and built according to *Feng shui* principles.

How does it work?

In the same way that acupuncture aims to balance the flow of vital 'life force' energy, or *Qi*, in the physical body, *Feng shui* aims to work with *Qi*, *yin* and *yang*, and the five natural elements in the surrounding environment in order to create harmony and flow. (For more about the meaning of all these terms, take a look at Chapter 4 on Traditional Chinese Medicine.)

JARGON ALERT

Geomancy

Geomancy, which comes from the Greek *geo* meaning 'earth' and *manteia* meaning 'divination', is a system for interpreting the shapes and patterns of grains of sands, scattered pebbles, or handfuls of dirt, or pencil markings on paper. The interpretation is based on both intuition and the actual positions of the pebbles and other materials and the patterns formed.

In the 19th-century, *Feng shui* was translated by missionaries as geomancy, but in fact the two are not the same because *Feng shui* is employed as a form of science, with complex calculations, to order environments rather than as a form of divination for answering questions.

Geomancy was popular in the Middle Ages as a form of fortune telling but was also sometimes used to decide the appropriate form of medicine for a sick person!

The state of flow, or *Qi*, is assessed by means of two special tools, the *Luo Pan*, a circular compass marked in rings with astrological, date, and other details, and the *Ba-Gua*, a diagrammatic chart based on elements from the famous divination book, the *I Ching*, or Book of Changes. The *Ba-Gua* is superimposed on the room, building, or plot of land being considered to see if any of its eight sections, each of which correspond to a different aspect of life (such as wealth, family, career), is missing. If so, steps are taken to put this situation right by changing the structure or moving furniture.

What's it good for?

Feng shui may be used for new or existing buildings, health centres, and clinics, and it is also used in the home.

What's the evidence?

No real scientific research exists on *Feng shui*. Anecdotal evidence suggests that people feel better in homes and rooms that have 'good' *Feng shui*, and some reported cases exist of people's health improving after their environment has been modified according to *Feng shui* principles.

How can I find a Feng shui practitioner?

Many different schools of *Feng shui* and different organisations representing practitioners exist. Check out the type and length of training that a person has had and their experience in actually applying *Feng shui* in a real-life setting.

One of the most reputable schools, whose practitioners offer consultations all over the world, is the Imperial School of Feng Shui (Tel: 0208 950 8282; www.imperial-fengshui.com).

For other UK and US *Feng shui* practitioners and associations, enter *Feng shui* practitioner into a computer search engine or consult www.fengshui directory.com or www.fengshui-usa.com. (Please note: I don't have any personal connection with these directories and am not endorsing them. I provide them simply as a resource and starting point in your search for a practitioner.)

For some self-help *Feng shui*, have a look at the tip at the end of this chapter.

Light therapy

Nature Cure practitioners and Naturopaths (see Chapters 8 and 13) have for centuries held that sunshine and natural daylight are essential for health. Modern science has shown that this belief is correct, for we now know that some daily light exposure is necessary to stimulate the body's production of Vitamin D (check out Chapters 8, 12, and 13 for other mentions of this) and also to maintain normal hormonal and mood balance. Recent studies have shown that lack of light during winter months can contribute to seasonal affective disorder (SAD), which triggers depression and lethargy.

In light therapy, you sit in front of a light box or underneath a full spectrum light, both of which emit bright, white, and usually full spectrum light that has been filtered of ultra-violet rays (the ones that cause damage to skin and eyes). Alternatively, in heliotherapy (sunlight therapy – see Chapter 8) you increase safe levels of exposure to natural sunlight.

How does it work?

As light passes through the eye, it travels along the optic nerve to stimulate the area of the brain linked to mood, appetite, sex drive, and so on. It also stimulates the pineal gland, which plays a role in regulating the body's hormones. Light therapy is thought to help reset the body's internal clocks and improve mood and hormonal balance. Natural sunlight also triggers Vitamin D production and has an anti-bacterial effect.

What's it good for?

Light therapy has been shown to improve SAD, thereby relieving depression, lethargy, and appetite and sleep disturbance. Sunlight therapy is used to strengthen bones and relieve skin infections and respiratory conditions (traditionally, it was used as a part of the treatment for tuberculosis).

Units of lux

Light is measured in lux units. A typical sunny day has a brightness of around 5,000 to 10,000 lux. A cloudy day, or the average home or office interior, has light of around 500 to 1,000 lux. Light boxes used in light therapy vary according to the amount of lux that they emit. 2,500–10,000 lux is needed for therapeutic effect. The higher the lux, the less time that you have to spend in front of the boxes. Proper UV filters are essential to protect your skin and eyes.

What's the evidence?

A small amount of research evidence exists on the use of light therapy in the treatment of SAD, and a few studies suggest that it may be helpful for skin conditions such as eczema and psoriasis. More research is needed.

How can I find a light box?

Light boxes may be purchased for home use from reputable suppliers such as Outside In (Tel: 01954 780 500; www.outsidein.co.uk).

Follow instructions with the light box carefully to avoid damaging your eyes. Also, don't use late at night as doing so can make sleep difficult. If you develop eye sensitivity to the light, then decrease or stop use.

Music therapy

Music is a part of every cultural tradition and has long been used to uplift the spirit and for pleasure and enjoyment. The therapeutic use of music began in the aftermath of the Second World War when traumatised and injured soldiers reported feeling better after listening to music. The music may be listened to, played, or sung on a one-to-one level or in groups.

How does it work?

Music in different keys and rhythms has been shown to have a beneficial effect on blood pressure, respiration, and brain waves, as well as to promote relaxation and mood.

What's it good for?

Music therapy has been widely used with children and adults with learning difficulties and mental, emotional, or physical health problems.

What's the evidence?

Research has confirmed some of the physical and psychological benefits of music therapy, including decreases in heart rate and blood pressure, boosting of the immune system, and improved ability and mood in children and adults with learning difficulties, depression, and so on.

How can I find a music therapist?

Music therapy has been an accepted profession in the UK, US, and Australia since the 1950s. In the UK, music therapy is quite widely available within the National Health Service (NHS). For more information in the UK, contact the British Society for Music Therapy (BSMT; Tel: 0208 441 6226; www.bsmt.org) or the Association of Professional Music Therapists (APMT; Tel: 0208 440 4153; www.apmt.org). In the US, contact the American Music Therapy Association, (AMTA; Tel: 00 (1301) 589 3300; www.musictherapy.org).

Within NHS settings, music therapy is free but some music therapists also work privately. Music therapy may also be offered as part of anthroposophical medicine (see the 'Anthroposophical medicine' sidebar earlier on in this chapter).

Play therapy

Play therapy uses a range of creative techniques, including art, story telling, dramatherapy, puppetry, masks, clay work, music and movement, creative visualisation, and sand play (known as the Tool Kit) used particularly with children with emotional, behavioural, and mental health problems. The therapy is based on principles developed since the 1960s, by Virginia Axline, Violet Oaklander, and others who were influenced by the work of different psychologists.

Playing with sand

British paediatrician Margaret Lowenfield, working in the 1920s, was responsible for developing sand play therapy as a tool in its own right. Her work was further developed in Switzerland by a Jungian therapist, Dora Kalff, in the 1950s. Basically, you're presented with a tray of sand and a host of toys and figurines and allowed, through free-play, to create any forms or patterns that you want in the sand and any arrangement of the toys and figurines. The therapist sees the end result as a reflection of your inner state and can analyse it. Both adults and kids can play! For more information, see www.sandplay.org and www.sandplay.net.

How does it work?

Through play, children can express their emotions and perspective of the world and can learn new ways of communicating and behaving.

What's it good for?

Play therapy may help children with emotional, behavioural, and mental health problems and adults with emotional and relationship issues.

What's the evidence?

Quite a body of research by psychologists and play therapists supports the use of these techniques.

How can I find a play therapist?

In the UK, contact the British Association of Play Therapists (BAPT; Tel: 01932 828638; www.bapt.info) and Play Therapy UK (PTUK; Tel: 01825 712312; www.playtherapy.org.uk). In the US, contact the Association for Play Therapy (Tel: 00 1559 252 2278; www.a4pt.org).

Sound therapy

Sound therapy uses sound waves at different frequencies for their reputed therapeutic effect on both the body and the mind. Devices may be used to apply these sound waves to the body's tissues. Alternatively, chanting may be used, as per the as Tibetan, Mongolian, and Hindu traditions.

Machines that emit sound waves for therapy have been in use since the 1950s. More recently, computer and sound recording technology have been used to create tapes and CDs that you can listen to at home as a form of sound therapy. Sound and listening therapies in use today include the following:

- ✔ **Tomatis method:** A type of listening therapy devised by French ear, nose, and throat specialist Alfred Tomatis in the 1950s, this therapy uses an *acoustic ear* that plays certain sounds into the ear via headphones, causing the muscles to contract and re-training the ear – a kind of ear gymnastics, if you like! For more information, see www.tomatis-group.com or www.tomatis.com.

- ✔ **Auditory integration training (AIT):** Devised by Dr Guy Berard, also a French ear, nose, and throat specialist, after working briefly with Alfred Tomatis. He went on to develop his own *ears education and retraining system*; see www.drguyberard.com. (For an interesting comparison of

Tomatis and AIT, see www.autismwebsite.com/ari/treatment/tomatis.htm.)

✔ **Johansen auditory discrimination training**: Known as *auditory discrimination training (ADT)* in Europe and *hemisphere specific auditory stimulation (HSAS)* in the US, this therapy was developed by Danish educationalist Dr Kjeld Johansen over the last 35 years. It involves listening to specially recorded tapes designed to stimulate nerve pathways to the areas of the brain concerned with language ability. For more, see www.johansen soundtherapy.com or www.dyslexia-lab.dk.

✔ **SAMONAS (spectrally activated music of optimal natural structure):** This type of listening training, devised by German physicist, sound engineer, and musician Ingo Steinbeck, involves listening to CDs (of music and natural sounds) at home to heal auditory dysfunction. For more, see www.samonas.com.

✔ **Cymatics:** This therapy developed out of work by the Swiss scientist Hans Jenny (he coined the term from the Greek *kyma*, meaning 'wave', and *ta kymatica*, meaning 'related to waves'), and his demonstrations of how sand crystals order themselves into beautiful patterns when vibrated on a metal plate by sound waves. Dr Peter Manners, a UK doctor who met Jenny, believed that sound waves could have a similar effect in ordering the function of human cells. He developed *cymatics therapy*, also known as *bioresonance*, which involves using sound to transform unhealthy tissue back into healthy tissue. This therapy is done by means of devices that emit a specific healing frequency over affected parts of the body. For more, see www.cymatics.org.uk.

✔ **Vibrational sound therapy:** This therapy was created by French musician and acupuncturist Fabian Maman, who devised a method for using tuning forks and coloured lights instead of needles on acupuncture points and along the spine. For more, see www.tama-do.com.

✔ **Physioacoustic methodology (PAM):** This therapy involves computer-generated sound waves played through speakers into a special chair in which you sit – basically musical furniture! – and was devised by Scandinavian music therapist Petri Lehikoinen. For more details, see www.soundwavetherapy.co.uk.

✔ **Functional orientated music therapy (FMT):** Devised by another Scandinavian music therapist, Lasse Hjelm, this therapy uses musical codes and patterns to improve physical and psychological function. For further information, check out www.fmt-metoden.se/engfmt/fmt.htm.

✔ **Overtone chanting:** This therapy comes from central Asia and is a form of throat singing using just one note to resonate through the cavities of the throat, mouth, and nose. It is widely used by Tibetan and Mongolian monks and was introduced to the West by the composer Karl Stockhausen. For more, see www.jillpurce.com.

Your fundamental note

I studied sound therapy with Fabian Maman when he first visited the UK many years ago. He gave us a series of lectures and had us all out in the park performing his unique form of *Qi gong* movement therapy, *Tao Yin Fa*, much to the bemusement of passers by! He also offered private sessions to find your 'fundamental note' – everyone is supposed to have one – by which he used a combination of tuning forks and intuition to find the note that most resonated with me and which would 'help empower the cells in my body'. To be honest this note didn't seem to make a huge difference to me and I was never quite sure what to do with it nor how much the note varies from person to person and what that may mean. However, several other versions of fundamental sound now exist and proponents claim that it can be a useful tool in therapy.

How does it work?

Sound frequencies are absorbed and reflected by various body tissues as well as received via the ears (for example, they're used in the making of ultrasound images). Practitioners believe that therapeutic frequencies can be used to improve physical and mental function and to affect certain physical systems such as slowing down the heart rate and lowering blood pressure.

What's it good for?

Sound therapy has been used extensively for children with autism, learning difficulties, and developmental delays. Listening therapies have also been used by actors and singers to enhance their voice and communication skills.

What's the evidence?

None of the above therapies have been conclusively verified in clinical trials, although quite a lot of research is available for review on Dr Guy Berard's auditory integration training Web site (`www.drguyberard.com`).

How can I find a sound therapist?

Refer to the list earlier in this section of therapy methods available, which includes Web links to direct you to practitioners of each therapy.

Experiencing Creative Therapies

The cost for the various types of creative therapy varies from free (such as art therapy or drama therapy available on the NHS in the UK) to several hundred pounds for some of the sound therapy trainings. The number of sessions varies from one-off to repeated sessions over some years.

If you're dissatisfied with your treatment, talk things over with your therapist or make a complaint to whatever professional body your therapist may belong.

Helping Yourself with Creative Therapies

Try applying some simple *Feng shui* principles to enhance your home or work environment.

- ✔ **Clear clutter as much as possible.** Clear work surfaces at the end of the day, empty waste baskets, remove debris from the floor, and hang clothes back in wardrobes. You're also supposed to sleep better if you don't keep things under your bed!

- ✔ **Position yourself well.** At work, try to place your chair against a wall to provide yourself with comfort and support, and seat yourself so that you have a good view of the door or overall office. Don't place high shelves or books above your desk as these will 'weigh you down'. At home, place your bed so that you have a wall behind you and a clear view of the door but make sure that your feet point towards a solid wall when you lie down.

- ✔ **Add plants and water to your surroundings.** Place living plants with rounded leaves in the room to enhance well-being. Avoid sharp-leaved plants as these are believed to create discord. Aquariums or water features, if placed correctly, can facilitate energy flow and prosperity.

- ✔ **Spread light.** Use mirrors cleverly to spread light through rooms and in dark corners. Avoid mirrors in bedrooms, however, unless they're on the inside of cupboard doors.

- ✔ **Repair broken items.** Don't keep broken items, cracked vases, and other damaged things in your home as these are believed to be damaging to the flow of vital energy. Repair them or get rid of them.

Part VI
The Part of Tens

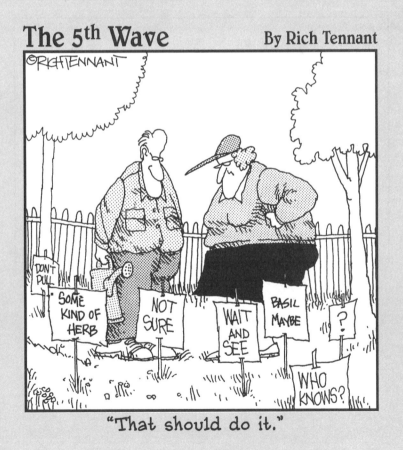

The 5th Wave   By Rich Tennant

"That should do it."

In this part . . .

The best things come in small packages, and these mini chapters are no exception. Every *For Dummies* book ends with an offering of condensed information that's easily digestible and fun to devour.

I give you some great tips for healthy living, the best superfoods to incorporate into your diet, and a list of herbal remedies to boost your health.

Also in this part is a handy A–Z list of therapies that you can use as a reference guide.

Chapter 24

Ten Complementary Medicine
Tips for Healthy Living

*M*ost of the complementary therapies covered in this book contain precious nuggets of self-care advice for optimising health.

In this chapter, I extract ten of the best, simple, self-care tips from these therapies that can help put you on the road to the best of health.

Be Aware

The traditional medical systems of China, India, Tibet, and Japan, as well as early European Nature Cure (see the chapters in Part II of this book for more about all these), all advocated body awareness and living in tune with the seasons. This awareness means getting to know your body well, being observant of changes, and learning how to read and interpret body signs of health and disease, such as in tongue and face analysis and urinalysis.

You've probably heard stories of people sometimes proving to be a better judge of what was wrong in their own bodies than their doctors, specialists, or even expensive diagnostic equipment.

Of course, in many cases early medical detection and treatment is accurate and effective. Yet developing the skill of body awareness, and learning to fully trust it, is surely good for your health – and in some rare cases may even turn out to be life-saving.

Take a look at the self-diagnosis skills described in Chapter 2 to help you increase your body awareness.

Remember to always seek medical advice if you have a cause for concern.

Eat Well

Practitioners of nutritional medicine are passionate about helping you to optimise your digestion and nutritional status by eating well.

Decide today to move away from consuming junk food, burgers, sugary foods, saturated and hydrogenated fats, and excess alcohol, tea and coffee and to replace these with lots of healthy whole grains; fresh fruit and vegetables; oily fish and lean meats (if not vegetarian or vegan); nuts, seeds, pulses; and even seaweeds, sprouted seeds, and grasses. And don't forget to add plenty of essential fatty acids from plant, nut, and seed oils (or fish oils if you eat oily fish) and oodles of water for adequate hydration.

For more comprehensive nutritional tips, go to Chapter 12.

Boost Immunity

Boosting your immune system is probably one of the best ways of staying healthy. We are all constantly exposed to bacteria and viruses, but if your immune response is good, you'll be most able to dispel these or render them harmless.

Herbalists have a range of herbs that they recommend to support the immune system. One of the most popular is the plant echinacea (also known as the purple coneflower), which you can take in tablet or liquid tincture form (available from health food shops). Echinacea has been shown to raise white blood cell count and reduce the likelihood of getting a cold or decrease its duration and severity if you already have one.

Other ways to boost the immune system include regular intake of bioflavonoids and other nutrients (see Chapter 26) or treatments such as acupuncture (more about this in Chapter 9).

For more on echinacea and other great herbal medicines, go to Chapter 11.

Balance Those Bones

Structural alignment and posture are also key to health. Years of bad habits such as balancing phones between the ear and shoulder, hours spent hunched over games consoles or computers, always carrying bags on one side of the body, sports injuries, and so on all take their toll on the bones, muscles, ligaments, and tendons. Gradually, the full range of movement of joints can be lost, wear and tear can occur, and repetitive strain is also a possibility.

Osteopaths and chiropractors can help rebalance the body and increase the range of movements as well as recommend exercises for practising at home to help maintain improvements. Therapies such as the Alexander Technique and Pilates can also help to improve posture and flexibility.

Give your body an indulgence and have one of these treatments, and learn some of their exercises to practise yourself everyday. For more on osteopathy and chiropractic, check out Chapters 14 and 15, while you can find details of the Alexander Technique and Pilates in Chapter 16.

Breathe

Ancient yogic sages have claimed over centuries that breathing is the key to life. They argued that each person has a finite number of breaths and that when you're stressed or angry your breath becomes shallower and more rapid, which means that your lifetime's supply will be used up more quickly!

This theory is unproven but it's certainly true that when you're relaxed and happy your breath is more relaxed and full and you breathe at a slower rate using your diaphragm more rather than restricting breathing mainly to your upper chest. On the other hand, lots of activities today, such as computing and gaming, which often involve stooped postures and intense concentration, lead people to hold or restrict their breathing, and thereby decrease the oxygen supply to the body.

Naturopaths and yoga practitioners recommend practising deep breathing in the fresh air every day in order to relax the body and oxygenate the tissues. Naturopaths also recommend taking air and sun baths for around 15 minutes daily whenever possible because moderate, sensible sunlight exposure facilitates the production of Vitamin D in the body and allows air to circulate around the body, which helps promote healthy skin.

Resolve to increase your breathing awareness from today and to get in some good full breaths of fresh air whenever and wherever possible. For more about naturopathy, read Chapter 13 and for more on breathing exercises check out Chapter 18.

Move It!

We all know that exercise is good for us but, as in all things, getting a balance is important. Overtly physical or aerobic exercise can increase oxygenation of the tissues and lead to the production of feel-good chemicals – the *endorphins* – in the brain. However, overdoing it can lead to long-term damage of joints and tissues, cell death, and even exercise addiction!

In Oriental medicine, the emphasis has been predominantly on therapeutic rather than aerobic exercise, with a focus on stretching, breathing, and co-ordination. Exercises such as yoga, *t'ai chi*, and *Qi gong* may look simple but they require stamina, precision, and good breath and muscle control. They are also said to facilitate the flow of 'vital energy', known as *qi* or *ki*.

Research has also shown that these exercises can have profound health benefits; for example, medical yoga treats such conditions as asthma, irritable bowel problems, and more.

Incorporating these types of exercise into your regular exercise routine can therefore be very helpful. Resolve to start discovering one of these therapeutic movement systems this year, or to deepen your practice, or learn a new form if you're already competent in one. For more about these movement therapies, check out Chapter 16.

Rest and Sleep Well

You cannot be in the best of health without incorporating adequate rest into your lifestyle and getting good sleep.

Famous politicians such as Winston Churchill and Margaret Thatcher are well known for having perfected the art of cat-napping in order to cope well with their busy lives and demanding schedules. Fatigue and insomnia (inability to sleep at night and wakefulness during the night) can grind you down, making it impossible to function effectively and leading to irritability, impatience, burn-out, and a myriad of health problems.

Oriental medicine practitioners advise you to build brief rest periods into every day; my *Qi gong* teacher in China always argued that taking short rests enables you to achieve more – not less – in your day overall. Acupuncturists also have a great remedy for insomnia using the acupoint Heart 7. This point is located on the inside of the wrist in the groove in line with the little finger when the hand is bent inwards. Clinical and research evidence suggests that massaging or applying pressure to this point can help facilitate a good night's sleep.

For more about acupuncture, see Chapter 9; for relaxation therapies head to Chapter 18.

De-stress

Moderate stress is actually good for you. It can stimulate the brain and lead to improved performance, production, and so on. But too much stress can set you on a downward spiral of anxiety, fatigue, burn-out, and stress-related disorders.

Psychological therapies such as psychotherapy, counselling, and hypnotherapy can make a difference by helping to identify areas of major stress and providing new coping strategies.

In the realm of self-care, even using positive affirmations and visualisations can make a difference. Many leading sports people now use these techniques to cope with pre-match nerves and to bring out their best performance.

Employing these techniques in everyday life is easy to achieve by increasing awareness of negative self-talk and then replacing such statements with healthier alternatives. For example, mental messages such as 'I'm useless at this' and 'I'm never going to finish this on time', which can rack up stress, may be replaced with repetition of 'I am capable of doing this' and 'I will be able to finish this on time'.

Homeopathic remedies (available over the counter and from qualified homeopaths) are also popular with some people to ease the strain. For example, the remedy Passiflora 30c is said to help to switch the mind off and reduce mental anxiety. Flower remedies are believed to increase mental positivity (check out Chapter 22) while some aromatherapy oils such as lavender and lime can be wonderfully relaxing and uplifting when you add them to bath water or room burners (more on aromatherapy in Chapter 19).

For more about homeopathy, see Chapter 10. Information about positive affirmations and creative visualisation is in Chapter 23.

Create and Express Yourself

Expressing yourself creatively is sometimes ignored as an aspect of health and seen more as a luxury or a leisure pursuit to be fitted in when time allows. Yet music, art, and drama therapies are established therapies that have been shown to be helpful for all types of people with various types of health problems.

Drama therapy, for example, can help adults work out emotional issues, sand play therapy can help children to non-verbally express their feelings about problem situations within their family, and art therapy has been successfully used in prisons enabling inmates to have an outlet for feelings of aggression and frustration.

On a more mundane level, incorporating some sort of creative activity into your daily life can be relaxing and enjoyable and can help you to release daily stresses. Just look at all the celebrities who've taken up knitting for this purpose! You also gain the satisfaction of looking at your finished 'masterpiece' and sharing it with others.

If you don't already then why not have a go incorporating sketching, painting, pottery, sewing, knitting, music playing, singing, amateur dramatics, or whatever turns you on into your life. Being creative is healthy and fun too! For more about creative therapies, take a look at Chapter 23.

Satisfy Your Soul

Health in body, mind, and spirit means paying a little attention to your spiritual needs too. For some doing so may mean following a particular religion but for others 'soul satisfaction' may be achieved through meditation, or through feeling a connection with 'universal energy and love'.

This satisfaction can come just through a special moment, meeting eyes with a loved one, catching sight of a beautiful flower, sensing the awesome power of nature, or through healing therapies.

Healing therapies such as Reiki claim to connect you directly with 'universal energy', thereby facilitating the body's own inherent healing power, while spiritual healers claim to channel 'divine energy' into the body. Many people enjoy these therapies and say that they lead to experiences of a deep sense of spiritual peace, calm, and well-being.

Try to find at least a few moments at the start and end of each day to 'tune in' and nourish your soul or find a personal or group spiritual activity that can have this effect on a regular basis. For more about healing therapies, visit Chapter 20.

Chapter 25

Ten Superfoods for Great Health

*I*n this chapter, I discuss some real superfoods that can be seriously health-ful! You'll have come across some of them before – such as garlic, water-cress, and ginger – but maybe haven't really considered their superfood status. Others may surprise you, such as the seaweeds, weeds, and sprouted seeds that I've included. Read on to find out how they can be superlatively good for you!

Garlic

Garlic is probably best known for its odour and for warding off vampires! This vegetable's part of the onion family and is used in Ayurvedic medicine for heart, digestive, and joint problems and in Traditional Chinese Medicine (TCM) for respiratory and digestive problems. Herbalists especially value its antiseptic and immune-boosting properties.

To make medicinal garlic syrup, dissolve two tablespoons of brown sugar in a pan over a gentle heat and then stir in the juice from one to four crushed cloves of garlic and a dash of lemon juice. Cool and seal in a sterilised jar or bottle. Take one teaspoon of the syrup at the first sign of a cough or cold.

Keep medicinal garlic syrup refrigerated and use within seven days after you open it. Keep away from the skin because garlic oil can cause skin irritation. Avoid excess garlic during pregnancy, because it can cause digestive upset or heartburn, and while breastfeeding because babies don't like the smell of it in breast milk!

Watercress

Watercress is a pungent, dark green plant that grows in running water and is packed with no less than 15 vitamins and minerals, most importantly iron. Nutritionists, herbalists, and naturopaths use watercress to treat skin problems, weakness, and fatigue.

For a nutritious summer cold soup, blend two generous handfuls of washed, organic watercress in a blender with half an avocado, some sprigs of parsley, some chopped cucumber, a squirt of lemon juice, and a glass of water until smooth. Add a dash of seaweed salt and eat immediately. Delicious!

Avoid excess watercress if you have kidney disease.

Ginger

Ginger is a superfood because it enhances circulation, contains valuable antioxidants that may help prevent cancer, is antiseptic, aids digestion, and stops nausea.

Simply add grated fresh ginger to porridge, soups, steamed vegetables, stewed fruits, or herbal teas to warm the body and boost circulation. You can also tie chunks of ginger in muslin in your bathwater for a warming bath in cold weather.

Don't take large quantities of ginger during pregnancy, if you're on any sort of blood-thinning drug such as Warfarin, if you have gallstones, if you suffer from heat and flushes, or if you have a fever.

Nettle

Nettle leaves are rich in minerals and high in fibre. Herbalists and nutritionists use them to treat skin, kidney, and heart problems and for detoxing the body.

To make nettle tea, don some thick gloves to avoid stinging, pick a handful of young nettle tops (the top 4 to 6 inches are best), and infuse in freshly boiled water in a teapot for 10 minutes. Strain, pour, and drink, sweetening with honey to taste if you like. Use several times a week to aid healthy skin, hair, and bones.

Always wear gloves when picking nettles to avoid stings. Use young leaves, preferably in the spring, and *never* consume them raw – always pouring boiling water onto them to kill off the sting before eating or drinking. Avoid leaves near roadsides because they may be polluted. Don't drink nettle tea every day because this can stress the kidneys.

Sunflower Seeds

Many types of edible seeds are now becoming part of people's everyday diets. Sunflower seeds (actually the kernel from sunflower hulls rather than the actual seed) contain healthy fatty acids, are a great source of dietary fibre and protein, are rich in minerals, and are packed with plant compounds called phytosterols that help maintain healthy cholesterol levels in the body.

These nutrients mean that sunflower seeds can help protect your heart, maintain good circulation, and regulate blood pressure and cholesterol levels, to name just a few of their benefits! Other excellent seeds with similar benefits are pumpkin seeds and sesame seeds.

Grind sunflower, pumpkin, and sesame seeds, plus a couple of nuts if wished (such as almonds, walnuts, or brazil nuts), for a few seconds in a small coffee grinder. Add this mixture to cereals, smoothies, rice, and so on for a nutritious, protein-rich boost.

Always try to get the freshest organic seeds that you can and store them in a cool, dark place to stop the oils in them going rancid.

Flax Seeds

Flax seeds are rich in fibre, essential fatty acids, minerals, and *lignans*, which are special compounds that may play a role in preventing breast cancer and other cancers and aid ovulation in women. Flax seeds help keep your bowels regular; can support heart, liver, and brain function; and aid hormonal balance and joint mobility.

Place two tablespoons of flax seeds in a coffee grinder together with a teaspoon of sesame seeds (black or white) and a dash of seaweed or herb salt. Then grind for a couple of seconds to make a fine condiment that you can use daily, sprinkled on any savoury dish or eaten directly as a healthy snack food.

Buy the seeds whole, and preferably organic, and store in an airtight container in a cool, dark place, or in the fridge, to keep them fresh.

Lecithin

Lecithin (*phosphatidylcholine*) is usually made from soybeans or eggs. It is a valuable source of choline, which is part of the family of B vitamins. Lecithin can aid memory and brain function, support your nervous system, help healthy liver and gall bladder function, and aid fat metabolism.

Add one to two tablespoons of lecithin granules to your food every day, such as in smoothies, on cereals, or on rice.

Buy organic and GMO-free (that is, made from non-genetically modified ingredients) lecithin when possible. Don't heat the granules because doing so destroys their health benefits, although you can add granules to warm food as a thickener. Fresh lecithin tastes pleasant and nutty. If it tastes nasty and bitter, the oil in it has gone rancid and it needs to be discarded.

Bioflavonoids

Bioflavonoids are plant compounds, found in fruits, vegetables, tea, and even red wine, which may help improve circulation and protect against cardiovascular disease and certain cancers.

To get more bioflavonoids in your diet, replace your usual black tea or coffee with health-giving green tea, which has higher levels of bioflavonoids. For great taste, place a heaped teaspoon of green tea leaves per person in a teapot and pour on freshly boiled (but not boiling) water. Allow to steep for only a few seconds and then pour off all the liquid into cups and drink. Don't leave to steep because the tea becomes bitter and unpleasant.

Seaweed

Seaweed is part of the staple diet in Asia and has also been eaten in Scotland and Ireland for centuries. Sea vegetables are incredibly nutrient-rich and contain special compounds that may bind with heavy metals and remove them safely from the body. Seaweed is a good source of the mineral iodine, which is important for the thyroid gland and for healthy teeth and bones.

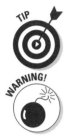

To incorporate seaweed in your diet, try using seaweed salt or dried sheets of *nori* seaweed, which may be shredded and added to rice as a topping, or laid flat, covered with rice and then rolled to make sushi rolls.

If you are hypothyroid and taking thyroxine, you should take your medication at least several hours apart from consuming seaweed, because its iodine content may interfere with the effective uptake of the drug.

Sprouted Seeds

Sprouting refers to the practice of germinating seeds, pulses, and nuts until they start to sprout. They can be grown easily and inexpensively year-round, even in small spaces with just a jam jar and some water and light. Sprouted seeds are rich in vitamins, minerals, protein, fibre, and live enzymes.

To sprout, put a heaped teaspoon of seeds (alfalfa, mungbean, and fenugreek are all good but any seed or pulse may be used) into a jam jar and cover the open end with mesh or cheesecloth held in place with a thick rubber band. Soak the seeds for a few hours, then drain and place the jar at an angle on a draining board or window sill. Rinse each night and morning with clean water until little shoots appear and then start to sprout. This process normally takes five to eight days, depending on the type and size of seed, and room temperature. The sprouts are then ready to rinse and eat as a snack or as a tasty, nutritious addition to salads, sandwiches, and so on.

For best results, use good quality, organic seed and good quality water, such as filtered water. Don't let your seeds become water-logged because they'll go mouldy. Make sure that all water is drained off after rinsing and that air can circulate in the jar at all times. Avoid direct sunlight and heat and keep sprouts in an even, warm temperature.

Chapter 26

Ten Great Herbal Remedies

In This Chapter

▶ Ten outstanding herbs and their uses in complementary medicine

▶ Simple teas, syrups, and other remedies to make and use at home

Certain herbs, easily grown in your garden or kitchen, have been used for centuries by herbalists, naturopaths, homeopaths, aromatherapists, and nutritionists. In this chapter, I pick out ten of my favourites and give you tips on how you can use them safely at home.

If you can't lay your hands on fresh herbs, have a go with dried herbs (available from any supermarket). Substitute one heaped teaspoonful of dried herb for one handful of fresh herb.

Where I've given no warning for any of the herbs in this chapter, these herbs are generally considered safe to use. If in doubt, consult a herbalist, naturopath, nutritionist, or aromatherapist as appropriate.

Camomile

This plant with daisy-like flower heads grows wild in many places and has been used by herbalists, naturopaths, and homeopaths for centuries for its wonderfully calming and anti-inflammatory effects.

For a calming drink at bedtime, infuse one tablespoon of camomile flower heads with freshly boiled water and steep for ten minutes before drinking. Add a teaspoon to baby's drinking water to relieve colic or teething. Soak two cotton wool pads in the cold leftovers and place over the eyes for ten minutes as a tonic for tired eyes. Homeopaths use the remedy Chamomilla 30c to ease painful teething, irritability, and colic in babies.

Camomile occasionally causes skin rash or irritation. If so, discontinue use.

Dandelion

This plant with its cheerful, bright yellow flowers grows everywhere. Its deep roots bring up nutrients from the soil and its mineral-rich leaves are prized by herbalists, naturopaths, and nutritionists who use them to treat liver problems, ease constipation, and relieve water retention.

Pick fresh dandelion leaves well away from roadsides and add to salads or simmer in a little water and strain and dilute the juice (one to two teaspoons of dandelion decoction per glass of water drunk twice daily) to ease constipation and improve liver function.

Only use clean dandelion leaves and not the flowers or stalks, the latter of which contain a bitter, milky fluid. Don't take dandelion without consulting a qualified practitioner if you have gall bladder, or intestinal blockage, or inflammation.

Elderflower

Elder is a shrub that grows throughout the countryside and in many gardens. Its attractive, large, white flower heads are great for aromatic cordials and its dark purple berries in autumn are rich in Vitamin C and immune-boosting bioflavonoids. Herbalists, naturopaths, and nutritionists use elderberry syrups to treat and prevent colds, flu, and sore throats, and to boost the immune system.

In summer, pour freshly boiled water over elderflower heads (around five times as much water as flower heads), steep, cool, and strain. Top up with sparkling water and sweeten to taste for a refreshing summer cordial or dab a little of the juice on the temples, said to ease headaches. In the autumn, place elderberries, a few slices of ginger, some cloves, and three teaspoons of demerara sugar in a pan and cover with water. Simmer gently for 30 minutes, then cool, strain, and bottle. Take one teaspoon every hour at first sign of a cold, flu, or sore throat and continue until better.

Consult a practitioner if you're pregnant or lactating.

Lavender

This fragrant woody shrub with purple flowers grows throughout Europe and is commonly used as a perfume and for food flavouring. Essential oil of lavender is one of the most popular aromatherapy oils and is used both to relax and to lift the spirits. Herbalists use lavender infusions to relieve headaches, nervousness, and depression.

Strew a large handful of lavender seeds into a bucket, or large bowl, of warm water to make a wonderfully invigorating foot bath for tired feet. Add a few drops of essential oil of lavender to your bath for a relaxing end to the day or place a couple of drops on a handkerchief next to your pillow to aid sleep.

Parsley

This green, leafy herb grows readily in pots and in the garden. Parsley's often used in cooking and was traditionally used to freshen rooms or chewed as a form of natural toothpaste! Herbalists value its ability to ease water retention and digestive wind; naturopaths use it in poultices to ease swellings; while nutritionists recommend it as a good source of iron and other minerals.

Chop a handful of fresh leaves and infuse in freshly boiled water for a refreshing, mineral-rich drink, or use a pestle and mortar to pulp some leaves and apply them to insect bites, stings, or swollen joints (held in place with clean gauze or a plaster) to bring relief. Chew parsley to banish bad breath.

Peppermint

Peppermint was used by the Greeks and Romans to crown themselves at banquets, to freshen breath, and to make sweets. Nutritionists often prescribe it for digestive problems such as wind or irritable bowel syndrome.

Pick a handful of fresh peppermint leaves, wash, and put through the juicer for added zing when making vegetable or fruit juices. If you don't have a juicer, simply add a sprig to any bought juice or infuse in a teapot for a stimulating tea that can ease tummy upsets.

Rosemary

This aromatic shrub, traditionally used at weddings as a symbol of love and fidelity, is a favourite amongst herbalists, naturopaths, and aromatherapists for its ability to calm anxiety and tension and relieve digestive upset.

Tie up some sprigs of rosemary and attach these under your bath tap as you fill the bath with water to create a wonderfully aromatic bath that can ease stress and tiredness. Infuse a handful of washed leaves with freshly boiled water in a teapot for 20 minutes. Herbalists recommend drinking one cup of this infusion daily to improve circulation and lower blood pressure. Add a few drops of rosemary essential oil to an aromatherapy vaporiser/burner, or onto a handkerchief, to ease colds, catarrh, and nasal congestion. Or add a couple of drops to your shampoo and massage into scalp for a great hair tonic.

Rosemary oil can irritate sensitive skin, so test on a small area of your skin first. The oil is not advised during pregnancy or if on medication for high blood pressure or epilepsy or if suffering from insomnia.

Sage

This Mediterranean herb has soft, pale green leaves with fabulous scent and flavour. Compounds in the leaves, called *phytooestrogens*, are believed to help ease menopausal symptoms, such as hot flushes. Herbalists and naturopaths use sage to treat sore throats and fevers.

Pick a handful of fresh sage leaves (red sage is best but any sage will do), soak in warmed cider vinegar (½ pint warmed cider vinegar to 1 ounce of sage leaves) for eight minutes and then strain and dilute with ½ pint of cold water. Gargle with this liquid every hour to ease sore throats. Alternatively, steep the leaves in freshly boiled water for ten minutes, sweeten to taste, and drink a cup daily to help balance hormones or hourly to cool a mild fever.

Sage isn't advised for long-term use and shouldn't be taken by anyone on the pill, HRT, Tamoxifen, or medication for epilepsy or diabetes. If you take it in supplement form, follow the dosages carefully. If fever is high, consult your doctor.

Thyme

This wonderfully aromatic Mediterranean herb contains a special oil, *thymol*, that is powerfully antiseptic and can help clear the airways. Herbalists use it to relieve respiratory complaints such as colds and flu, chest infections, and bronchitis. Thyme can also be used to clear mucus.

Infuse a handful of fresh thyme leaves in some freshly boiled water for ten minutes, then sweeten to taste. Drink a cup daily to ward off coughs and colds. Make a syrup by steeping leaves in a little water and sugar in a pan and simmering until a syrup is produced. Bottle and take one teaspoon every hour at the first sign of a cold or chest infection. For a chemical-free antiseptic wipe, soak a teaspoon of crushed thyme leaves in a little warm water for 15 minutes, then strain and use the liquid to cleanse wounds, wipe down kitchen surfaces, and so on.

Valerian

This summer-flowering plant used to be called *Heal All* in medieval times. Herbalists use it to treat insomnia, anxiety, nervousness, spasms, and cramps. The famous herbalist Culpeper used the leaves to treat headaches.

Infuse a handful of fresh valerian leaves in boiled water, sweeten to taste, and drink an hour before bedtime to aid peaceful sleep. Rub the leaves between the fingers and apply the juice to the temples to ease headaches.

Valerian can cause drowsiness. Don't use it if you're taking medication for insomnia or depression. If valerian is ineffective as a sleep remedy, try passionflower or hops instead.

Appendix

An A–Z Guide to Complementary Therapies

• •

*T*his appendix contains an A–Z of every complementary medical therapy that I can fit in these pages!

All the main therapies that feature in this book have chapter references so that you can nip directly to the chapter if you want to find out much, much more. All the jargon words, such as *meridian* and *acupoint*, are explained in the relevant chapters, too.

The A–Z also contains lots of other, perhaps lesser known, therapies that I wasn't able to squeeze in anywhere else in the book. If a single, main contact link for the therapy exists, then I've tried to include that, too.

Mention of these less well-known therapies in the A–Z list doesn't necessarily mean that they're effective or have been scientifically validated or are even safe. However, neither can you necessarily assume they're no good. Many of these therapies are relatively new and have not yet been investigated independently. For all we know, some of these therapies may even become mainstream in the future.

If you want to try out any of these therapies, find out as much as you can about the therapy and the practitioner's level of skill and experience before treatment. Take a look at Chapter 1 and the individual chapters on all the main therapies for guidance on how to select a therapy, how to know if it's effective, and the type of questions you may want to ask.

If I've missed out any therapy in this A–Z through oversight or ignorance, then please let me know about it and I'll consider including it in future editions of this book.

I hope you find this handy reference guide useful.

Acupressure: The application of finger-tip or thumb pressure to different points on the body in order to balance the meridian (vital energy) system. For more, see Chapter 9 on acupuncture and Chapter 17 on massage.

Acupuncture: The insertion of fine needles into points on the skin, said to balance the flow of *Qi* (vital energy) that is believed to flow in invisible channels known as *meridians*. For more, see Chapter 9 on acupuncture.

Alexander Technique: A technique for realigning posture devised by Australian actor, F. M. Alexander. For more, see Chapter 16 on bodywork therapies.

Allergy testing: A range of diagnostic approaches used to determine which food or inhaled substances may cause body imbalance or illness. For more, see Chapter 12 on nutritional medicine and Chapter 22 on energy medicine.

Amatsu: A modern-day synthesis of *anma* massage with Japanese bodywork techniques. For more, see Chapter 17 on massage.

Anma: An ancient Japanese massage technique using fingers, thumbs, and hands, or sometimes elbows and feet, to apply pressure to acupoints and stimulate flow in the acupuncture meridians. For more, see Chapter 17 on massage.

Anthroposophical medicine: A system of medicine based on creative therapies, herbal medicine, homeopathy, and healthy eating of foods grown biodynamically. For more, see Chapter 23 on creative therapies.

Applied kinesiology: See 'Kinesiology'.

Aqua detox: A therapy involving placing the feet in an electrically operated footbath supposedly designed to remove toxins from the body. Regarded by some as a scam but others swear by it! For more, see www.aquadetoxuk.com or www.devicewatch.org/reports/aquadetox.shtml.

Aqua touch: A whole body treatment given in water.

Aromatherapy: The use of essential oils, extracted from plants, in massage, inhalations, and so on. For more, see Chapter 19 on aromatherapy.

Art therapy: The use of art (painting, drawing, collage making, sculpture, clay modelling, and so on) to promote physical, mental, and emotional well-being. For more, see Chapter 23 on creative therapies.

Auricular acupuncture: Acupuncture treatment for the whole body using just the ear! For more, see Chapter 9 on acupuncture.

Auro-soma: See 'Colour therapy'.

Autogenic training/therapy (AT): A relaxation technique to ease mental and physical stress. For more, see Chapter 21 on psychological therapies.

Ayurveda: Traditional Indian system of medicine with treatments that include diet, yoga, and meditation. Also includes Marma massage, Panchakarma purification techniques, Chavutti Thirumal, and Indian head massage. For more, see Chapter 5 on Ayurveda and Chapter 17 on massage.

Baby massage: Gentle massage strokes and stretches to stimulate the baby's immune system and aid digestion and relaxation. For more, see Chapter 17 on massage.

Bach flower remedies: Flower remedies developed by Dr Edward Bach for the treatment of emotional conditions. For more, see Chapter 22.

Bates method: Exercises to improve eye health and vision developed by Dr William Bates in the US. For more, see Chapter 16.

Bi-aura therapy: A system of bio-energy healing used to remove blockages in energy flow. See Chapter 22 for more.

Bibliotherapy: The therapeutic use of literature, through books, film, and theatre, to help resolve trauma or emotional problems. For more, see Chapter 23 on creative therapies.

Biodynamic massage: A form of massage therapy to release physical and energetic blockages. For more, see Chapter 17 on massage.

Bio-energetics: A therapy involving holding various physical positions and exploring feelings to release inner blockages. For more, see Chapter 16 on bodywork therapies.

Bio-energy therapy: A system of gentle hand movements to increase the flow of vital energy, or *Qi*, in the body and remove blockages. See Chapter 22 and www.bioenergyhealing.net.

Biofeedback: The use of electronic devices to feed back information on body functions with the purpose of bringing them under voluntary control. For more, see Chapter 21 on psychological therapies.

Biorhythm therapy: Calculating biorhythms, supposed cycles of emotional, physical, and mental 'highs' and 'lows' calculated mathematically on the basis of your birth date, to determine the best day for activities, operations, and so on. For more, see Chapter 21 on psychological therapies.

Bowen technique: A soft-tissue therapy developed by Tom Bowen involving light finger and thumb movements over the body to relax and release tension. For more, see Chapter 16 on bodywork therapies.

Buteyko breathing technique: A system of breathing exercises devised to promote relaxed breathing and relieve asthma. For more, see Chapter 18.

Chelation therapy: A treatment designed to remove heavy metals from the body that has also been used to help clear blockages in the arteries. For more, see Chapter 12 on nutritional therapy.

Chinese medicine: Also known as Traditional Chinese Medicine (TCM), a system of medicine that for thousands of years has incorporated acupuncture, herbal medicine, massage (*Tui na*), therapeutic exercises (*Qi gong*), and dietary and lifestyle regimes. For more, see Chapter 4.

Chiropractic: A system of spinal manipulation and therapy for joint and muscular problems. See also McTimoney chiropractic. For more, see Chapter 15 on chiropractic.

Chua Ka: An ancient form of Mongolian massage originally used by warriors preparing themselves for battle. For more, see Chapter 17 on massage.

Clinical ecology: Also known as environmental medicine, this involves assessment with electronic devices to detect sensitivities to foods, chemicals, moulds, pollens, and so on. For more, see Chapter 22 on energy medicine and Chapter 12 on nutrition.

Colonic hydrotherapy: Involves the therapeutic cleansing of the colon using water, or other liquids, which can be done by machine or manually. For more, see Chapter 13 on naturopathy.

Colour therapy: The use of coloured light, with different wavelengths and frequencies, or exposure to coloured materials, liquids (auro-soma), and so on, to affect the body therapeutically. For more, see Chapter 23 on creative therapies.

Cranial osteopathy: A subtle form of osteopathy that focuses on the ebb and flow of cerebro-spinal fluid and slight movements within the cranial bones. For more, see Chapter 14 on osteopathy.

Cranio-sacral therapy: A system of light pressure techniques on the cranium (skull) and sacrum (tailbone) that is designed to release tension and promote free flow of the fluid in the spinal cord. For more, see Chapter 14 on osteopathy.

Crystal healing: Healing via different types of crystals designed to balance energy in the body. For more, see Chapter 20.

Dance therapy: The use of movement and dance to promote mental and physical well-being. For more, see Chapter 23 on creative therapies.

Darkfield microscopy: A form of live blood analysis that uses powerful microscopes to illuminate the blood cells and is claimed to detect internal health problems and disease risk. For more, see Chapter 22 on energy medicine.

Deep-tissue massage: A form of massage that uses slow, deep finger pressure to break down scar tissue and release toxins, tension, and pain. For more, see Chapter 17 on massage.

Do-In: A traditional Japanese system for personal and spiritual development that combines self-massage, acupressure, and shiatsu stretches with a macrobiotic diet, breathing exercises, and meditation. For more, see Chapter 7 on Japanese medicine.

Dolphin therapy: Swimming with dolphins has been found to be therapeutic for various conditions such as depression and autism. For more, see www. idw.org/html/about_idw.html.

Dowsing: The use of a pendulum, branch, or rod to detect water or diagnose imbalance in the body. For more information, see Chapter 22 on energy medicine.

Dramatherapy: The use of theatrical techniques to increase self-awareness and promote mental and physical health. For more, see Chapter 23 on creative therapies.

Dream therapy: Analysing dreams for insights into current problems. See Chapter 21 on psychological therapies.

Emotional freedom technique (EFT): Involves light tapping with the fingers on 11 acupressure points to release emotional blockages. For more, see Chapter 21 on Psychological Therapies.

Feldenkrais technique: A system of gentle movements devised by Moshe Feldenkrais, an Israeli physicist and Judo expert, to reduce patterns of muscular tension and pain and promote ease of movement and vitality. For more, see Chapter 16 on bodywork therapies.

Feng shui: Various techniques used to rebalance energy flows in order to create harmonious environments and increase health, happiness, and prosperity. For more, see Chapter 23 on creative therapies.

Flotation: Floating in salt water in an enclosed tank to promote deep relaxation. This therapy grew out of American physiologist and psychoanalyst

John C. Lilly's work on sensory deprivation in the 1950s. For more, see Chapter 18.

Gerson Diet: A form of nutritional therapy based on raw food, devised by German army surgeon Max Gerson in the 1950s, to control his migraines and now used as a therapeutic regime for cancer. For more, see Chapter 12 on nutritional medicine.

Healing: The use of the hands, heart, and mind to transfer healing energy and promote healing in another being. For more, see Chapter 20 on healing.

Hellerwork: A form of deep tissue massage combined with psychotherapy and postural realignment developed by Joseph Heller, a pupil of Dr Ida Rolf (creator of Rolfing). For more, see Chapter 16 on bodywork therapies.

Herbal medicine: The use of the stems, roots, leaves, branches, and fruits of different plants to promote healing and relieve illness. Herbal traditions exist in both Eastern and Western traditions. For more, see Chapter 11 on herbal medicine.

Holographic re-patterning: Now renamed resonance patterning, this therapy synthesises polarity therapy, kinesiology, and acupuncture to 're-pattern body frequencies causing dissonance'. For more on polarity therapy and kinesiology see Chapter 16 on bodywork therapies.

Homeopathy: A therapy based on treating 'like with like' using infinitesimal doses of diluted plant, mineral, human, and animal substances to enable the body to repair itself. For more, see Chapter 10 on homeopathy.

Hot stone massage: The application of stones, heated or cooled to different temperatures, to different parts of the body to promote circulation and relaxation. For more details, see www.lastonetherapy.com.

Hydrotherapy: All kinds of therapeutic treatments using water. For more, see Chapters 8 and 13 on Nature Cure and naturopathy.

Hydrotherm massage: A massage performed while you lie on a mattress filled with warm water. For more, see Chapter 17 on massage.

Hypnotherapy: The introduction of therapeutic suggestions to the mind during a receptive and relaxed state to facilitate healing of mental, physical, and emotional problems. For more, see Chapter 21 on psychological therapies.

Indian head massage: See 'Ayurveda'.

Indonesian massage: A form of deep-tissue massage that uses the thumbs to work deep into the muscles and surrounding tissues. For more, see Chapter 17 on massage.

Iridology: Diagnosis of the iris in the eye, viewed under magnification. For more, see Chapter 13 on naturopathy.

Jin Shin Do: A synthesis of acupressure, *Qi gong* exercises, and psychology for releasing physical and emotional tension. For more, see Chapter 17 or www.jinshindo.org.

Johrei: A healing approach involving the channelling of 'universal energy' or 'divine light' through the giver to the receiver. For more, see Chapter 20 on healing therapies.

Kahuna: A Hawaiian form of deep-tissue massage for the whole body, sometimes called Lomi Lomi. For more about massage, see Chapter 17.

Kinesiology: A system of muscle testing to detect and regulate body imbalances. For more, see Chapter 16 on bodywork therapies.

Kum nye: Poses and breathing exercises designed to increase awareness and still the mind, a part of Tibetan medicine. For more, see Chapter 16 on bodywork therapies.

LaStone therapy: See 'Hot stone massage'.

Laughter therapy: Using humour and laughter to boost mental and physical well-being. For more, see Chapter 21 on psychological therapies.

Light therapy: Therapy that involves exposure to sunlight, full-spectrum light, or coloured light. For more, see Chapter 23 on creative therapies.

Magnet therapy: The use of fixed magnets or pulsed magnetic field devices to stimulate tissue healing, improve circulation, and aid muscle relaxation. For more, see Chapter 22 on energy medicine.

Manual lymphatic drainage: A gentle massage approach designed to stimulate the flow of lymph in the tissues. For more, see Chapter 17 on massage.

Massage: Gentle pressure applied with the fingers and hands and sometimes other body parts (such as knuckles, elbows, or feet) to relax and heal, performed with or without oil. For info on all types of massage, see Chapter 17.

McTimoney chiropractic: A gentle form of manipulation therapy devised by British engineer and chiropractor John McTimoney. For more, see Chapter 15 on chiropractic.

Metamorphic technique: A gentle touch technique designed to release emotional, mental, and physical blocks created while in the womb. For more, see Chapter 16 on bodywork therapies.

MORA therapy: A type of 'bio-resonance' therapy using an electro-acupuncture device to test for allergies and imbalances. For more, see Chapter 22 on energy medicine.

Music therapy: The use of musical sounds and sound frequencies to stimulate healing. For more, see Chapter 23 on creative therapies.

Myofascial massage: A type of massage that stretches the tissues to release tension and pain. For more, see Chapter 17 on massage.

Naturopathy: A system of natural medicine incorporating nutritional and herbal medicine, homeopathy, acupuncture, and Nature Cure and designed to stimulate the body's innate healing ability. For more, see Chapter 13 on naturopathy.

Neuro-linguistic programming: A set of techniques for modifying language, behaviour, and experience. For more, see Chapter 21 on psychological therapies.

Neuromuscular therapy: Also known as trigger-point therapy or myotherapy, this involves direct thumb or finger pressure on tender points, known as trigger points, to improve circulation and release pain. For more, see Chapter 17 on massage.

Nutritional therapy: Also called nutritional medicine, this therapy uses foods and sometimes nutritional supplements to improve digestion and ease common ailments. For more, see Chapter 12 on nutritional medicine.

On-site massage therapy: Mobile massage therapists take a portable chair into workplaces and perform 15- to 30-minute massages on the head, neck, upper back, and arms. For more about the different types of massage, see Chapter 17.

Orthomolecular therapy: The treatment of disease using concentrated doses of vitamins and minerals. For more, see Chapter 12 on nutritional therapy.

Osteopathy: A type of manipulation therapy that uses mobilisation and massage techniques to improve mobility and restore structural balance. For more, see Chapter 14.

Oxygen therapy: The use of oxygen, either inhaled or introduced into extracted blood as in ozone therapy, which is believed to oxygenate the tissues and help limit the spread of bacteria and cancer cells.

Photodynamic therapy (PDT): The application of light-sensitive substances to increase oxygenation at cancer sites, which is believed to help trigger cancer cell death. For more information, see Chapter 22 on energy medicine or www.doveclinic.com.

Pilates: A system of exercises for increasing body awareness, improving posture and alignment, and increasing flexibility. For more, see Chapter 16 on bodywork therapies.

Play therapy: The use of sand play, art, story telling, drama, puppetry, music, movement, and so on to help children with emotional, behavioural, and mental health problems. For more, see Chapter 23 on creative therapies.

Polarity therapy: A system using massage techniques, touch, and healing to rebalance the body's 'energy field'. For more, see Chapter 16 on bodywork therapies.

Pranayama: See 'Yoga'.

Pregnancy massage: Massage technique specially designed for use with pregnant women to ease discomfort and facilitate blood flow to the unborn child. For more, see Chapter 17 on massage.

Psionics: A form of dowsing similar to radionics. For more, see the discussion on radionics in Chapter 22.

Psychic healing: Healing given by someone while in a trance-like or meditative state, involving the transfer of energy and sometimes even 'surgery', where the body is apparently entered by hand or cut open without anaesthetic or surgical instruments. For more, see Chapter 20 on healing therapies.

Psychosynthesis: A form of psychological therapy that emphasises self-awareness and *soul* knowledge. For more, see Chapter 21 on psychological therapies.

Qi gong: Part of Traditional Chinese Medicine (TCM), this form of movement therapy is designed to free the flow of *Qi* (vital energy) and promote flexibility and healing. For more, see Chapter 4 on TCM and Chapter 16 on bodywork therapies.

Quantum touch: A form of energy healing using such elements as hand healing and breathing techniques. For more, see www.quantumtouch.com.

Radionics: A form of dowsing, using a hand-held pendulum or a radionic device to detect energetic imbalances in the body and 'broadcast' healing at a distance. For more, see Chapter 22 on energy medicine.

Rebirthing: The use of breathing and other physical techniques to 're-enact' your birth and resolve birth traumas that can impact on later life. For more, see Chapter 21 on psychological therapies.

Reflexology: A form of foot massage using finger-tip and thumb pressure to nerve reflex points on the feet. For more, see Chapter 17 on massage.

Regression therapy: Sometimes called past-life therapy or past-life regression therapy, this therapy involves deep relaxation and then being taken back supposedly to specific times in your early life or even past lives. For more, see Chapter 21 on psychological therapies.

Reiki: A Japanese healing approach involving the transfer of healing energy. For more, see Chapter 20 on healing.

Remedial massage: A form of soft tissue massage often used for healing joint pain and sports and other injuries. For more, see Chapter 17 on massage.

Rolfing: Also called structural integration, a bodywork system for correcting misalignment developed by Ida Rolf in the 1950s. For more, see Chapter 16 on bodywork therapies.

Self-massage: Simple do-it-yourself massage techniques, using finger-tip and hand pressure and kneading to release tension and promote circulation. For more, see Chapter 17 on massage.

Shamanic healing: The use of rituals, singing, dancing, drumming, fasting, consciousness-altering plants, and trance-like states for self-development and healing. For more, see Chapter 20 on healing therapies.

Shiatsu: A Japanese massage system, often performed through clothing, involving pressure from fingers, elbows, feet, and knees to rebalance the body. For more, see Chapter 17 on massage.

Sonodynamic therapy: This therapy uses low-level ultrasound in an attempt to destroy tumour cells. For more, see Chapter 22 and www.doveclinic.com.

Spiritual healing: The channelling of universal healing energy or 'life force' via a trained healer intended to promote mental, physical, and spiritual well-being. For more, see Chapter 20 on healing therapies.

Sports massage: A combination of massage techniques designed to enhance sports performance and promote healing of injuries. For more, see Chapter 17 on massage.

Swedish massage: A popular form of massage developed in Sweden and sometimes called therapeutic massage, Swedish massage is based on kneading, stroking, and pummelling movements designed to stimulate circulation and promote relaxation. For more, see Chapter 17 on massage.

Ta'i chi: Part of Traditional Chinese Medicine, this movement therapy involves slow, flowing sequences of movements and breathing techniques to stimulate and regulate the flow of *Qi* energy. For more, see Chapter 16 on bodywork therapies.

Thai massage: A thorough form of deep-tissue massage with muscle stretching and pressure techniques designed to ease tension and pain and promote relaxation. For more, see Chapter 17 on massage.

Therapeutic touch: A type of laying-on-of-hands therapy. For more, see Chapter 20 on healing.

Thought field therapy (TFT): A form of psychological treatment designed to ease emotional problems, stress, and anxiety rapidly. For more, see Chapter 21 on psychological therapies.

Tibetan massage: An ancient Tibetan medical technique involving oil massage and pressure to particular points on the body to ease pain and obstructions and promote healing. For more, see Chapter 6 on Tibetan medicine.

Touch for Health: Developed out of applied kinesiology by US chiropractor John Thie, who believed simple techniques for body balancing could be learnt and used by anyone. See also 'Kinesiology'.

Traditional Chinese Medicine (TCM): See 'Chinese medicine'.

Tragerwork: A system of gentle, rhythmical movements, devised by one-time chronic back-sufferer Milton Trager, to ease tension and pain and improve mobility. For more, see Chapter 16 on bodywork therapies.

Trigger-point therapy: See 'Neuromuscular therapy'.

Tsubo therapy: Therapy involving stimulation of *tsubo*, acupoints, using massage, heat treatment, or electrical stimulus. For more, see Chapter 17 on massage.

Tui na: *A Traditional Chinese Medicine (TCM) form of massage that uses fingers, hands, arms, elbows, and knees to rub, knead, and roll the skin. Tui na is designed to release blockages in the acupuncture meridians and to release muscular tension. For more, see Chapter 17 on massage.

Visualisation: Sometimes also called mental imagery, guided imagery, or creative visualisation, this therapy involves creating positive images, while in a relaxed state, to help resolve mental or physical problems. For more, see Chapter 21 on psychological therapies.

Watsu: Shiatsu performed in the water! The idea is that the body is relaxed and weightless to aid stretches. See also 'Shiatsu'.

Yoga: A system of therapeutic exercises and breathing (*pranayama*) and meditation techniques that are a part of Ayurveda. For more, see Chapter 5 on Ayurveda and Chapter 16 on bodywork therapies.

Zero balancing: A light manipulation therapy designed to rebalance the 'energetic body'. For more, see Chapter 16 on bodywork therapies.

Zone therapy: See 'Reflexology'.

Index

• *I* •

• T •

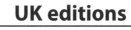

DUMMIES®

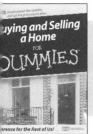

Do Anything. Just Add Dummies

UK editions

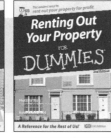

Buying and Selling a Home
978-0-7645-7027-8

Renting Out Your Property
978-0-470-02921-3

Buying a Property in Eastern Europe
978-0-7645-7047-6

PERSONAL FINANCE

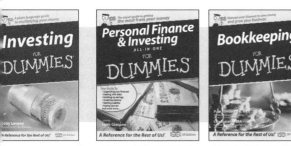

Investing
978-0-7645-7023-0

Personal Finance & Investing
978-0-470-51510-5

Bookkeeping
978-0-470-05815-2

BUSINESS

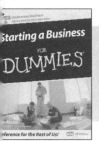
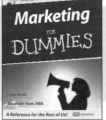

Starting a Business
978-0-7645-7018-6

Marketing
978-0-7645-7056-8

Business Plans
978-0-7645-7026-1

Answering Tough Interview Questions For Dummies
(978-0-470-01903-0)

Arthritis For Dummies
(978-0-470-02582-6)

Being the Best Man For Dummies
(978-0-470-02657-1)

British History For Dummies
(978-0-470-03536-8)

Building Self-Confidence For Dummies
(978-0-470-01669-5)

Buying a Home on a Budget For Dummies
(978-0-7645-7035-3)

Children's Health For Dummies
(978-0-470-02735-6)

Cognitive Behavioural Therapy For Dummies
(978-0-470-01838-5)

Cricket For Dummies
(978-0-470-03454-5)

CVs For Dummies
(978-0-7645-7017-9)

Detox For Dummies
(978-0-470-01908-5)

Diabetes For Dummies
(978-0-470-05810-7)

Divorce For Dummies
(978-0-7645-7030-8)

DJing For Dummies
(978-0-470-03275-6)

eBay.co.uk For Dummies
(978-0-7645-7059-9)

English Grammar For Dummies
(978-0-470-05752-0)

Gardening For Dummies
(978-0-470-01843-9)

Genealogy Online For Dummies
(978-0-7645-7061-2)

Green Living For Dummies
(978-0-470-06038-4)

Hypnotherapy For Dummies
(978-0-470-01930-6)

Life Coaching For Dummies
(978-0-470-03135-3)

Neuro-linguistic Programming For Dummies
(978-0-7645-7028-5)

Nutrition For Dummies
(978-0-7645-7058-2)

Parenting For Dummies
(978-0-470-02714-1)

Pregnancy For Dummies
(978-0-7645-7042-1)

Rugby Union For Dummies
(978-0-470-03537-5)

Self Build and Renovation For Dummies
(978-0-470-02586-4)

Starting a Business on eBay.co.uk For Dummies
(978-0-470-02666-3)

Starting and Running an Online Business For Dummies
(978-0-470-05768-1)

The GL Diet For Dummies
(978-0-470-02753-0)

The Romans For Dummies
(978-0-470-03077-6)

Thyroid For Dummies
(978-0-470-03172-8)

UK Law and Your Rights For Dummies
(978-0-470-02796-7)

Writing a Novel & Getting Published For Dummies
(978-0-470-05910-4)

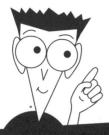

FOR DUMMIES®

Do Anything. Just Add Dummies

HOBBIES

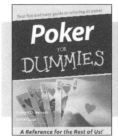

Poker
978-0-7645-5232-8

Sewing
978-0-7645-6847-3

Drawing
978-0-7645-5476-6

Also available:

Art For Dummies
(978-0-7645-5104-8)

Aromatherapy For Dummies
(978-0-7645-5171-0)

Bridge For Dummies
(978-0-471-92426-5)

Card Games For Dummies
(978-0-7645-9910-1)

Chess For Dummies
(978-0-7645-8404-6)

Improving Your Memory
For Dummies
(978-0-7645-5435-3)

Massage For Dummies
(978-0-7645-5172-7)

Meditation For Dummies
(978-0-471-77774-8)

Photography For Dummi
(978-0-7645-4116-2)

Quilting For Dummies
(978-0-7645-9799-2)

EDUCATION

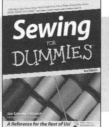
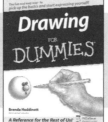

Cooking Basics
978-0-7645-7206-7

The Koran
978-0-7645-5581-7

Anatomy & Physiology
978-0-7645-5422-3

Also available:

Algebra For Dummies
(978-0-7645-5325-7)

Algebra II For Dummies
(978-0-471-77581-2)

Astronomy For Dummies
(978-0-7645-8465-7)

Buddhism For Dummies
(978-0-7645-5359-2)

Calculus For Dummies
(978-0-7645-2498-1)

Forensics For Dummies
(978-0-7645-5580-0)

Islam For Dummies
(978-0-7645-5503-9)

Philosophy For Dummies
(978-0-7645-5153-6)

Religion For Dummies
(978-0-7645-5264-9)

Trigonometry For Dumm
(978-0-7645-6903-6)

PETS

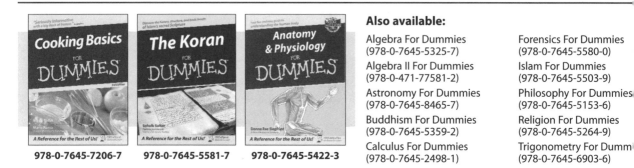

Puppies
978-0-470-03717-1

Dog Training
978-0-7645-8418-3

Cats
978-0-7645-5275-5

Also available:

Labrador Retrievers
For Dummies
(978-0-7645-5281-6)

Aquariums For Dummies
(978-0-7645-5156-7)

Birds For Dummies
(978-0-7645-5139-0)

Dogs For Dummies
(978-0-7645-5274-8)

Ferrets For Dummies
(978-0-7645-5259-5)

Golden Retrievers
For Dummies
(978-0-7645-5267-0)

Horses For Dummies
(978-0-7645-9797-8)

Jack Russell Terriers
For Dummies
(978-0-7645-5268-7)

Puppies Raising & Trainin
Diary For Dummies
(978-0-7645-0876-9)

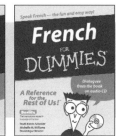
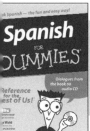
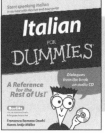
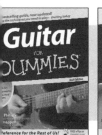
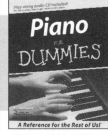
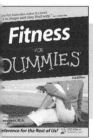
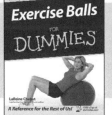
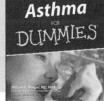

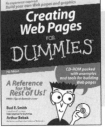
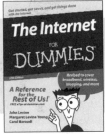
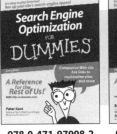
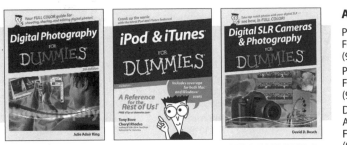
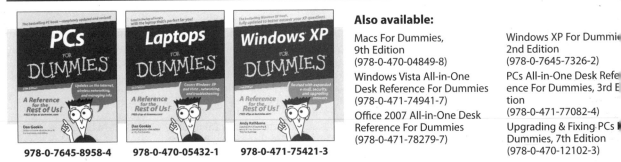